*Dedicated to my parents, who first interested me in people, to **Rhian, Bethan** and **Catrin**, whose unique take on the world keeps me on my toes and of whom I am immensely proud.*

Essential
Revision Notes
in Psychiatry
for MRCPsych

Edited by

Chris Fear MBChB, MD, MRCPsych

Consultant General Adult Psychiatrist

Gloucestershire Partnership Trust and Honorary Clinical Teacher

University of Bristol

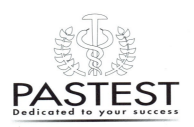

PASTEST
Dedicated to your success

© 2004 PASTEST Ltd
Egerton Court
Parkgate Estate
Knutsford
Cheshire
WA16 8DX

Telephone: 01565 752000

First published 2004

ISBN 1 904627 03 X

A catalogue record for this book is available from the British Library.

The information contained within this book was obtained by the authors from reliable sources. However, while every effort has been made to ensure its accuracy, no responsibility for loss, damage or injury occasioned to any person acting or refraining from action as a result of information contained herein can be accepted by the publishers or authors.

Text prepared by Saxon Graphics, Derby
Printed and bound by Page Bros, Norwich

Contents

Preface

One of the fascinations of psychiatry is the fuzziness of its boundaries. As well as covering the whole of physical medicine and its effect on the mind, it includes psychology, sociology, jurisprudence, philosophy, statistics and an unspecified eclectic knowledge allowing communication with mentally ill individuals whose life experiences are encompassed within their psychopathology. While fascinating, it is also daunting, particularly when one is preparing to face the examiners for either part of the MRCPsych examination. The breadth and depth of knowledge required is demonstrated by the MRCPsych curriculum. The large number of textbooks of psychiatry that claim to be comprehensive, in attempting to cover everything, are difficult to assimilate for examinations so that most candidates will rely upon a number of shorter books covering different aspects of the syllabus.

This addition to the PasTest Essential Revision Notes portfolio does not claim to be comprehensive. In editing it, I have chosen the authors on the basis of their knowledge of their subject but, more importantly, my knowledge of them as clinicians or researchers and my confidence in their ability to put their subject across in a succinct and exam-friendly way. There is a smattering of eminent academics, such as Professors Owen, Lloyd and Onyett, a large number of jobbing clinicians, such as myself, and Specialist Registrars, who have recently gained MRCPsych and are therefore well-versed in its rigours. Each author has been asked to write their chapter in response to the question: What would you want to know to pass the MRCPsych? More than one chapter draft has already been used as a study aid by local candidates.

I have made the decision to devote more space to those topics that are most likely to be examined, or are generally poorest understood by candidates. Nevertheless, the essentials of each topic are covered in the order in which they appear in the curriculum. While the written part of the examination may examine little of some of these topics, they are an essential background to the clinical part of the Part II in which candidates are judged both on their clinical knowledge and the impression they create as credible senior colleagues.

The result is a volume that is sufficiently detailed to provide a primary study aid for both parts of the MRCPsych and to cover the territory between books of short notes, and detailed tomes. The style is informal, comprising succinct notes, bullet points, diagrams and tables. Aimed at MRCPsych candidates, it is likely to appeal to a variety of mental health professionals, as well as medical students who are sufficiently interested to want to know more about the compulsive topic of psychiatry.

I would like to thank the authors for their perseverance through a number of anankastic revisions and for accepting the extremely tight original brief. My PA, Dawn Pearman, has provided considerable support in finding and chasing the past and present colleagues who became authors. Jeff James was invaluable in researching the chapter on management. Jane Janaway and Liz Kerr at PasTest have shown immense patience and have kept the faith through a lengthy project, with gentle encouragement and sparing use of the whip. We can all be proud of the result.

Chris Fear

Contributors

Alka Ahuja MRCPsych
Research Specialist Registrar
Division of Child and Adolescent Psychiatry
Department of Psychological Medicine
University of Wales College of Medicine
Heath Park
Cardiff
CF14 4XN

Peter Aitken MRCGP MRCPsych DCH DRCOG
Consultant Liaison Psychiatrist
Liaison Psychiatry Team
Devon Partnership NHS Trust
Wonford House Hospital
Dryden Road
Exeter
EX2 5AF

Tim Amos MA (Oxon), MSc, MRCPsych, DPMSA
Senior Lecturer in Forensic Psychiatry, University of Bristol
Consultant Forensic Psychiatrist
Fromeside Clinic
Glenside Hospital
Blackberry Hill
Stapleton
Bristol.
BS16 1ED

Nicholas Ardagh-Walter MRCPsych, MRCP(UK)
Consultant Psychiatrist
Holly House,
6 West Lodge Drive,
Gloucester
GL4 4QH

Robin Balmer MBChB MRCPsych MRCGP
Consultant Adult Psychiatrist
Long Fox unit
Western General Hospital
Grange Road
Uphill
Weston-super-Mare

Nicholas J Bray MRCPsych
Lecturer in Psychology
University of Wales College of Medicine
Heath Park
Cardiff
CF14 4XN

Alan Butler BA MA MScDip Psychother
Director of Postgraduate Studies
Leeds School of Medicine
Division of Psychiatry and Behavioural Science
Leeds School of Medicine
15 Hyde Terrace
Leeds
LS2 9LT

Andrew Clark MA, MBBS, MRCPsych, MInstGA.
Consultant Psychotherapist,
Avon and Wiltshire Mental Health Partnership Trust
Blackberry Hill Hospital
Manor Road
Bristol
BS16 2EW

Matt Crawford, Ph.D. in Social Psychology
Lecturer
Department of Experimental Psychology
University of Bristol
Bristol
BS8 1TN

Eric Davis PhD, MSc Clinical Psychology, BSc Hons Psychology, Thorn Diploma, Thorn
Advanced Diploma, Certifcate in Management
Consultant Clinical Psychologist, Gloucestershire Early Intervention Project Lead and
NIMHE Southwest Associate for Early Intervention in Psychosis
GRIP Early Intervention Team
Cheltenham Community Projects
Grove Street
Cheltenham
Gloucestershire
GL50 3LZ

Mhairi Duff BSc(Econ), MClin Psych, MB, ChB, MRC Psych
Consultant in the Psychiatry of Learning Disabilities
Gloucestershire Partnership NHS Trust
Heathfield
30 Denmark Road
Gloucester
GL1 3HZ

Sanju George MBBS MRCPsych
SpR in Psychiatry
Sandwell Outreach Team
6-6a The Cottage
Simpson Street
Old Bury
West Midlands
B69 4AL

Trevor Hicks MB ChB MRCGP DRCOG MRCPsych LLM
Consultant in Adult Mental Health
Department of Community Psychiatry
RAF Brize Norton
Carterton
Oxfordshire
OX18 3LX

Katie Kelly MBBCh MRCPsych
Specialist Registrar Avon, Gloucester & Wiltshire Psychiatry Training Scheme
Charlton Lane Hospital
Charlton Lane
Cheltenham
GL53 9DT

Nick Kosky MBBS MRCPsych
Consultant Psychiatrist and Clinical Director
North Dorset Primary Care Trust
West Haven CMHT
Radipole Lane
Weymouth
Dorset
DT4 0QE

Anne Lingford-Hughes, MA PhD BM BCh MRCPsych
Senior Lecturer in Biological Psychiatry & Addiction
Academic Unit of Psychiatry,
University of Bristol,
Cotham House
Cotham Hill,
Bristol
BS6 6JL

Keith Lloyd MD MSc(Econ) MSc MRCPsych
Professor of Psychological Medicine
Swansea Clinical School
University of Wales Swansea
SA2 8PP

Rob MacPherson MB ChB MRCPsych MD
Consultant Psychiatrist
Wotton Lawn Hospital
Horton road
Gloucester
GL1 3PX

Jan K Melichar BSc MB BS MRCPsych MD
Clinical Lecturer & e-Learning Teaching Fellow
Academic Unit of Psychiatry
University of Bristol
Cotham House
Cotham Hill
Bristol
BS6 6JL

Steve Onyett
Senior Development Consultant at National Institute for Mental Health in England –
South West Development Centre, and visiting professor at Faculty of Health and Social
Care, University of the West of England
NIMHE-SW
Hebron House
Sion Road
Bedminster
Bristol
BS3 3BD

Professor Mike Owen
Head of Department of Psychological Medicine
UWCM Neuropsychiatric Genetics Unit
Tenovus Building
Heath Park
Cardiff
CF14 4XN

Sarah Price MB ChB MRPsych
Specialist Regstrar in Psychiatry
Southmead Hospital
Bristol
BS10 5NB

Hugh Rickards MD MRCPsych
Consultant in Neuropsychiatry
Hon Senior Lecturer in Psychiatry
Queen Elizabeth Psychiatric Hospital
Mindelsohn Way
Edgbaston
Birmingham
B15 2QZ

Sandy Robertson MB BCh FRCPsych
Member of Mental Health Tribunal
Honorary Clinical Senior Lecturer at Birmingham University
Previously Consultant Psychiatrist
Kidderminster Hospital
Worcestershire
DY11 6RJ

Mark Scheepers MRC Psych, MB, ChB
Consultant in the Psychiatry of Learning Disabilities
Gloucestershire Partnership NHS Trust
Heathfield
30 Denmark Road
Gloucester
GL1 3HZ

Jane Scourfield PhD MRCPsych
Senior Lecturer/Honorary Consultant in Child & Adolescent Psychiatry Dept
Psychological Medicine University of Wales College of Medicine
Heath Park
Cardiff
CF14 4XN

Manfusa Shams, C.Psychol AFBPsS
Chartered Health Psychologist
Luton
Bedfordshire

Arden Tomison MB ChB FRCPsych
Consultant Senior Lecturer in Forensic Psychiatry, University of Bristol
Consultant Forensic Psychiatrist
Fromeside Clinic
Glenside Hospital
Blackberry Hill
Stapleton
Bristol
BS16 1ED

Karen J Williams MBChB MRCPsych
Lead Consultant Psychiatrist
County-wide Specialist Substance Misuse Service
44 London Road
Gloucester
GL1 3NZ

Paul Winterbottom MB, ChB, MRC Psych
Consultant in the Psychiatry of Learning Disabilities/Medical Director
Gloucestershire Partnership NHS Trust
Heathfield
30 Denmark Road
Gloucester
GL1 3HZ

Chapter 1

Basic Psychology

Manfusa Shams

CONTENTS

1

Basic Psychology

LEARNING

What is learning?

A manifested, relatively permanent change in behaviour, thoughts, or feelings of an individual as a result of past experiences.

Principles of learning theory

The principles of learning are based on four major learning models:

1 Classical conditioning
2 Operant conditioning
3 The clinical application of behavioural treatments
4 The impact of reinforcement schedules on behaviour

Classical conditioning

The learning process whereby a neutral stimulus elicits a positive or negative emotional/physiological response in the absence of an original stimulus which has caused such responses through the mechanism of pairing neutral and original stimuli to obtain a conditioned response. For example, secretion of saliva at the sound of a bell (neutral stimulus) and without the presence of food (original stimulus).

Major components of classical conditioning

- **Unconditioned stimulus** (UCS) is a stimulus that elicits a response naturally, eg food/smell of food in hungry state.
- **Unconditioned response** (UCR) is an unlearned response to an original stimulus, eg salivation at the sight of food/smell of food in hungry state.
- **Conditioned stimulus** (CS) is a neutral stimulus that elicits a response naturally as a result of its pairing with the UCS, eg salivation at the sound of a bell.
- **Conditioned response** (CR) is a learned response to a CS similar to the UCR but responding to a CS rather than a UCS, eg salivation at the sound of a bell.

Phases of classical conditioning

The process of classical conditioning involves four phases:

- **Acquisition**: Learning process during which the occurrence of CR strengthens, eg the learned response (salivation) to the sound of a bell.

3

- **Extinction**: When the CS and UCS are uncoupled, the probability of CR decreases, eg in the absence of food, continuous presentation of a bell sound may extinguish the salivation response.
- **Spontaneous recovery**: Reappearance of CR without the presence of UCS, eg after a period of extinction, when the bell sound is resumed, the salivation response reappears (caused by the memory of previous conditioned learning).
- **Savings**: When the CS is paired with the UCS after a period of extinction and briefly, the CR returns to its level in the acquisition phase, eg the sight of food with a bell sound elicits salivation response.

Causes of conditioning

- **Temporal contiguity**: Cognitive explanations suggest the importance of the proximity in time between CS and UCS for the conditioning effect.
- **Contingency explanation**: There is a dependent relationship between CS and UCS.

Applications of classical conditioning theory to understand pathogenic behaviours

- **Fear**: A conditioned emotional response towards a particular object/situation/person even in the absence of the UCS.
- **Garcia effect**: Withdrawal at the sight of an unpleasant food previously experienced.
- **Neuroses**: Failure to identify if a UCS will bring a desired UCR in the presence of vicarious CS.
- **Addictions**: A behavioural pattern as a result of the pairing of UCS (alcohol intake) with the CS (alcohol shop) to elicit UCR (psychological dependencies on alcohol). The principles of learning to fight addiction are the use of extinction and counter-conditioning.

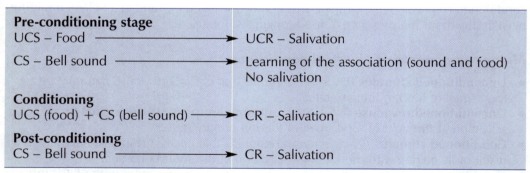

Pre-conditioning stage
UCS – Food ⟶ UCR – Salivation

CS – Bell sound ⟶ Learning of the association (sound and food)
No salivation

Conditioning
UCS (food) + CS (bell sound) ⟶ CR – Salivation

Post-conditioning
CS – Bell sound ⟶ CR – Salivation

Table 1.1 Schematic representation of classical conditioning

Graphical representation of phases:

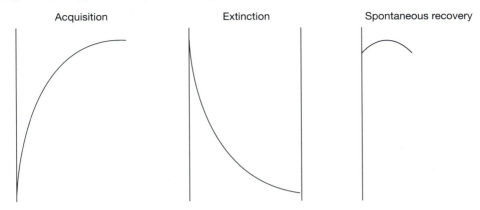

Figure 1.1 Graphical representation of phases

Operant conditioning

Learning concerning a stimulus–response connection operated by rewards and punishment. The classic experiment was conducted by Thorndike (1989, 1911) using a cat in a puzzle box (Thorndike's puzzle box).

The **Law of effect** suggests that over time those behaviours which are rewarded are likely to occur again in the future and those behaviours which are punished are unlikely to occur again in the future.

Processes in operant conditioning

- **Extinction** occurs when reinforcement ceases to exist in the learning of a behaviour, eg a toddler will continue to say 'hello' when sweets are provided and the likelihood of saying it is at a minimum as soon as the sweet is withdrawn when the word is said.
- **Reinforcement** is a process of increasing the probability of a given response associated with the stimulus.
  - **A positive reinforcer** is a rewarding stimulus that follows a behaviour (operant) and strengthens the associated behaviour.
  - **A negative reinforcer** is an unpleasant stimulus, withdrawal of which results in the increased probability of the desired response.
  - A reinforcer can acquire strength through learning.
  - **Conditioned reinforcer**: a positive reinforcer can become a conditioned reinforcer for behavioural responses.
  - **Premack principle** of reinforcement hierarchy – the more preferred activity can be used to reinforce a less preferred activity. For example, an outgoing patient will eat fast if that is followed by a guided stroll in the garden.
  - **Secondary reinforcers** are stimuli which are less satisfying and less tangible to elicit a desired response than the primary reinforcers.

Generalisation

When a response is elicited to a stimulus similar to the original stimulus/unconditioned/conditioned stimulus, it is called stimulus generalisation.

Incubation

Learning is incomplete for a certain period of time but with appropriate delivery of a cue the learning is completed.

Stimulus preparedness

Stimulus preparedness is part of the biological determinism of learning for survival needs. It is more apparent in animals, eg birds living on steep cliffs learn to make their nests in such a way that their eggs will not roll out.

The clinical application of behavioural treatments: applying learning principles

- **Reciprocal inhibition** suggests that a particular behaviour can be suppressed from both stimulus presentation and response elicitation contexts. For example, if the sound of a bell at a dinner time does not bring food for patients, they will not look for food when a bell is rung.
- **Habituation** occurs when a strong association is built between a stimulus and a response; it takes the form of a habitual response as a result of previous reinforced trails.
- **Chaining** is the use of a conditioned reinforcer after responses to a sequence of actions, followed by a primary reinforcer after a final response, eg learning to use a spoon to eat.
- **Shaping** is a learning process to change behaviour in small steps for which reinforcers are used until the final desired response occurs, which is then reinforced.
- **Escape and avoidance conditioning** is a learning process to avoid a response with the use of a negative reinforcer, eg abusive behaviour is controlled by a verbal warning from the police.

The impact of reinforcement schedules on behaviour

- A **fixed ratio** reinforcer is delivered after a fixed set of responses.
- A **variable ratio** reinforcer is delivered intermittently after a fixed set of responses.
- A **fixed-interval** reinforcer is delivered for the first response after a fixed period of time.
- A **variable-interval** reinforcer is delivered intermittently for the first response.

The psychology of punishment

Punishment in the learning process is used to decrease the probability of the occurrence of a desired response. Positive punishment is the application of an unpleasant stimulus and negative punishment is the removal of the pleasant stimulus.

Observational learning

In observational learning the learning occurs by observing others without any reinforcers and active engagement to elicit a desired response. The classic experiment was conducted by Bandura (1963).

Cognitive models of learning

These suggest that learning involves an understanding of the learning situation as a whole (cognitive map), and an expectancy about the consequences of one's own actions (Tolman, 1948).

Insightful learning

Learning occurs when a meaningful relationship is found between stimulus and response, it is more than a 'trial and error' situation (Kohler, 1925).

Connectionist learning model

Learning involves interconnections between different features of physiological (sensation and thoughts) and behavioural elements.

VISUAL AND AUDITORY PERCEPTION

What is perception?

Perception is the meaningful interpretation of sensations; it is a set of processes by which we recognise, organise, and make sense of our environment.

What is visual perception?

Visual perception is the process of encoding information received by the visual senses of the human body.

Theories of perception

- **Bottom-up processing** is the encoding of information directly from the external stimuli (Gibson's theory of direct perception; Gibson, 1950, 1966, 1979) with the use of sensory data.
  - **Optical flow patterns**: The perceptual effects of the movement from the point of standing, eg the movement perceived by a pilot.
  - **Optical array**: Natural processing of light into the eye.

- ○ **Invariants**: Stability of the optical array, eg understanding size constancy.
- ○ **Resonance**: The process with which to detect optical array, eg the workings of a radio.
- ○ **Affordances**: Potential uses of objects are directly observed, eg a chair affords 'sitting'.
- **Top-down processing** involves perception as the encoding of information from the environment taking into account knowledge, past experiences and expectations (Gregory, 1970)
- **Neisser's cyclic theory** states that perception is the outcome of both bottom-up and top-down processes (Neisser, 1976).

Perceptual organisation

Using the Gestalt principle of 'whole'/'form', various types of perception are presented.

Form perception

The use of rules to encode sensory information into wholes.

Figure and ground

A stimulus can bring more than one perception on the basis of prior knowledge about the figure–ground relationship.

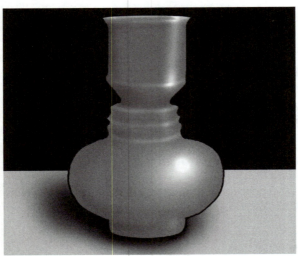

Figure 1.2 Reversible perception

Grouping

A collection of stimuli is perceived as a group according to the rules of proximity (grouping by distance between stimuli), similarity (grouping by similarity between stimuli), continuity (perception of an object in terms of continuity), closure (perception of a complete object although the stimulus presents it as incomplete), connectedness (perception as a single unit when stimuli are interlinked).

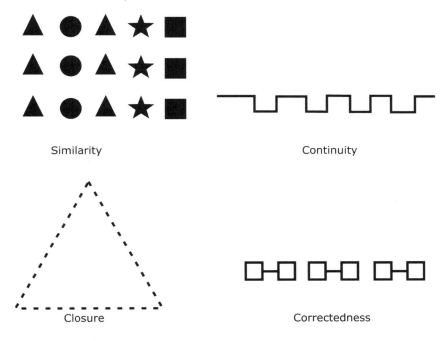

Figure 1.3 Grouping

Depth perception

Depth perception allows us to perceive objects in three-dimensions although a two-dimensional object is presented to the retina.

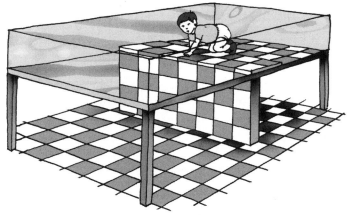

Figure 1.4 Depth perception

9

Processes in depth perception

- **Binocular cues**: Depth disparity and convergence created by both eyes give different interpretations of the stimuli presented.
- **Monocular cues**: Linear perspective and overlap occur when using only one eye. The cues used are, relative size of the object (smaller size is perceived as nearer), interposition (the longer the distance an object is from our sight, the smaller its image is on the retina), relative height (distance is perceived by length), relative motion (objects beyond the fixation period appear to move slowly, eg views from a train window), linear perspective (parallel lines appear to converge with distance, eg railroad tracks), relative brightness (bright light appears nearer than a faint one).

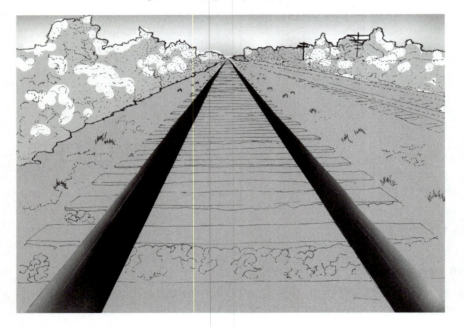

Figure 1.5 Linear perception

Perceptual constancy

Objects are perceived as constant, even if the sensory data are changing as a result of past experiences, knowledge and expectancies (top-down theory).

Perceptual distortions

Errors in perception occur despite the incoming sensory data coming correctly.

- **Muller-Lyer illusion** (error in judging the length of two same-length lines).
- **Ponzo illusion** (illusion created by depth and distance cues, railway tracks), ambiguous figures (perceptual shift between a vase and figures).

The Muller-Lyer illusion

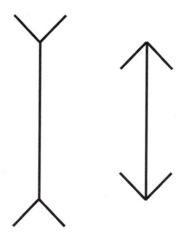

Variant on the Muller-Lyer illusion

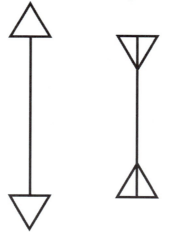

Figure 1.6 Illusions

Is **hallucination** an error in perception? Hallucination is not an error in perception because the sensory responses occur without any sensory stimulus being presented.

Auditory perception

What is auditory perception?

Auditory perception is the process of encoding information received by the auditory senses of the human body.

Selective attention

Selective attention is the tendency to attend to only one message while simultaneously ignoring others, ie the Cocktail party phenomenon (the ability to follow one conversation amid the disruption from numerous conversations, Cherrie, 1953).

Theories of selective attention

Filter theories: the process of filtering auditory data (Broadbent, 1958), conversation in a running train.

Attentional resource theory

Attention is limited as a result of the allocation of a fixed amount of auditory resources to the perceived requirements of a task.

Perception, social and cultural context

Perceptual set: perceptual responses vary according to individual and sociocultural factors (social constructivist theory).

- **Field dependence**: A perceptual style in which perception is distorted by contextual factors (Witkin, 1967).
- **Trait anxiety**: An individual high in trait anxiety will perceive incoming stimuli and encode them more negatively than people with low trait anxiety.
- **Social deprivations**: Deprivation may distort perception, eg economically deprived people perceive the value of an object more than those who are economically better off (Bruner & Goodman, 1967).
- **Social systems**: People from individualist and collectivist cultures perceive various things differently, eg depression after childbirth is not always recognised as a postnatal depression by collectivist culture but it is in an individualistic culture.

MEMORY AND FORGETTING

What is memory?

Memory is the dynamic mechanisms associated with the retention and retrieval of information about past experience (Crowder, 1976).

Stages in memory

Encoding →	Storage →	Retrieval
(the mechanism by which information is processed to enter memory)	(short-term and long-term memory/explicit and implicit)	(forgetting, interference)

Table 1.2 Stages involved in memory

Types of memory

Sensory memory

Sensory memory has the smallest capacity for storing information for the shortest duration.

- **Iconic store**: Limited capacity store for visual information for half a second.
- **Echoic store**: Limited capacity store for auditory information for two seconds after the presentation of an auditory stimulus.

Short-term memory

Short-term memory is very limited and is a fragile capacity which disappears if not well practised. The processes involved in short-term memory are the following:

- **Chunking**: A process of recording single items by grouping them on the basis of similarity/other organising principles.
- **Rehearsal**: The process of repeating is **maintenance rehearsal** and the process of actively analysing to store information is **elaborative rehearsal**.
- **Primacy effect**: The tendency to recall the first few words.
- **Recency effect**: The tendency to recall the last few words.

Working memory

Working memory has been described by Baddley & Hitch (1974).

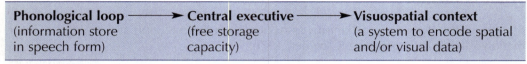

Phonological loop (information store in speech form)	**Central executive** (free storage capacity)	**Visuospatial context** (a system to encode spatial and/or visual data)

Table 1.3 Working memory

Long-term memory

Long-term memory is a permanent store of all information according to meanings, importance and usability.

There are various types of long-term memory:

- **Episodic memory**: Storage of information about particular events, situations.
- **Semantic memory**: Organised way of storing information about various things in the world; activation at the posterior region of the cortex.
- **Flashbulb memory**: Accurate retrieval of an emotionally significant event.

How do we retrieve information?

- **Explicit memory**: Conscious recollection of stored information (episodic and semantic memory).
- **Implicit memory**: Natural recollection without any conscious effort (cognitive, perceptual, motor skills).
- **Recall, recognition and relearning**.
- **Retrieval cues**: Activation of associations unconsciously (priming).
- **Mnemonic techniques**: Aid to improve memory.
- **Method of loci**: Retrieving information with the aid of associated materials.

Strategies to enhance retention and recall

The following strategies can be used to enhance retention and recall.

- **Improve encoding**: Ensure information is understood, make information meaningful, make information interesting, go into subject more deeply than necessary.
- **Improve storage**: Rehearse information, repeated learning of a subject.
- **Improve retrieval**: Encourage frequent recall.

Forgetting

Failure to retrieve information from long-term memory causes forgetting.

Theories of forgetting:

- **Trace decay theory**: Gradual decay of the memory traces as a result of the natural processes within the brain.
- **Interference theory**: Previous learning interferes with recent learning (proactive interference) or recent learning interferes with previous learning (retroactive interference).
- **Cue-dependent forgetting**: Information cannot be retrieved because of an absence of a suitable cue.
- **Mood-state-dependent forgetting**: If the mood state at retrieval remains similar to the state of learning.
- **Repression**: Motivation and conscious efforts to forget unpleasant events.

Memory deficiencies

Amnesia is a partial loss of memory from accidental injuries to the brain, strokes, encephalitis, alcoholism, electroconvulsive shock and surgical procedure.

Types of amnesia

Anterograde amnesia ↓	Retrograde amnesia ↓
Inability to acquire new factual information and day to day events → extensive memory loss	Inability to remember events that occurred before the injury and disease

Table 1.4 Types of amnesia

THINKING AND PROBLEM SOLVING

What is thinking?

Thinking is comprised of the cognitive processes of perception, thinking, remembering and forgetting.

Functions of thinking

- **Concepts**: Identifying objects that are common in properties.
- Processing of concept can be subdivided as follows:
  - ○ **Critical feature**: Listing of critical features that are sufficient to include a concept in that category
  - ○ **Prototype**: Features are structured around an ideal or most representative category

- ○ **Schemas**: A general conceptual framework of knowledge about objects/people/situations
- ○ **Scripts**: An event schema, a cluster of knowledge about sequences of inter-related, specific events and actions expected to follow a certain direction in a particular context.

Defining problem solving

Problem solving can be defined as a process in thinking that involves three stages – an initial stage, a set of operation and a goal stage.

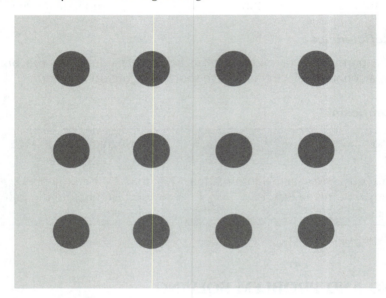

Figure 1.7 Problem solving: Draw a triangle

Stages in problem solving

An **algorithm** is a methodical procedure used to solve a problem using heuristic (an informal rule of thumb to problem solving using judgemental operations) methods.

Obstacles to problem solving

- **Confirmation bias** is a tendency to search for information that confirms one's preconceptions.
- **Fixation** is a tendency to perceive and solve a problem from one perspective only.
- **Functional fixedness** is the failure to acknowledge the diverse and changing functions of objects.
- **Representative heuristic thought** is the tendency to solve a problem from a prototype.

Reasoning

Reasoning involves a realistic thinking process that draws on evidence to solve a problem. There are two types of reasoning:

- **Deductive reasoning** draws a conclusion from established rules using syllogism (deductive arguments that lead to a conclusion).
- **Inductive reasoning** draws on available evidence to solve a problem towards a goal.

PERSONALITY

What is personality?

Personality is an individual's enduring characteristics of thinking, feeling and behaving in response to environmental stimuli.

Approaches to personality

There are two approaches to personality: The **idiographic approach** focuses on the unique characteristics of an individual; this approach calls for a person-centred approach to the study of personality. The **nomothetic approach** focuses on shared characteristics of individuals and accepts universal features in personality.

Personality theories

Trait theory

Trait theory states that there are generalised predispositions that cause certain behaviours.

- **Allport's theory** recognises three types of traits:
  - **cardinal trait**: A trait around which a person's life evolves
  - **central traits**: Major characteristics of a person
  - **secondary traits**: Specific characteristics of a person.
- **Cattel's factor-analytic theory** recognises:
  - **surface trait**: Superficial characteristics without any basis for true existence
  - **source trait**: Underlying traits that generate surface traits.
- **Extroversion** is a cluster of traits representing outgoing, sociable individuals. The opposite of these traits is called **introversion**.
- **Neuroticism** comprises traits representing emotional vulnerability and unstable social dispositions.
- **Psychoticism** describes the characteristic traits of social withdrawal, apathy and sensitivity.
- **Big five personality theory** (Norman,1963; Costa & McCrae,1992) recognises the following traits:
  - neuroticism

○ extroversion
○ openness (imagination, intelligence, inquisitiveness)
○ agreeableness (pleasant dispositions, empathy and friendliness)
○ conscientiousness (reliability, hard work, righteousness, sense of time).

The Integrationists' theories

These theories state that personality is the outcome of the interaction between the characteristics of a person and the environment.

- **Rotters' theory of locus of control** recognises a degree of personal control over the environment.
- **Bandura's social learning theory** states the influence of environment in shaping personal characteristics.

Psychoanalytic theory

This theory states that inner motivational factors shape personality.

Humanistic theory

This theory states that there are learned tendencies to develop and change in a positive direction to achieve self-actualisation.

- **Roger's person-centred theory** describes the client's goal and personal initiatives to achieve personal development and growth.

Measurement of personality

Four major types of assessment have been in use.

- **Questionnaires** are a standardised technique which assesses personality using a set of questions covering various aspects of personality.
- **Ratings** are a method of assessing personality using personality characteristics. The Q-sort technique is a type of rating using self-concepts.
- **Objective tests** involve a clinical process of assessing personality disorder, eg the Minnesota Multiphasic Personality Inventory (MMPI; Hathway & Makinley, 1943) and Cattell's 16-PF scale (Cattell *et al.*, 1970) using standardised questionnaires.
- **Projective tests** are a technique used to assess personality using unstructured tasks, eg the Rorschach inkblot test (Rorschach, 1921), and the Thematic Apperception Test (TAT; Murray, 1943).

Cultural issues in personality measurement

Culture-mediated experiences influence test performance and so the validity of a test score is questioned. One possible solution is to develop 'culture-fair' tests (that can be applied equally well to all cultures) and 'culturally-adapted' tests (modifications of an original test that adapt it to the needs of a culture).

MOTIVATION

What is motivation?

Motivation is the arousal of a need to activate a behaviour.

Mechanisms in motivation

- **Intrinsic motivation** is the desire to satisfy personal needs such as seeking enjoyment, pleasure.
- **Extrinsic motivation** is the desire to seek external recognition and avoid punishments, eg the desire to excel in a competition.
- **Achievement motivation** is the desire to have outstanding accomplishments and reach high standards, eg accomplishment of new musical notes by a student musician.
- **Drive** is the arousal state created by physiological needs.
- **Homeostasis** is the regulation, by internal mechanisms, that maintains a balance in the drive reduction stage, eg feeling cold is resolved by warm clothes and heating.
- **Incentives** are when motivation is influenced by positive or negative stimuli, eg the arrival of a physician may motivate a patient to take medicine.
- **Optimum arousal** describes some motivated behaviours that reach an arousal level beyond the satisfaction level, eg climbing a mountain driven by curiosity and achievement motivation.

Levels of motivation

- **Maslow's need hierarchy** identifies eight levels of needs – biological, safety, attachment, esteem, cognitive, aesthetic, self-actualisation and transcendence.
- **McClelland's need for achievement** describes the need to achieve that is varied in strength for different people across cultures.
- **Cognitive motivation theory** states that cognition is a central process in motivation.
- **Cognitive consistency theory** describes how a discrepancy between one's beliefs and the goal to be attained results in tension and arousal. The resulting outcome is to maintain a consistency between the two cognitions with the accomplishment of the task.

EMOTION

What is emotion?

An emotion is a response comprising physiological arousal, expressive behaviour and conscious experiences.

Emotional components

Emotion has various components.

- **Physiological arousal**: Expressed behavioural responses to an external stimuli activated by the autonomic nervous system.
- **Expressive behaviour**: Emotion expressed in non-verbal behaviour (absence of language in emotional expression), and in facial expression (communicate, amplify and regulate emotions).
- **Conscious experience**: When emotions are experienced at various magnitudes and levels. The most common/basic five emotions recognised across cultures are happiness, fear, anger, sadness and disgust.

Theories of emotion

The **James-Lange theory** states that emotion involves three stages:

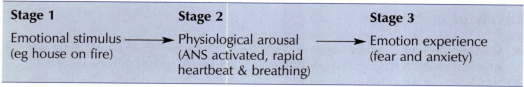

Stage 1	Stage 2	Stage 3
Emotional stimulus (eg house on fire)	Physiological arousal (ANS activated, rapid heartbeat & breathing)	Emotion experience (fear and anxiety)

Table 1.5 James-Lange theory

The **Canon–Bard theory** states that experiences of emotion occur before bodily changes.

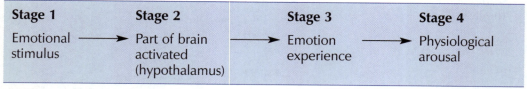

Stage 1	Stage 2	Stage 3	Stage 4
Emotional stimulus	Part of brain activated (hypothalamus)	Emotion experience	Physiological arousal

Table 1.6 Canon–Bard theory

Cognitive labelling theory includes the **Schachter–Singer theory** that emotion is the labelling of physiological arousal. The cognitive process of labelling physiological arousal leading to an experience of emotion is called the 'emotional feedback loop'.

Lazarus's cognitive appraisal theory states that emotion is the cognitive appraisal of an emotional experience. It involves three stages:

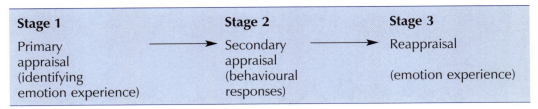

Stage 1	Stage 2	Stage 3
Primary appraisal (identifying emotion experience)	Secondary appraisal (behavioural responses)	Reappraisal (emotion experience)

Table 1.7 Lazarus's cognitive appraisal theory

CONSCIOUS AND UNCONSCIOUS PROCESSES

What is consciousness?

Consciousness is an awareness of ourselves and the world we live in.

Levels of consciousness

The preconscious level is the readiness to make information available at the unaware stage, eg driving a car (automatic behaviours). The **unconscious level** is the mechanism to keep information that cannot be readily available to awareness (repression), eg forgetting a painful surgery.

Unconscious processes: sleep and dreaming

Sleep is a reduced state of awareness and serves two functions: conservation and restoration. Five **stages of sleep** are recognised (Dement & Kleitman, 1957).

- Stage 1: Alpha waves – awake stage
- Stage 2: EEG waves – drowsy stage
- Stage 3: EOG and EMG waves – asleep
- Stage 4: Slow delta waves – deep sleep stage
- Stage 5: Low EMG waves – rapid eye movement (REM) sleep.

Sleep deprivation and disorders

Irregular patterns of sleep, including complete loss of sleep, can cause sleep disorders, such as:

- **Insomnia**: Lack of sleep
- **Narcolepsy**: Sudden uncontrollable sleep
- **Sleep apnoea**: Breathing difficulties during sleep

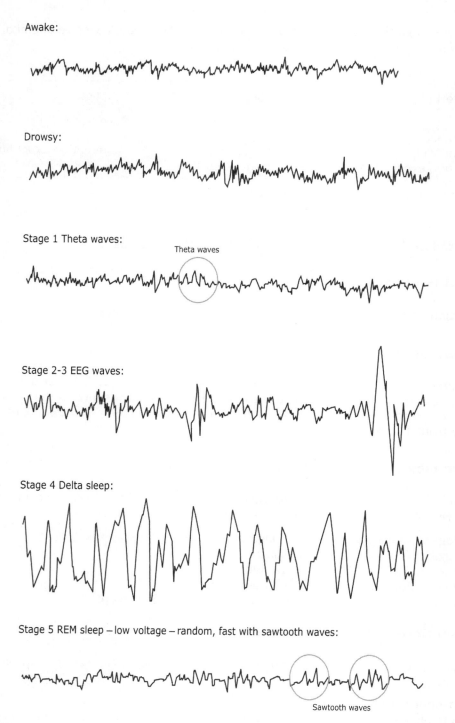

Figure 1.8 Brain waves in sleep

- **Somnambulism**: Walking, talking during sleep stages and not remembering the sleep-walking stage during the waking stage.

What is a dream?

Dreams are brain activities during rapid eye movement (REM) stage.

Four major theories of dreaming are discussed below.

- **Freud's wish fulfilment theory**: A dream is the portrayal of repressed feelings and thoughts kept at the unconscious level.
- **Activation-synthesis theory** (Hibson & McCarley, 1977): A dream is the high level of random brain activation and processing of information during this neural activity.
- **Reverse learning theory** (Crick & Mitchison, 1983): A dream is the process of unloading excessive and useless information stored in the brain.
- **Cognitive theories**: A dream is a symbolic representation of current concerns (Foulkes, 1990), the creative reshuffling of what has happened during the day.

NEUROPSYCHOLOGICAL PROCESSES

(For a more detailed account see Chapter 7.)

Organisation of the brain

The brain hemispheres are each divided into four regions or lobes:

- **Frontal lobes** form the area behind the forehead that are responsible for planning and control of movements. They are also used for the highest thought processes and reasoning.
- **Parietal lobes** are situated at the top of the rear part of the brain and are the seat for sensations such as pressure, pain and temperature.
- **Occipital lobes** are situated at the back of the brain and regulate visual processing.
- **Temporal lobes** form the area behind the ear and are mainly responsible for auditory processing and speech perception.

Lower level brain structures

- **Brainstem**: The lowest part and central core of the brain. It begins where the spinal cord enters the brain and functions as a natural control of arousal (reticular formation – network of neurones).
- **Medulla**: The base of the brainstem. It controls heartbeat and breathing.
- **Thalamus**: The top of the brainstem. It serves as a control centre for incoming and outgoing neural messages.
- **Cerebellum**: The rear of the brainstem. It is responsible for voluntary movement and balance.

- **Amygdala**: Two neural clusters at the border of the brainstem. It controls emotional responses (mainly rage and fear) as well as perception of others' emotion.
- **Hypothalamus**: A neural structure below the thalamus. It directs primary needs (hunger and thirst) and governs emotion.

Chapter 2

Social Psychology

Matt Crawford

CONTENTS

Social Psychology

ATTITUDES AND PERSUASION

Defining attitudes

An attitude is any cognitive representation that involves the evaluation (either positive or negative in valence) of an object or class of objects.

Attitude formation

The tripartite model of attitudes maintains that there are three components of attitudes.

- **Cognitive**: Knowledge that people have about an attitude object.
  - Formation involves the consideration of relevant facts and evaluation is based on beliefs about the properties of an object. Cognitively based attitudes serve an object-appraisal function.
- **Affective**: Feelings or evaluations that the attitude object arouses.
  - Based on emotional, sensory, or aesthetic reactions to an object. These reactions are not governed by logic or knowledge about the object and are often linked to people's values (eg religious and moral beliefs).
  - **Classical conditioning**: By pairing a neutral stimulus with one that elicits a positive or negative evaluation, eventually the neutral stimulus will come to elicit the same evaluation.
- **Behavioural**: Knowledge of past, present, or future interactions.
  - **Operant conditioning**: Positive interactions with an object result in positive evaluations of that object, whereas negative interactions result in a negative evaluation of the object.
  - **Observational learning**: Individuals form attitudes based on observation of others' interaction with an object.
  - **Self-perception theory**: Individuals can sometimes determine personally held attitudes by observation of their own behaviour. This is most likely to be the case when the attitude is somewhat new or ambiguous (ie not strongly held).

Attitude measurement

- **Thurstone scale** uses the fact that the extent to which one object is evaluated more positively than another object is related to the distance in their scale values on the psychological dimension of favourability. To measure one's attitude toward a specific object, that object must be paired with other objects for comparison. This scale is cumbersome and time-consuming.

- **Likert scale** presents a series of statements that participants respond to using a five-point scale: 1 = strongly disagree, 2 = disagree, 3 = undecided, 4 = agree, to 5 = strongly agree. Comparison between items is not necessary.
- **Semantic differential** is a measure that generally consists of a series of bipolar adjective scales, separated into seven categories. Participants rate each attitude object on the bipolar scales (eg beautiful–ugly, bad–good, pleasant–unpleasant, dirty–clean, wise–foolish) and generally yield three evaluative dimensions: evaluation, potency and activity.

Attitudes and behaviour

Attitude–behaviour consistency depends on several factors including the qualities of the behaviour, the person, the attitude and the situation.

- **Qualities of the behaviour**: It is important to measure both attitudes and behaviours at equivalent levels of specificity. Both behaviours and attitudes range from very specific to very general. To increase the behavioural prediction power of attitudes, it is important to measure both at the same level. That is, specific attitudes better predict specific behaviours, and more general attitudes predict general behaviours better than specific behaviours.
- **Qualities of the person**: There are individual differences in attitude–behaviour correspondence; some people show more attitude–behaviour consistency than others.
  - **Locus of control**: Individuals with a high internal locus of control (ie those who feel that their behaviours are under their own internal control) show more attitude–behaviour consistency.
  - **Self-monitoring**: Low self-monitors exhibit much higher consistency between their attitudes and their behaviours than do high self-monitors.
- **Qualities of the situation**: Situational norms can suppress behaviour consistent with held attitudes.
  - **Time pressure**: More attitude-consistent behaviour is exhibited when individuals are placed in situations involving time constraints.
- **Qualities of the attitude**: Stronger attitudes (not necessarily more extreme) lead to more consistent behaviours than do weaker attitudes.
  - Direct experience with the attitude object results in stronger attitudes than secondary attitude experience.
  - Amount of information: the more information one has about an attitude object, the more consistency between that attitude and behaviours toward that object will be shown.

How attitudes guide behaviour

The **Theory of Reasoned Action** assumes that people deliberate about the wisdom of a given course of action, and that behavioural intention (not the attitude itself) is the best predictor of behaviour. Forming a behavioural intention depends on two factors:

- attitude toward the behaviour; and
- subjective norms regarding the behaviour.

The **Attitude–Behaviour Process Model** posits that attitudes guide behaviour without conscious deliberation. The attitude defines the situation as pleasant or unpleasant and the individual acts upon this feeling or impulse.

How behaviour affects attitudes

When freely chosen behaviours are at odds with personally held attitudes, the inconsistency produces uncomfortable arousal, known as **cognitive dissonance**. To alleviate this arousal, individuals may change their initial attitudes to be more consistent with the behaviour. Four steps are necessary to produce dissonance and attitude change:

- The behaviour must be perceived to be inconsistent with the attitude.
- Personal responsibility must be taken for the behaviour. If an external attribution of cause can be made, then no dissonance will be aroused.
- The individual must experience physiological arousal.
- The arousal must be attributed to the inconsistent behaviour.

Models of persuasion

There are two models: the **Elaboration Likelihood Model** and the **Heuristic Systematic Model**; both models posit two routes to persuasion.

- **Peripheral (or Heuristic) route**: Processing persuasive messages peripherally relies on cognitive shortcuts (or heuristics) that allow judgements to be made with little or no effort.
  - **Messenger characteristics**: Competence, trustworthiness, expertise (even mere perceptions of expertise), and speed of speech all serve as heuristic cues to persuasion.
  - **Message characteristics**: Longer messages are more persuasive than shorter messages, and a higher number of arguments (not the quality of arguments) results in greater persuasion than shorter messages or fewer arguments.
- **Central (or Systematic) route**: The central route to persuasion requires conscious and logical consideration of the quality of the argument in the persuasive message. Persuasion in this case involves four steps:
  - attending to the message
  - understanding the message
  - elaboration (eg production of counter-arguments)
  - acceptance.

When are individuals more likely to process messages systematically?

- **Motivation**: When individuals are motivated by a concern with being **accurate** in judgement and/or when the persuasive message is **self-relevant**, they are more likely to consider message quality.
- **Cognitive capacity**: Individuals require **cognitive resources** to be available to process information deeply. In addition, the individual also needs the **ability**, **knowledge** and **concentration**.

THE SELF

Self-concept is what one knows about the self (ie self-knowledge).

Self-esteem is how the self is evaluated (positive or negative).

How is the self unique?

People have greater knowledge about the self than about other people. There is greater affect and motivation involved with the self (eg self-enhancement, self-protection, etc).

Perception of others is based primarily on observations of their behaviour. For the self, aside from behaviour, people also have access to thoughts and feelings.

People have extremely rich and well-developed representations of the self.

Sources of self-knowledge

- **Behaviour**: People learn about the self by observing their own behaviour (Self-Perception Theory).
- **Thoughts and feelings**: Our own reactions to the world provide a great deal of information about who we are. In addition, external pressures do not influence these internal reactions.
- **Labelling body states and emotions**: People use internal physiological cues in determining beliefs and attitudes.
- **Physiological–cognitive theory of emotion**: Both the arousal and the interpretation of the arousal matters when interpreting internal physiological cues. All emotions/arousals are the same in terms of physiological state, it is how this arousal is interpreted that determines what is felt.
- **Other people's reactions**: To some extent, we are who others perceive us to be (Looking-glass Self).
- **Social comparison**: To gain accurate self-evaluation, people compare the self to similar others (Social Comparison Theory).

Measuring the self-concept

The self-concept can be measured traditionally or using more modern approaches.

Traditional approaches include:

- **Q-sort** involves sorting 100 statements/adjectives into categories that describe actual and ideal selves (Rogers, 1951).
- **Adjective ratings** involve rating the self on relevant traits or characteristics (eg How well does 'intelligent' describe you?).
- **Self-report** invites an open-ended response: describe yourself.

Modern approaches include:

- **Self-schematics and aschematics** which state that just because an item is self-descriptive does not mean that it is part of the self-concept.

○ **Schematic**: Highly descriptive and of high importance to self-definition.
○ **Aschematic**: Moderately descriptive but unimportant to self-definition.
- **Possible selves** posits that the self can better be understood in terms of multiplicity rather than as a single unitary concept. So, the self-concept involves many selves, including good selves, bad selves, hoped-for selves, feared selves, not-me selves, ideal selves, ought selves.
- **Self-complexity** represents differences in the extent to which people perceive themselves as playing different roles.
- **Self-discrepancy theory** posits that the actual self exists as well as two primary self-guides that provide comparison. Discrepancies between the actual self and the self-guides have implications for emotional wellbeing.
  ○ **Ideal self** is the self that one would ideally like to be.
  ○ **Ought self** is the self that one feels one should be.

The self and behaviour

- **Self-expression** is the attempt to convey self-concept through actions. This serves to reinforce the sense of self. People choose situations in which one can act consistently with self – even when that situation is negative.
- **Self-presentation** is an attempt to create a desirable impression of the self, ie to gain power, influence, or approval through positive self-presentation.
- **Self-monitoring** is shaping behaviour to project an impression consistent with what one thinks the current audience or situation demands.
- **Self-evaluation maintenance**: One's self-concept can be threatened by the behaviour of others – especially when outperformed on some task/ability. The level of threat is determined jointly by the closeness of the comparison other and the personal relevance of the behaviour.
- **Self-enhancement**: People rate themselves above average on virtually all positive dimensions and below average on negative dimensions (Lake Woebegone Effect). This effect is stronger for more abstract characteristics or abilities (eg loyalty vs creativity or friendly vs punctual).

INTERPERSONAL ISSUES

Person perception: basis of impressions

Expectations guide perceptions of social targets in that people see in others what they expect to see.

Salient features are those features that 'stick out' in the visual array, ie attractiveness and appearance.

- **Physical appearance** is often the first, and sometimes only, information we have about someone else. Appearance is believed to indicate the personality of observed others because people project, to some extent, how they wish to be seen by others.

- **Physical attractiveness** is governed by the idea that 'What is beautiful is good.' We infer that attractive others are more intelligent, sociable, friendly, warmer, interesting, outgoing, etc, 'the halo effect'. Teachers rate attractive children higher in intelligence and academic potential than less attractive students. Children view unattractive peers as more aggressive and unfriendly. Strangers are more likely to help attractive others. Attractive defendants receive lower bail recommendations in criminal cases. If convicted, they also receive shorter, or less severe, sentences.

Non-verbal communication, such as standing, speaking distance, gait, posture, habits, are recognised.

- **Emotional expression**: there is a 'Universality' of emotional expression recognition, ie there are six primary emotions that are both recognised and elicited across all cultures: anger, fear, happiness, surprise, sadness, and disgust.

Inferring traits from behaviour, ie 'What people do is what they are like,' leads to:

- **Fundamental Attribution Error** (aka correspondence bias): people over-infer the degree of correspondence between a given behaviour and the dispositional implications of that behaviour – even when the behaviour in question was not freely chosen.
- **Consequences of inferring a trait**:
  - the perceiver infers other psychologically related traits according to Implicit Personality Theories
  - new behaviours are interpreted in terms of traits already inferred (especially when subsequent behaviours are ambiguous)
  - behaviour toward others is guided by trait inferences, which, in turn, affects their behaviour (ie self-fulfilling prophecy).

Attribution theory

The **Theory of Mind** represents a specific cognitive ability to understand others as intentional agents, that is, to interpret their minds in terms of theoretical concepts of intentional states such as **beliefs** and **desires**. Normally developing children develop Theory of Mind around 4 years of age.

Naïve Psychology (Heider) describes the conceptual frameworks by which people interpret, explain, and predict the behaviour of others. Intentional concepts (eg beliefs, desires, trying, purpose) play a central role in the interpretation of behaviour. Additionally, the distinction between person (internal) and situation (external) causes is used in the explanation of behaviour.

Correspondent inference (Jones and Davis) posits that people make dispositional inferences based on the behaviours of others by focusing only on those behaviours that are likely to be the most informative.

- **Free choice**: Freely chosen behaviours are more informative than behaviours that are constrained by the situation.
- **Social desirability**: Perceivers weigh behaviours that are low in social desirability as providing more diagnostic information about others' dispositions than behaviours that are high in social desirability.

- **Non-common effects**: Careful attention is paid to outcomes that can be achieved by one action, but not by others. That is, the chosen action produces distinctive, non-common effects.

Kelley's Theory of Causal Attributions can be described as follows. A behaviour occurs: 'John yells at Michelle'. This raises the question: *why?* Is it:

- … something about John (internal)?
- … something about Michelle (external)?
- … something about the situation?

To answer this question, of why John yelled at Michelle, one must examine three types of evidence before making an accurate attribution.

- **Consensus**: Do other people respond in the same way to the stimulus?
- **Consistency**: How does the actor usually respond to the stimulus?
- **Distinctiveness**: How does the actor respond to other stimuli?

A problem with this is that the model is **Normative** rather than **Descriptive**, ie the model describes what people 'should' do rather than what people actually do. Some behaviours lead to stronger trait inferences than others because they are more diagnostic (eg immoral or illegal acts; high ability/talent behaviours; freely chosen behaviour).

The trait inferred is based, not on some objective standard, but depending on expectations, recent, frequent, or chronic activation of concepts. That is, whatever is accessible to the mind of the perceiver drives the interpretation of the observed behaviour.

Affiliation and friendship

The first step in getting to know someone is sparked by feelings of attraction or liking.

- **Physical attractiveness**: People like attractive others, and beauty itself is aesthetically pleasing. There are, however, cultural, temporal, and individual differences in what is seen as attractive.
- **Interaction**: Interaction spells liking … usually.
  - Proximity can lead to liking (eg people who live near each other, friendships in the classroom, cubicle neighbours). Why? It may be **Mastery**, ie we compare our feelings with other people to understand ourselves and to test the truth of our views; there may be feelings of connectedness with others; or familiar others seem likable (a mere exposure effect).
  - The valence of the interaction matters, ie more interaction with a disliked other results in greater dislike and annoyance.
- **Similarity and liking**: People tend to interact with similar others. There is an assumption that similar others will like us. Similar others are more likely to validate our beliefs/attitudes.
- **Similarity, liking and interaction** form a mutually reinforcing relationship. People interact with similar others and discover similarities when interacting with others. People interact with those they like and people like those with whom they interact. People like similar others and think that those whom they like are similar to themselves.

SOCIAL INFLUENCE

Social norms

Social norms represent spoken, or unspoken, rules indicating how one should or ought to behave. These can be explicit (eg written laws, regulated rules) or implicit ('unwritten' rules of conduct) guides to appropriate behaviour.

Conformity is the convergence of individual thoughts, attitudes, or behaviour to the norm associated with a given social group. There are two bases for conformity.

- **Normative Social Influence** represents a need for social identity and acceptance by others. Conformity can maintain or improve individual status within a group. Normative social influence is based on anonymity and the ability of the group to deliver rewards and punishments (eg ostracism). Any disagreement with the group unanimity can decrease individual levels of conformity.
- **Informational Social Influence** represents a need for accurate and correct information in an attempt to understand and master the world. Informational social influence is based on ambiguity and uncertainty and is based on the difficulty of the task, the expertise of the others making judgements, and the self-confidence of the individual group member.

When **Conformity** goes awry there may be:

- **Polarisation** which is the process by which a group moves from a more moderate position to a more extreme position following interaction within the group.
- **Deindividuation** which is the feeling that one's personal identity has become lost in the crowd. This occurs when group membership dominates thought and behaviour to the point of blindly following group norms and ignoring personally held attitudes or beliefs (eg riot or mob mentality).

Compliance is the use of norms to influence others. These norms are:

- **Norm of Reciprocity**: We should try to repay, in kind, that which another person has given us.
- **Norm of Social Commitment**: One should fulfil obligations and stand by agreements.
- **Norm of Social Proof**: People determine what is correct by finding out what other people think is correct. A behaviour is correct in a given situation to the degree that we see others performing it.

Obedience to Authority is most likely to work when the authority figure is perceived to have legitimate authority and that figure accepts personal responsibility for the actions of the individual.

However, it is possible to move from obedience to atrocity. Simple obedience can become tragedy by **Gradual escalation**.

- **Self-justification**: The action, if against personal beliefs, is likely to evoke cognitive dissonance. However, this dissonance can be eliminated by focusing on the positive implications of the behaviour or by blaming the victim.

Majority and minority influences

In the **Majority influence** there are a greater number of people holding a particular view-point, therefore there are more arguments favouring that position.

- When people believe that others share their views, they are more likely to mention them, and these majority views receive more discussion (and may lead to group polarisation).
- Majority arguments seem more compelling because they receive multiple endorsements from members of the group. Additionally, majority arguments are presented more compellingly because their views are raised earlier in group discussions.

For **Minority influence** minorities can successfully influence the majority, but must follow a few basic rules.

- Because majorities are unlikely to be swayed quickly, minorities are most influential when they agree among themselves and provide a consistent argument (ie they provide an alternative consensus).
- Minority group members must present themselves as different from the majority, but not too different, or they may not be perceived as members of the in-group, so will be less influential.
- Minority groups are likely to be more influential if they can manage to motivate other group members to consider the arguments systematically (ie effortful processing).

Leadership

Leadership generally involves two types of behaviours:

Task-focused behaviours are focused on achieving the goal(s) set out by the group or situation.

Socio-emotional behaviours are aimed at enhancing both group cohesion and positive relationships among members of the group.

- An effective leader is one whose personal characteristics match the demands of the situation. That is, if the task requires interpersonal interactions and co-operation, a leader who is socio-emotionally oriented may be more effective than a task-oriented leader.

Gender differences and leadership effectiveness. Although it is believed that males make better group leaders than do females, the research indicates that females are just as likely as men to be successful leaders when it comes to task performance, but that women are much better than men at creating connectedness and cohesion within the group.

INTER-GROUP BEHAVIOUR

Inter-group behaviour is affected by:

Stereotype, the cognitive component, the schematic representation of a group that contains information about:

- What the group looks like.
- What the group is like (eg personality traits, attributes, abilities). This information can be both positively and negatively valenced. Additionally, the information can be accurate or inaccurate.

People tend to overestimate uniformity. Even accuracies in knowledge representation become exaggerated and applied to all members of the group.

Prejudice, the affective or evaluative component, covers feelings about the group or about group members.

Discrimination, the behavioural component, covers actions toward group members based on thoughts and feelings about the group. Discrimination can lead to **Racism**.

- **Institutionalised racism**: The majority of people hold racist attitudes because prejudice and discrimination are the norm in the larger society.
- **Modern racism** is a more subtle form of racism that is represented by outward non-prejudiced actions (to avoid being labelled a racist), paired with the maintenance of prejudicial attitudes. These prejudicial attitudes may manifest themselves in situations in which prejudicial responding is considered 'safe'.

Basis of stereotype knowledge

Categorisation: People categorise objects (both social and non-social) in an attempt to simplify the world. So, stereotypes provide an efficient way to parse the social world.

- **Inductive potential**: Stereotype knowledge allows social perceivers to 'go beyond' the information given and provides a basis for making inferences about social targets. This, in turn, provides a perception of both prediction and control over the social environment.
- **Social Identity Theory** maintains that individual self-esteem is determined by group membership and that to assess the self accurately, one must compare the groups to which one belongs (in-groups) with relevant comparison groups (out-groups).

Personal Experience: Interaction can become the basis of stereotype.

- **Illusory correlation**: Salient group members plus distinctive information become highly associated (and accessible) in memory. Perceivers overestimate the co-occurrence of these types of information represented in the real world.
- **Social roles** are not considered. As roles change, so do stereotypes (eg German ruthlessness becomes German efficiency once the conflict has been removed).

Emotion has two affects:

- **Incidental affect** is the mood that one brings to the interaction. Mood interferes with ability to do tasks because it is a distraction and reduces cognitive capacity, which results in greater stereotyping.
- **Integral affect** is the mood caused by interaction. Interaction with members of another group can cause anxiety. With repeated exposure, the anxiety and frustration become associated with the group (ie classical conditioning) and the group is viewed negatively.

Social Learning: People learn about other groups in the absence of first-hand experience from a variety of sources, including parents, teachers, peers and the media. These others provide social norms for behaviour. Children observe and imitate, even if they do not understand.

Role Justification: Societies produce and maintain inequalities; stereotypes can serve to justify these differences (Subjective Essentialism).

'Just-World' beliefs: The idea that people get what they deserve and deserve what they get. This belief system maintains perceptions of a controllable world.

Stereotypes and information processing

- **Interpretation**: Stereotype knowledge affects how the behaviours of group members are interpreted (ie consistent with stereotype). This is especially true for ambiguous behaviours that may have more than one interpretation.
- **Attribution**: People tend to attribute behaviours that are consistent with stereotypic knowledge as representing the dispositional characteristics of group members, whereas stereotype-inconsistent behaviours are attributed to external (or situational) factors.
- **Memory**: People show better memory for behaviours that are consistent with a stereotype than for behaviours that contradict the stereotype. This is especially true when processing information under capacity constraints (eg time pressure).

Membership in stigmatised groups

Negative Social Identities: What effect does being a member of a disliked group have on individual members? There will be decreased self-esteem and emotional well-being as a result of:

- Unequal employment opportunities; less access to good education, medical care; poor living conditions.
- Stereotype threat, ie apprehension felt by members of a minority group when placed in a situation in which their performance has the possibility of confirming the stereotype. The arousal causes poorer performance, which, subsequently, does confirm the stereotype (ie self-fulfilling prophecy).

There are various methods for **Defending Self-Esteem**.

- **Attribution**: Members of a stigmatised group can attribute any failures to the prejudice of others. This serves the benefit of protecting the self from the potential negative impact of the evaluation; however, the costs can be quite severe. Attribution of success may be attributed to others' attempts to appear non-prejudiced. If failures are attributed to prejudice, then one cannot learn from mistakes made. Over time, this may result in a sense of hopelessness.

- **Social mobility** allows psychological escape from the group.
- **Disidentification**: Minimising of personal connections to the group and avoidance of reminders of membership in the group (eg dressing, language).
- **Dissociation**: Actual physical separation between the self and the group. In some cases it is possible to conceal membership in the group (eg homosexuals 'in the closet'). The benefits include freedom from discrimination, but the costs are isolation and loneliness because the person does not belong to the group that he or she is attempting to pass the self off as a member of.

Inter-group contact

The **contact hypothesis** (Allport, 1954) posits that mere interaction between members of different groups can decrease stereotyping and prejudice between members of those groups. However, subsequent research has indicated that mere contact is not enough, and that certain situational requirements must be met to decrease negative perceptions of the groups involved. Specifically, authority must support the interaction, the groups must be of equal status, and the interaction should involve co-operative tasks for contact to be successful in decreasing prejudice between the groups.

There are several cognitive mechanisms that allow individuals to maintain stereotypes in the face of disconfirming information.

- Explaining away inconsistencies.
- **Subtypes**: Creating special, narrower groups within the larger category, which do not have an impact on perceptions of the group.
- **Exceptions to the rule**: Very inconsistent members have no impact on perceptions of 'typical' members of the group.

Members of stigmatised groups can counter these cognitive processes by presenting repeated inconsistency or widespread inconsistency, and by presenting themselves as typical as well as inconsistent.

Alternatively, members of stigmatised groups can bring about social change by:

- **Social creativity**: Emphasise dimensions of superiority of the group
- **Social competition**: Build solidarity and oppose the dominant group
- **Recategorisation**: Creation of new, inclusive in-groups.

AGGRESSION

Origins of aggression

Freud (1930) viewed aggression as an instinctive response and the expression of aggression as both natural and cathartic. He divided aggression into:

- **Inward**: Self-destructive and
- **Outward**: Violence against others.

Lorenz (1966) stated that aggression serves an evolutionary advantage. In animals, most violence is male–male and serves the function of determining mating success. So, aggression serves the evolutionary function of increasing the likelihood of passing on genes.

The **Frustration–Aggression Theory** of Dollard & Miller (1940) defines frustration as the blocking of a goal. Their strong hypothesis was that aggression always stems from frustration and frustration always produces aggression. However, neither of these statements is always correct.

Defining aggression

Aggression can be defined as any action that is intended to hurt others. A key component of this definition involves intentionality. Aggression can be further broken down into two types of aggression depending on the goal of the aggressive action.

- **Instrumental aggression** is aggression as a means to an end (eg hurting another person to steal property from them). It involves considerations of the costs and rewards associated with the aggressive action. Several factors that determine the perceived costs and benefits are:
  - **Personal abilities**: If aggression is easy for the individual or the person has experienced previous success with aggressive actions, then aggression becomes more likely.
  - **Gender differences**: In general, aggression is less risky for males.
  - **Impact of models**: Exposure to aggressive social models provides evidence for when and how aggression can be used successfully.
- **Emotional aggression** is aggression as an end in itself. It occurs in response to provocation (eg 'Was that bump an accident?' ... or ... 'Was that person intentionally trying to provoke me?').
  - **Intentionality**: If the action against the self is perceived as an intentional provocation, then aggression as retaliation is more likely.
  - **Controllability**: If the action against the self is perceived to be outside the control of the other person, retaliation becomes less likely as a response.
  - **Individual differences**: Aggressive people are more likely to interpret ambiguous behaviours as intentional and respond accordingly.

Exposure to violent media

Psychological research has shown several major effects of exposure to violent television on children.

- Children become less sensitive to the pain and suffering of others.
- Children become more fearful of the world around them.
- Children become more likely to behave in aggressive or harmful ways toward others because they believe, for a short while at least, that aggression is fairly common and often appropriate.
- Violent scenes arouse less those children who watch a lot of television, ie they become desensitised to the violence that they see through repeated exposure.

However, there are important mitigating factors that attenuate the relationship between exposure to media violence and actual aggressive behaviour.

- Group or family discussions of the social implications of the viewed violence decrease the likelihood of subsequent aggressive behaviour in children.
- Training children to think about the reasons why viewed violent behaviours are bad decreases subsequent aggressiveness by creating an unfavourable attitude toward the violence.

HELPING, ALTRUISM AND CO-OPERATION

Pro-social behaviour is any act performed with the goal of benefiting another person. In layman's terms, this is helping.

Altruism is any act that benefits another person but does not benefit the helper (and often involves some personal cost to the helper).

Why do people help?

Socio-biology would state that helping may give an evolutionary advantage.

- **Kin selection**: Helping blood relatives serves the evolutionary purpose of ensuring that our own genes (because of the shared genes in relatives) are likely to be passed on to future generations.
- **Norm of reciprocity**: People help others so as to get help at a later point in time, if necessary. Learning societal norms are adaptive.

Social Exchange Theory describes the calculation of costs and rewards of helping behaviour (ie determining self-interest). According to the Social Exchange Theory, the decision to help is incumbent upon the personal benefits outweighing the potential costs of the helping behaviour. So, according to this theory, true altruism does not exist.

- **Maximise rewards**, ie increase in reciprocal helping, relief of personal distress (others' suffering causes distress), gain of social approval, increased feelings of self-worth.
- **Minimise costs**, ie physical danger, pain; embarrassment; waste of time and/or effort.

Empathy–Altruism Hypothesis maintains that altruism does exist, but only when the potential helper feels **empathy** (experiencing some of the pain and suffering of another person) for the person in need. When empathy is not felt for the person in need, an individual is likely to help only if it is in his or her self-interest.

Personal determinants of helping

There are individual differences in determinants of helping.

- **Developmental**: If, at an early age, children receive rewards or praise for helping, then they are more likely to be helpful later in life. However, the reward itself cannot be too large or too much emphasis placed on the actual reward (eg overjustification effect).
- **Modelling helping behaviour**: Children observe and imitate what they see – this works for helping as well as aggressive behaviours.

There is an effect of mood on helping. **Positive moods** increase helping behaviour.

- Good moods make one look on the bright side of life; subsequently one is more likely to give people the benefit of the doubt.
- Helping others is a way of prolonging/maintaining positive feelings. Not helping may serve to decrease positive mood upon reflection.
- Positive mood increases self-attention and focus on values and ideals (eg altruism = good).

However, **negative moods** can also increase helping behaviour.

- The **Negative-state Relief Hypothesis** states that when sad, people are motivated to do things to make themselves feel better. This is especially true with guilt.

Situational determinants of helping

There are five steps that are necessary for an individual to provide helping behaviour.

- noticing the event
- interpreting the event as an emergency (this involves perception of the person in need as deserving of assistance)
- assuming personal responsibility
- knowing how to help (does the potential helper know what the problem is and what needs to be done to offer assistance?)
- deciding to implement the help (involves both a determination of costs as well as perceptions of ability to give the necessary help).

Co-operation and social dilemmas

A **Social dilemma** is a situation in which personal interests are in conflict with the interests of either another person, or a group.

- **Prisoner's Dilemma** is a situation in which co-operative responding is in the best interest of each individual, regardless of their partner's choice. However, if one individual co-operates and one competes, the competitive individual receives the maximum benefit and the co-operative partner receives the maximum cost. The optimal strategy over repeated games is tit-for-tat.

- **Replenishable resource dilemma** involves conflicts regarding the consumption of renewable resources in which it is in each individual's interest to take as much as possible, but if every member of the group acted in his or her self-interest, the resource would be depleted.
- **Public goods dilemma** involves public goods that are available to all or none of the group. This promotes 'free riders', those who use the resource without paying for it.
  - Overcoming the dilemma involves identification with the group. When members feel connected to the group (and its outcomes) they are more likely to forego personal self-interest for the benefit of the group.
  - These feelings of connectedness can be maximised by: encouraging communication among group members, providing equal opportunities and outcomes among the group members, making certain that group norms of co-operation and other related values are accessible to group members, and providing feedback that shows how individual efforts affect the group as a whole (ie increasing individual responsibility to the group).

Chapter 3

Human Growth and Development

Manfusa Shams

CONTENTS

Human Growth and Development

PRECONCEPTUAL AND PRENATAL INFLUENCES ON DEVELOPMENT

Developmental processes

Human development is a lifelong process starting from birth and continuing to old age. However, debates persist around three major issues:

- **Nature/nurture**: Developmental irregularities may result from genetic (nature) and/or environmental (nurture) deficiencies.
- **Continuous/discrete**: Development may go through continuous/separate stages.
- **Stable/flexibility**: Our characteristics change as we grow or remain stable.

Subjects of different
ages observed at a single point in time

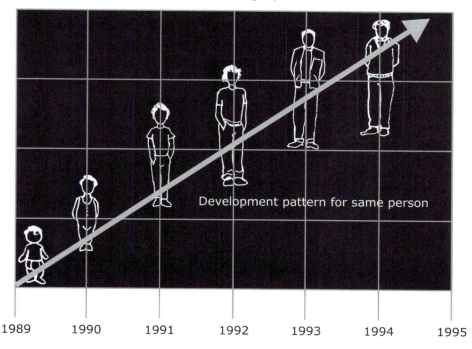

Figure 3.1 Human development

Prenatal development

The characteristic features of prenatal development are:

- **The prenatal development of the brain:** Higher brain regions develop from five months' gestation and this continues until birth. Complex control of neural activity emerges, at the same time anomalies in the brain may occur as a result of external toxication, ie alcoholic mothers bring the risk of birth defects and mental retardation. This is called fetal alcohol syndrome (FAS) and presents as an infant with a small head and mental retardation.
- **Maternal conditions and prenatal development:** The fetus is influenced by the biochemical changes in mothers caused by emotions, illnesses, diet, and stress. In addition attitudes towards pregnancy can also have an effect on the biochemical changes in mothers affecting the fetus's health.
- **Social context and prenatal development:** Mothers from low socio-economic backgrounds may suffer from malnutrition and their babies can be born prematurely, and suffer from birth defects and illnesses. Prenatal mortality rate is high among mothers from low socio-economic backgrounds.
- **Environmental factors and parental development**: External environmental factors affecting mothers can lead to defects in normal development and to premature death of infants, eg
  - drugs (tobacco, alcohol, cocaine, methadone and heroin)
  - infections (rubella, AIDS)
  - rhesus incompatibility
  - radiation
  - pollution.
- **Other medical conditions and injury:** Babies may suffer from a variety of problems if they experience the following during the prenatal stage or at birth:
  - asphyxiation or head injury during delivery can lead to brain damage
  - acute difficulty breathing at birth
  - difficulty digesting food because of an immature digestive system.
- **Use of medication at childbirth:** The administration of analgesics during labour and heavy use of other obstetric drugs may cause the following problems for babies after birth:
  - difficulty in breathing
  - lower attention and greater irritability
  - poorer muscle tone
  - slow sucking responses
  - learning disorders.

Genetic vs environmental outcome on developmental outcome

Genetic influences

- **Polygenic**: human characteristics are determined by a combination of genes.
- **Constitutional factors**: genetically determined physical and psychological characteristics, eg temperament.

- **Genetic or chromosomal abnormalities**, eg
  - ○ sickle-cell anaemia (serious abnormalities of the red blood cells)
  - ○ phenylketonuria (PKU; a metabolic disorder interfering with nervous system and brain development)
  - ○ Down's syndrome (mental and physical retardation).

Environmental influences

There is debate on whether developmental sequences occur in stages or are continuous.

- **Continuous**: development is the cumulative action of the same continuing processes.
- **Stages**: development is subject to a stepwise progression towards an expected completed developmental stage. The major stage theories are proposed by Freud (see pages 47–48), Piaget (see page 50), and Erickson (see pages 54–55).
- **Critical period**: a sensitive time in development in which certain behaviour occurs naturally with the environmental stimulation.
- Modern psychologists place emphasis on the influences of both nature and nurture on normal development and growth.

INFANCY AND CHILDHOOD

Development is a lifelong process and encompasses several major stages in life: infancy and childhood, adolescence, and adulthood/old age. Maturation is systematic changes in development that are influenced both by genetic and environmental factors.

Stage period	Major features
Prenatal stage (conception to birth)	Physical development
Infancy (birth to 18 months)	Locomotion, preliminary language-usage, emotional attachment
Early childhood (18 months to 6 years)	Cognitive, social and language development, moral reasoning
Late childhood (6 years to 13 years)	Higher-order cognitive abilities, spatial and reasoning abilities

Table 3.1 Stages in early life-span development

Major theories of psychological development

Psychosexual development

Proposed by Freud in 1905, this theory draws attention to four major stages, each characterised by major psychosexual functions, failure of which can lead to serious maladaptive behaviours and psychiatric problems in later life.

These stages are:

- **Oral**: The first developmental stage for infants when pleasure comes mainly from the use of the mouth.
- **Anal**: The second developmental stage when pleasure comes from retaining and expelling excrement.
- **Phallic stage**: The third developmental stage when pleasure principles suggest the use of the genitals.
- **Genital/latent stage**: The fourth developmental stage when sexual energy is diverted towards the opposite sex.

Cognitive development

Piaget (1977) proposed four stages of development based on three approaches:

- **Schemas:** Mental structures, predispositions and enduring abilities to carry out specific tasks
- **Assimilation:** External sensory data are adjusted with existing internal, cognitive structures
- **Accommodation:** Restructuring/modifying the child's existing schemas to accept new external information.

- **Sensorimotor stage** (0–2 years): characterised by development of Sensor–Motor cognitive sequences and **Object Permanence** (awareness of the existence of objects and their functions).

- **Pre-operational stage** (2–7 years): mental representation of objects; the important features are egocentrism, ability to distinguish mental and physical worlds and centration (ability to focus on central features of objects).

- **Concrete-operational stage** (7–11 years): mental functions to examine properties of an object and to understand that a change in the appearance of an object does not necessitate the change of physical properties in it (**conservation**).

- **Formal operational stage** (11+ years): development of abstract thinking.

Table 3.2 Stages of cognitive development

Language development

Early stages of language development are those of **receptive language** (language comprehension) and **productive language** (language expression/speaking).

Language development involves four types of knowledge about language:

- **Phonology**: The sound system of a language
- **Semantics**: The meaning underlying words and sentences
- **Syntax**: Grammatical rules
- **Pragmatics**: Principles to modify language in a context.

Name of the sequence	Major features
Shared rhythms/early vocalisations (1–9 months)	Babbling and echolalia (frequent repetition of sounds)
One-word stage (until 18 months)	use of single-word only

Table 3.3 Sequences in language development

Mistakes

- **Over-extension**: Using the same word to generalise objects/person, eg using Daddy for every man.
- **Under-extension**: Under-use of a word, eg the name fruit is used only for orange.
- **Holophrastic period**: To apply one word to cover a wide range of objects, eg pointing to a ball means playing with a ball.
- **Telegraphic period**: Predominant use of nouns and verbs only.

Regular speech

Use of grammatical morphemes (meaningful units) and pragmatics develops from 2 years to 5 years.

- **Transformational grammar**: Chomsky (1965) used this term to refer to the transformation of the meaning of a word into another word.
- **Echoic response**: Learning by imitation.
- **Tact**: Use of reward for correct pronunciation of a word.
- **Mand**: Learning a word that is significant to a child.
- **Critical period hypothesis**: Language learning depends on biological maturation and it is much easier to learn one's own language before puberty (Lenneberg, 1967).
- **Aphasia**: Some loss of language as a result of brain injury, most can be recovered if the loss occurs before puberty.
- **Dyslexia**: Failure to attain minimum level of language skills.

Social and moral development

Moral development refers to the development of an ability to distinguish between right and wrong.

Components of moral development

- **Emotional component**: Feelings associated with moral thoughts and behaviour
- **Cognitive component**: Thinking about moral issues and information processing regarding right and wrong acts
- **Behavioural component**: Understanding of how we behave morally.

Theories	Stage of development
Piaget's stages of moral judgement	**Premoral** (0–5 years): vague understanding of rules and judgements **Moral realism** (5–10 years): Heteronymous morality **Moral relativism** (10+ years): Autonomous morality
Kohlberg's theory	**Preconventional** (under 9 years): understandings of moral reasoning by reward and punishment, arrived at via two stages of development. **Conventional** (10+ years): conformity to the existing social justice, mutual respect and social approval seeking behaviour carried out in two stages. **Post-conventional** (20+ years): abstract notion of justice and universal ethical principles carried out in two stages.
Gilligan's theory	Gender differences in moral judgement: Boys develop morality of justice Girls develop morality of care
Bandura's social learning theory	Moral behaviour is developed by two types of learning: **Direct tuition**: learning with the use of reward and punishment **Observational learning**: imitating rewarded moral behaviour.
Erickson's psycho-initiative–social theory	Development of : Trust in self and others (0–1 years), Independence (2–3 years), Initiative (4–5 years), Industry (6–12 years).

Table 3.4 Theories of moral development

Parent–child relationships

A special bond is created immediately after a baby is born that eventually becomes an attachment in late childhood. The psychosocial factors helping to develop the parent–child bond/attachment are:

- **Body contact**: The classic experiment by Harlow *et al.* (1971) showed that warmth is more wanted than feeding only without warmth.
- **Familiarity**: Exposure to certain stimuli during a certain period after birth is crucial for development. This is called the 'critical period'. The process of developing an attachment during the critical period is called imprinting.
- **Temperament**: Responding to a child's temperament in an appropriate way helps to develop a secure attachment.
- **Responsive parenting**: Parenting styles are crucial determinants of types of attachment children form with their parents. Baumrind (1980) suggests two types of parenting styles:
  - **permissive–demanding**: Degree of parental control over children
  - **accepting–rejecting**: Degree of parental affection towards children.

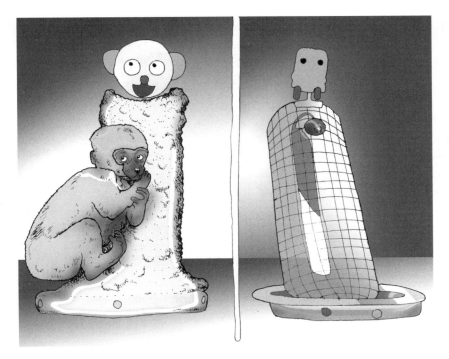

Figure 3.2 Attachment: warmth vs primary needs

Deprivation of attachment

There are severe short-term and long-term consequences of maternal deprivation (Bowlby, 1952).

- **Short-term effects** include:
  - **Protest**: Crying and panic-stricken phase
  - **Despair**: Apathetic and withdrawal tendency
  - **Detachment**: Loss of interest and less emotion.
- **Long-term effects** include:
  - **Anaclitic depression**: Seen with the complete deprivation of maternal attachment, eg orphans, showing resigned helplessness and loss of appetite.
  - **Affectionless psychopathy**: A mental disorder characterised by lack of remorse and guilt, eg juvenile delinquency.
  - **Privation**: Failure to form any attachment with anyone, leads to extreme disturbed behavioural and emotional problems which are long-lasting and severe.

Cross-cultural differences

Significant differences are reported between various cultures regarding cross-cultural practices in developing an attachment and child-rearing practices. So, individualistic societies practise a parenting style different from collective societies.

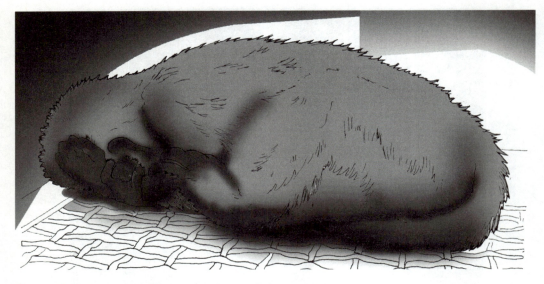

Figure 3.3 Emotional distress at maternal deprivation

Gender and child rearing

Social learning theory (Bandura, 1960) and social cognition theory suggest that children learn gender-linked behaviour by observing and imitating important people in their lives as well as by making sense of the experiences of being a member of a gender group, eg boy or girl.

The role of play in a child's development

Play is an active behaviour and has significant influence on a child's development.

Stages in play

In fantasy and socio-dramatic play three elements are noted:

- **Decentration**: Incorporating others in the pretend activities, eg pretending to drink from empty cup at around the age of 1–2 years.
- **Decontextualisation**: Ability to use less realistic substitute objects, eg using 'wooden block' as 'cake' at around the age of 2 years.
- **Integration**: Spontaneous sequence of activities at around the age of 3–4 years.

Types of play

- **Language play**: Starts as early as 2 years of age and is characterised by presleep monologues or dialogues.
- **Rough-and-tumble play**: Vigorous activities in play, usually imitating parents, friends and from the media (video/TV), starts from 3 years onwards.

- **War toys and war play**: Aggressive play with the use of toy guns, combat figures etc, starts from 2 years onwards.
- **Video and computer play**: More co-ordinated play starts as early as 6 years.

Play sequences

Piaget (1951) proposed a developmental sequence from: practice play (early sensory–motor play in infants), then symbolic play, and finally play with rules. Constructive games are also identified, a transitional period between play and intelligent work.

Developmental issues in play

- Role-learning and socialising
- Elaboration and extension of skills
- Development of sensory discrimination, learning about real-life
- Cognitive development, accommodation and assimilation with the environment
- Emotional development, creative thinking
- Skill acquisitions, confidence and a sense of mastery.

Methodology in child development research

Self-reports

Self-reports are used to record the responses of individuals about themselves.

- **Advantages**: Obtain detailed accounts of personal childhood experiences.
- **Disadvantages**: Self-report is inaccurate and less reliable.

Naturalistic observation

Naturalistic observations involve recording children's developmental processes in a natural context using a diary, eg the recordings made by Darwin (1877) and Piaget (1954) of their own children's developmental processes are of enduring scientific value.

- **Advantages**: Most effective in understanding developmental niche (the contextual factors in which the child lives, the culturally determined child-rearing practices and educational training, the psychological characteristics of the child's parents).
- **Disadvantages**: Subjective reports and less scientific, so difficult to establish causal connections.

Clinical interview

A clinical interview is a structured session used mainly to examine developmental irregularities, eg Freud used this method to treat psychologically disturbed people.

- **Advantages**: Focuses on dynamics of individual development.
- **Disadvantages**: Restricted use and difficult to establish causal connection.

Experimental methods

Experimental methods involve introducing a change in the environment to see an effect on the child's behaviour in a controlled environment using cross-sectional and longitudinal designs.

- **Advantages**: Effective in finding causal connection, and enforcing control to minimise the effects of external factors on the developmental process.
- **Disadvantages**: It can be applied in all situations for ethical reasons, and provides limited findings making it difficult to generalise.

Ethics and professional issues

Strict ethical principles need to be endorsed in all research design and studies must adhere to the guidelines for research with children provided by the appropriate organisations. The British Psychological Society has provided a guideline on this (1998).

Theoretical framework used to examine developmental process

There are various theoretical frameworks used in the study of development.

- **The biological-maturation framework** places emphasis on biological factors.
- **The environment-learning framework** places emphasis on environmental factors.
- **The constructivist framework** places emphasis on children's ability to construct their development using both biological and environmental factors.
- **The cultural-context framework** places emphasis on the contextual factors in conjunction with biological and environmental factors.

ADOLESCENCE

Adolescence is the period between childhood and adulthood. It is marked by sexual maturity and a sense of psychosocial independence.

Psychological effects of puberty

Emotional and cognitive changes are apparent, such as, depression, anorexia, apathy, social deviancy, and egocentrism caused mainly by hormonal imbalance.

Cognitive development

The **reasoning power of adolescents**: with the use of a psychological process and formal operations, adolescents can work on abstract logic, can reason hypothetically and can deduce consequences.

Social development

Erickson (1968) proposed eight psychosocial developmental stages. Each stage is characterised by normative crisis and conflicts.

Stages Normative crisis	Age	Major characteristics
Trust vs Mistrust	0–1 years	Primary social relations with mother/carer, trust in life-sustaining care
Autonomy vs Shame	1–2 years	Primary social interaction with parents, toilet training and autonomous will
Initiative vs Guilt	3–5 years	Primary social interaction with immediate family, language and locomotion development, conscious development
Industry vs Inferiority	6 years	Primary social interaction with peers and teachers, task ability
Identity vs Role confusion	Adolescence	Primary social interaction with peers, identity crisis, consolidation of early stages and constitution of coherent self
Intimacy vs Isolation	Early adulthood	Primary social interaction with opposite sex, sense of adult commitment
Generativity vs Stagnation	Middle age	Primary social interaction with next generation, productivity and creativity
Integrity vs Despair	Old age	Primary social interaction is indirect reflective

Table 3.5 Psychosocial development stages of Erickson (1968)

Gender and sexuality

Gender-role identity

Gender-role identity involves the acquisition of a set of masculine and feminine behaviours within a particular culture. The onset of learning gender-role identity occurs in the middle of childhood with an apparent marked development in adolescence. Cultures vary as to the onset and primary characteristics of gender-role identity (Mead, 1935). The dimension of masculinity and femininity is usually measured on a social inventory scale (Bem, 1975).

Sexual knowledge, attitudes and behaviour

Interest in sexual knowledge generates during puberty for both boys and girls, and with informed knowledge from educational institutions and the media, the processes of reproduction become known. Parents play a major role in development of sexual behaviour.

Parent–child relations

Major problems in the family	Effects of problems
Divorce/separation	Depression, anxiety, suicidal tendency, aggression, truancy, homelessness
Conflict with parents	Withdrawal, communication difficulties, behavioural and psychiatric problems
Over-excessive parental bond	Depression and anxiety, psychosomatic disorders, social isolation
Marital discord and domestic violence	Negative peer interaction, juvenile delinquency
Child neglect and abuse	Long-term effects on mental health, adolescent criminal behaviour
Parenting styles (authoritarian, authoritative permissive)	Psychological problems and social maladjustment

Table 3.6 Psychosocial problems that may arise from parent–child relations

AGEING (see also Chapter 22)

The study of all psychological aspects in ageing is called **behavioural gerontology**.

Perspectives on ageing

- **Age changes**: The ways in which people change as they grow older.
- **Age differences**: The ways in which people differ within the same age group as a result of their exposure to different life experiences.
- **Ageism**: Negative attitudes towards old people and discrimination against them.

Major changes in ageing

Physiological

Major changes in physiology caused by ageing include:

- **Vision**: Lenses become more rigid resulting in impaired vision, especially at night, usually after 65 years of age.
- **Hearing**: Loss of hearing, usually after 60 years of age, can bring behavioural problems such as mild paranoia, suspecting conversation at a level not audible for an old person.

- **Sexual function**: Less sexual activity as a result of the declined functions of the reproductive organs; however, pleasure associated with sexual activities is not diminished by age.
- **Brain function**: Slower neural processes cause learning and memory loss, gradual loss of brain cells (approximately 5% by the age of 80). Active neural connection can

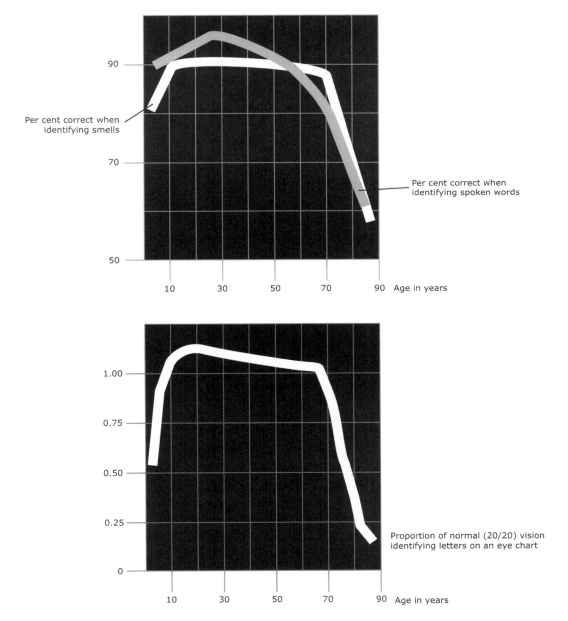

Figure 3.4 Ageing and physiological functions

compensate for the loss of brain cells. Active old people will therefore have fewer problems in memory and retention.

- **Organic brain disease**: Strokes, tumour, alcoholism and dementia.
- **Other major physical disease**: Eg longstanding diseases such as diabetes, cancer, heart diseases, weakened immune system.

Cognitive

Major cognitive changes occurring with age include the following:

- **Intelligence**: Ageing brings a decline in some cognitive functioning
- **Crystallised intelligence**: Vocabulary and analogies increase with ageing
- **Fluid intelligence**: Quick problem solving and abstract reasoning decrease with age
- **Memory**: Deficits occur in areas of short-term and working memory.

Psycho-social

Depression may be precipitated by physiological disorders such as eating problems, high blood pressure, social isolation and insomnia.

Ageing makes family relationships more important, with greater dependency on children and spouses. Erickson referred to the major areas dominating adult life as **intimacy** (close relations with family) and **generativity** (productive and supporting future generations).

Empty nest syndrome is the term used to describe a feeling of distress focusing on a loss of purpose and relationship.

Social contact

Ageing can lead to selectivity about social relations which may lead to loneliness and depression. However, selective social relations may also help older people to gain rewarding relations.

Disengagement is the notion that elderly people voluntarily withdraw from social contact to prepare for death.

Work and retirement

Ageing may pose a threat to the stability of working life as retirement comes closer. Various psychological problems, eg anxiety and stress-related symptoms, are prevalent during this transition in life.

Death and bereavement

The immune system of old people undergoes a change at the loss of their partners and the bereaved elderly are therefore more likely to have increased rates of illness. There are several stages of mourning (Kalish, 1985): shock stage, longing stage, depression stage and recovery stage.

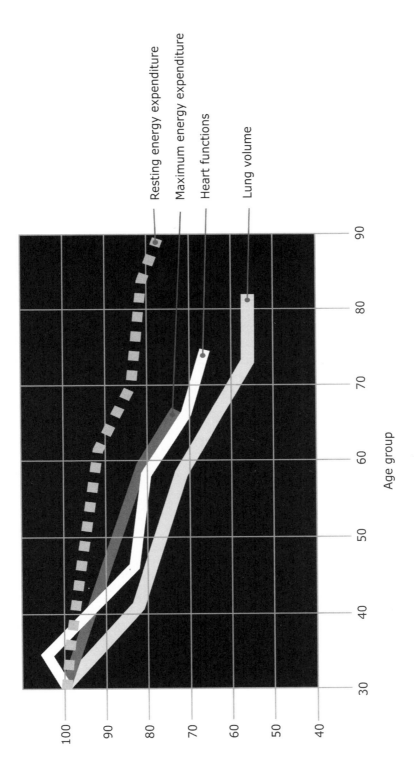

Figure 3.5 Memory and ageing

Chapter 4

Psychological Assessment and Psychometrics

Eric Davis

CONTENTS

Psychological Assessment and Psychometrics

PSYCHOLOGICAL ASSESSMENT

Systematic psychological assessment comprises two stages: gathering of clinical information and making decisions about patients' difficulties.

- **Comprehensive information gathering**: The clinician develops hypotheses (clinical formulations) about the triggering and maintenance of difficulties.
- **Selective data collection**: Data are used for greater precision in hypothesis – testing which continues throughout treatment.

Types of data

Numerical data assume two forms.

- **Measurement data** equates to the result of a given measurement, eg the score on a memory test or the time taken to run 100 metres.
- **Frequency data**, conversely, embraces statements such as '18 people like lime jelly, but 16 do not', or 'the Labour party has 284 MPs, and the Conservative Party has 167 MPs'.

Counting things means that data consist of totals or frequencies.

A United Kingdom election would encompass many thousands of people, but the results (data) would consist of relatively few numbers – the number of votes for each candidate. Thus, with measurement data, measuring these same thousands of people would derive thousands of numbers – one for each person. If data represent one or more measurements for each participant this results in measurement data. In contrast, whenever data represent total (or subtotal) counts, this equates to frequency data.

Difference and relationships

The majority of statistical questions can be examined in terms of difference and relationships.

- **Difference**: One experiment might be primarily interested in whether there is a difference between people given a diagnosis of schizophrenia compared to people with no such diagnosis on a given task.
- **Relationship**: A different experimenter might be interested in whether there is a relationship between the experience of auditory hallucinations and score on this same task.

Numbers of groups or variables

A fundamental distinction concerns the number of groups or the number of variables to which the statistical techniques apply. Therefore consideration of types of data, differences and relationships and numbers of groups or variables allow for statistical procedures to be sorted into specific categories. One further criterion used in categorising tests involves the scale of measurement that applies to the data.

Scales of measurement

The choice of statistical procedure is influenced by the different types of scales of measurement. These have been defined as: nominal, ordinal, interval and ratio.

Nominal scales

Nominal scales are something of a misnomer. They are not really scales because items are not viewed along a scalar dimension. A typical example would include numbers that are assigned to rugby players. The numbers are purely symbolic and used simply to differentiate one player from another.

Ordinal scales

Ordinal scales represent the true fundamental properties of a scale in which people, elements, or events are depicted along a continuum. One example of an ordinal scale might be the intelligence quotients (IQs) obtained for a given class of pupils. The scale tells us who has achieved scores along a continuum. Such a grading system can lead to controversy: it is debatable whether a person with an IQ of 99 can truly be said to be more intelligent than a person with an IQ score of 98.

Ordinal scales do not give information about the relationship between different points on a scale. We do not know if the difference between IQ scores of 100 and 90 is comparable to the difference between IQs of 90 and 80.

Interval scales

The Fahrenheit scale is commonly cited as a good example of an interval scale. Here, there are legitimate differences between scale points. Thus, the difference between 5 and 15 degrees is the same as the difference between 45 and 55 degrees. Interval scales also incorporate the integral properties of nominal and ordinal scales but cannot reliably differentiate ratios. Thus 45 degrees cannot be said to be three times hotter than 15 degrees or half as hot as 90 degrees.

Ratio scales

Ratio scales must contain a true zero point, for example, length. They incorporate the properties of the above scales but ratios can also specify ratio. Thus 20 cm is twice as long as 10 cm.

In psychology and psychiatry it is not always clear what particular scale is involved. An IQ test might be viewed as a ratio scale in which a zero score equates to zero intelligence and a score of 80 indicates twice the intelligence of a score of 40. Many people would, however, reject this view. Perhaps the most appropriate approach would be to consider the IQ scores to represent an ordinal scale. Here, 80 > 70 > 60 but the differences do not represent equal differences in intelligence.

Norm-referenced and criterion-referenced approaches

Two further forms of testing used in psychometrics are norm- and criterion-referenced approaches.

- **Criterion-referenced testing**: The ability of an individual to attain satisfactorily a criterion. For example, a school may set its entrance criterion at 76%, the result that must be achieved to gain entry. The mark establishes an absolute standard of quality.
- **Norm-referenced testing**: Individuals are ordered relative to their test performance. The Standard Assessment Tests (SATs) used in schools grade pupils according to achieved scores. The pupils are ordered in relation to other pupils so that the standard of quality is relative. Similarly, in A-level examinations, students' grades are based upon their relative ordering within the cohort of students taking the examination. The assigned grades are norm-referenced.

INTELLIGENCE

Intelligence is defined as 'the capacity of the individual to act purposefully, to think rationally, and to deal effectively with his/her environment'.

Nature and components

Intelligence is a controversial concept. Many psychologists and psychiatrists conceive of intelligence as a multidimensional construct. An overall derived score for a given individual equates to an Intelligence Quotient or IQ. As well as being considered a general (behaviour as a whole) entity, it can be construed as an aggregate of specific abilities (dimensions/abilities qualitatively different from one another).

Testing and measurement

The Wechsler Adult Intelligence Scale III (WAIS-III, 1997) has evolved through a number of previous test batteries (Wechsler Intelligence Scale for Children (WISC) is the child-related form) through:

- reviewing existing items and developing new items and subtests
- piloting to investigate psychometric characteristics
- national and international data collection to examine item difficulties, bias, subtest functioning and factor structure

- a national standardisation study to collect normative information, examine bias, and make final item and subtest decisions
- concurrent and multiple studies with standardisation to gauge reliability, concurrent validity, construct validity and clinical use of the test.

The WAIS-III measures IQ in different ways. A global score is measured from full-scale IQ (FSIQ), derived from a combination of performance IQ (PIQ) and verbal IQ (VIQ) which are, in turn, derived from an aggregate of five and six specific subtest scores, respectively. An average FSIQ score for the population as a whole would represent a score of 100.

The concept of IQ and stability (WAIS-III)

WAIS-III development and evolution has been necessary because the measurement of IQ at an individual and societal level is dynamic. A number of changes have been incorporated through time:

- **Updating of norms**: IQ-score inflation over time is about 0.3 points per year. Key demographic variables (age, sex, education level, geographical regions) are also updated.
- **Extension of age range**: To include adults 75–89 years of age.
- **Item modification**: Items such as the WAIS-III Information subtest (a type of general knowledge subtest) can become chronologically remote. Such subtests can also discriminate against certain cultural groups, eg Native American population of USA.
- **Artwork stimuli**: Items are re-sized to accommodate the visual acuity needs of older adults.
- **Extension of floor and enhancement of clinical use**: Items are added to measure particularly low IQs and provide meaningful observations about neurologically compromised populations.
- **Decreased reliance on timed performance**: Time constraints for older adults were problematic.
- **Enhancement of fluid reasoning measurement**: 'The ability to perform mental operations, such as manipulation of abstract symbols'. Usually contrasted with 'crystallised intelligence' (eg knowing that London is the capital of England).
- **Strengthening the theoretical basis**: Inclusion of new subtests to ensure that the four main hypothesised intelligence constructs were covered: verbal comprehension, perceptual organisation, working memory and processing speed.

Concept formation tests in verbal formats

- **Proverbs Test:**
  - three forms, each containing 12 proverbs of equal difficulty
  - elicits more concrete responses from subjects over 60
  - poor performance by patients with bilateral frontal lobe lesions.
- **California Proverbs Tests (CPT):**
  - uses proverbs that are less and more familiar
  - ten proverbs administered in an oral, free-response trial, and printed, four-choice format (two choices correct – abstract and concrete)

- incorrect phonemic response (similar sounding words have semantically different meanings or an incorrect response).
- **Stanford–Binet Subtests (SBS):**
  - items are scored on a pass–fail basis
  - similarities subtests contain questions such as, 'In what way are wood and coal alike?'
  - differences subtest contain questions such as, 'What is the difference between a bird and a dog?'

Concept formation tests in visual formats

- **Category Test (CT):**
  - examines abstracting ability for 208 visually presented items
  - six sets, each organised on the basis of a specific principle, followed by a seventh set made up of previously shown items
  - subject must work out the principle underpinning each set and respond accordingly
  - score is the number of observed errors
  - sensitive to age (steep increase in errors after age 40)
  - measures abstract concept formation, sustained attention, and visuospatial ability
  - sensitive to frontal lobe problems and chronic alcoholism.
- **Identification of Common Objects (ICO):**
  - colloquially referred to as '20 questions'
  - subject is shown an array of 42 objects, such as animals or clothing, and must find out which object the experimenter is thinking of by asking a series of questions
  - Korsakoff patients' pattern of questioning is deficient
  - patients with frontal lobe dysfunction perform slightly better than the alcoholic groups, but less well than controls.
- **Ravens Progressive Matrices (RPM):**
  - paper and pencil multiple-choice format
  - the subject must identify the correct shape or design missing from a visuospatial series, high level of validity as a measure of general ability
  - correlates well with other tests of ability
  - limited as a screening tool for brain damage
  - tends to identify more severe organic impairment (moderate – severe dementia of Alzheimer type, chronic alcoholics).

OTHER COGNITIVE PARAMETERS

Memory: Wechsler Memory Scale III (WMS III)

Designed to complement the WAIS-III, scores obtained on the WMS III can be cross-referenced with intelligence scores obtained on the WAIS-III. Clinical psychologists can deduce relative areas of strength and weakness. Scores can provide useful feedback to the patient and assist in clinical decision-making with regard to rehabilitation and treatment.

They can also be used for medico-legal and research purposes. The WMS III assesses immediate and delayed auditory and visual memory, general and working memory.

Visuo-perceptual dysfunction: the Visual Object and Space Perception (VOSP) Battery

A series of tests that examine visual and perceptual functioning, including pattern recognition, laterality and ability to recognise common objects from degraded levels of stimulus information. As for the Wechsler scales, results can be compared across population norm-derived scores. The battery can also be repeated to assess potential clinical change accruing from, for example, neurological disorder.

Assessing facial processing deficits: the Benton Facial Recognition Test (BFRT)

The BFRT is a face-matching test. The subject is required to find a target face from among a set of six alternatives exposed simultaneously. Patients with right posterior lesions produce the highest proportion of defective scores.

Unilateral neglect

This is characterised by the patients failure to orientate, respond to, or report salient stimuli appearing on the side contralateral to a cerebral lesion.

- **Copying/Drawing Tests**: The patient copies line drawings (eg a four-pointed star, Greek cross, butterfly, or cube). In most cases, the patient exhibiting neglect demonstrates a striking omission of the left side of an object or group of objects.
- **Visual Search and Cancellation Tests**: Alberts' Line-crossing Test requires the patient to cross out 40 apparently random lines (2.5 cm long). It is a sensitive indicator of hemispatial neglect.
- **Line Bisection**: Another sensitive test of neglect, this requires the patient to estimate and select the midpoint of a group of horizontal lines of varying length.
- **Behavioural Inattention Test (BIT)**: The BIT pinpoints potentially disruptive aspects of functioning. It enables resources to be directed to functionally relevant areas. The BIT was standardised on 80 stroke patients and 50 controls. Validity, parallel form and rater-reliability are all high.

Language dysfunction: the Psycholinguistic Assessment of Language Processing in Aphasia (PALPA)

PALPA is a norm-referenced series of subtests that assess expressive (ability to produce) and receptive (ability to understand) language. Certain subtests are very sensitive to left fronto-temporal lesions.

Frontal lobe dysfunction

Patients are characterised by a range of potential difficulties:

- starting or stopping behaviour
- planning
- monitoring potential plans
- shifting from one intellectual task to another
- inappropriate social behaviour.

Controlled Oral Word Association Test (COWAT)

The COWAT is quick and easy to use. There are clinical norms and it can reliably discriminate frontal from non-frontal patients.

The patient is given 60 seconds to produce as many words as possible beginning with F, then A, then S. Proper nouns, numbers or changing word suffix are not allowed. The total score is adjusted for age, years of education and gender. The 'FAS' version is very sensitive to bilateral frontal damage.

Wisconsin Card Sorting Test (WCST)

Four stimulus cards showing one red triangle, two green stars, three yellow crosses and four blue circles, respectively, are placed in a row before the subject, who is required to sort a set of response cards on the basis of criteria determined by the examiner. Subjects are given a pack of 128 response cards made up of two sets of 64 cards. These two sets contain all possible combinations of colour, shape and number. The subject must place each response card underneath one of the four stimulus cards. They are required to judge where to place each card as the examiner will only issue feedback in terms of 'correct' or 'incorrect'. Once the subject has worked out the card sorting criterion (on the basis of colour, shape, or number), ten correct responses are required before the examiner (unknown to the subject), changes the card sort rule. The test is discontinued if, or when, six correct categories (of ten responses) are achieved.

DEMENTIA

The neuropsychological assessment of dementia typically occurs within the wider context of the clinical evaluation of patients' neurological, psychiatric and physical disability. Most clinical psychologists assume that no test or test battery by itself can reliably differentiate dementing from non-dementing patients. However, the collection of systematic psychiatric, psychological and medical information (including brain scanning) can considerably enhance functional and diagnostic accuracy.

The **Cambridge Index of Mental Disorder in the Elderly** (CAMDEX) incorporates a history from the relative or carer as well as patient physical examination.

A brief neuropsychological assessment using the **Cambridge Cognitive Examination** (CAMCOG) provides a means of quantifying severity of impairment using several potential scales, a 'cut-off' point for diagnosing dementia and guidelines for classifying patients with regard to various dementia subtypes.

DESIGN OF INVESTIGATIVE STUDIES (see also Chapters 11 and 17)

Variables

Different events or objects can exhibit different values. These are referred to as variables, eg eye colour is a variable because the eye can have different 'values' (ie blue, brown, green). Other variables include weight and height. A variable can be discrete or continuous and independent or dependent.

- **Discrete variables**: The identified variable can register few possible values (eg gender, employment).
- **Continuous variables**: A given value could occur between the lowest and highest points on a scale (eg engine torque, time).
- **Independent variables**: Variables are manipulated by the experimenter. In psychology and psychiatry common examples would be behavioural schedules of reinforcement, prescription of specific medicine, or methods of teaching and clinical supervision.
- **Dependent variables**: These variables are not under the experimenter's control. They represent the data. Common examples would be scores on a test, degree of concordance or compliance with medication or outcomes derived from specific methods of teaching or supervision.

Studies are concerned with the interaction between independent variables and the study results (data) in the form of dependent variables.

Hypothesis testing

An experiment is designed to test a hypothesis. For example, different groups could be compared with respect to some specific attribute or variable. Thus verbal achievements of boys and girls at a certain age could be compared, or reading behaviour of children with television sets in their homes versus those without television sets. In the latter example, one prediction might be that children without television sets in their homes spend significantly more hours reading per week than their counterparts who possess television sets. This would be termed the **experimental hypothesis**. It proposes a specific, measurable discrepancy between the two groups. However, it is important to consider other potential experimental outcomes.

The concept of the **null hypothesis** is of critical importance in the testing of hypotheses. The null hypothesis for the above example would be that there is no difference in weekly hours spent reading between the two groups of children. The main reason, philosophically, for constructing a null hypothesis is that we cannot prove something to be true but we can prove something to be false. Therefore, absence of evidence does not constitute evidence of absence for null hypothetical alternative experimental results.

Control subjects

A number of years ago a study in the USA was designed to test the hypothesis that cerebral damage in the fetus and perinatally was a contributory factor to later behavioural abnormality in the child. The major difficulty for the experimenters in their experimental design was to find, within the child population, samples on which the hypothesis could be tested with great accuracy. On the one hand, an experimental group, a sample of children with known abnormal behaviour problems, for whom credible hospital records of pregnancy, birth and operative delivery procedures was required. On the other, a control group was needed for comparison. The control group should match as closely as possible the experimental group on factors such as age, socio-economic status, educational experience, home background and so forth. They should differ from the experimental group in one regard – no observed later abnormality of behaviour. Reliable hospital records should also be available for the control group. Experimentally it is difficult to meet the stringent requirements of such a design. From this study, an initial sample of 1800 children exhibiting behavioural abnormality was reduced by approximately 75% because selection-matching criteria could not be obtained for the two groups.

Study design

Repeated measures

A repeated measures design ensures that the same subject is measured under all levels of one or more independent variables. One advantage of this design is that overall variability is reduced by using a common set of subjects for all treatments, thereby allowing for the removal of subject differences. The statistical test used is **analysis of variance** (ANOVA).

Matched subjects

There are two related (dependent or matched) samples and the hypothesis under scrutiny is that the difference between their corresponding population means is zero. The statistical test is a **matched-sample *t*-test**.

The experimenter might examine subjects under one condition, introduce a treatment (to produce a particular effect), then examine the subjects again. The *t*-test would examine the presence or absence of different mean scores when comparing the first session with the second.

Independent groups

The most likely result for two independent groups is that the sample means differed by some amount. The **two-sample *t*-test** allows determination as to whether any observed difference is sufficiently large to merit the conclusion that the two samples were drawn from different populations.

Case–control

A sample of patients with, for example, a specific disease are examined to determine whether they have been exposed to a specific risk factor more often than a number of control subjects without the disease who are matched for age, sex and relevant medical history. The subjects who have been exposed are the cases and the others are the controls.

Cohort

A cohort is any subdivision of the population. One definition for such studies is, 'a group of people marching together through time'. Cohorts can be defined in terms of particular birth weeks or years, school leavers or marriage cohorts. Cohort studies use the development of such groups to answer specific questions, such as gathering epidemiological data. Early lifestyle and life opportunities can be cross-referenced with the population's characteristics later in life, shedding light on developmental potentiators as well as hindrances. Inferences can be drawn for different domains (eg income, health, education etc).

Clinical trial procedures

Randomisation

Randomisation is the arbitrary method of dividing subjects into groups. It is done so as to avoid experimenter bias which might otherwise influence the interpretation of trial results. Subjects are allocated to groups by chance. Randomisation can also be used to determine the treatment received by different subjects. Thus, receiving a new (experimental) or existing treatment would similarly be left to chance.

Blinding

To avoid experimental bias it is important to ensure that both patients and treatment administrators do not know which treatment is being received by whom. Where both patients and treatment administrators/evaluators have no knowledge of which treatment is being received by whom, then the term **double-blind** is used. In practice, this can be virtually impossible to achieve (eg surgery, specific forms of psychotherapy).

Comparison groups

The experimental group (for example, students attending a specific intensive education group) is matched to other comparison groups. Thus, comparison Group 1, might match children with the experimental group of students for age, gender, educational attainment and level of social, emotional and behavioural difficulties in the same mainstream schools, but who do not receive input from a specific intensive educational group. Comparison Group 2 could contain a group of children matched for age and gender with the experimental group but without emotional and behavioural difficulties. The study would aim to demonstrate experimental efficacy for the intensive educational group as measured against the comparison groups.

Placebo groups

Groups do not receive active treatment (eg medicine), or a specific intervention (eg psychotherapy), but are included in clinical trials for comparative purposes.

Sequential design

If there are more than two treatments being compared in a clinical trial, administering them sequentially to the same group of subjects may require far fewer subjects than a fixed-sample design while ensuring that the same error probabilities are achieved.

Crossover design

Two groups of people repeat experimental tests in a different order. Crossover designs are used in an attempt to eliminate inter-subject variability.

Factorial design

Every level of every variable is paired with every level of every other variable so that all combinations are explored. This usually applies to designs wherein separate groups of subjects receive the different treatment permutations. The advantage of factorial designs over one-factor-at-a-time experiments is that they are more efficient and they allow inter-actions to be detected.

QUALITATIVE RESEARCH

Discourse analysis

This approach is concerned with language and its role in the make-up of social and psychological life. It asks questions about the relationship between discourse and subjectivity (thinking or feeling), and practices (what people do, and the conditions in which such experiences occur). Thus, the way in which people talk about things has implications for how the world is perceived, physically and psychologically.

Participant observation

This usually takes place in natural settings (a bar, a football stadium etc). The observers can be covert or overt, known or not known to those around them. The observer/researcher engages in a variety of activities which include participation, documentation, semi-structured interviewing and reflection. Recording of data should take place as close as possible to its original occurrence, and will usually contain the actual observations that have been made.

Case studies

Individual cases are studied for a number of reasons. Either as a result of the intrinsic interest associated with a case, or because it is representative of a wider context. Cases can be compared to generate wider understanding. Different designs include:

- intrinsic versus instrumental
- simple versus multiple
- descriptive versus explanatory.

Triangulation

Different qualitative researchers may wish to examine a certain concept, for example self-identity, by use of different qualitative methods. The aim of triangulation within this context would be to cross-reference findings with regard to self-identity. The degree of convergence obtained from different methods would allow for a statement of 'reality'.

SINGLE-CASE DESIGNS

Single-case studies are conducted for a variety of reasons including the following.

- Social scientists experience great difficulty in generalising results obtained from groups of people to individuals in clinical settings.
- Clinical versus statistical significance. Group studies may yield findings that are statistically significant but that are individually clinically meaningless.
- Highlighting variability in the individual. Detecting intrapsychic change experimentally can be facilitated by planned changes in within-study design.

A-B-A-B

This has also been referred to as an **equivalent time-samples design**. It ends on a treatment phase (B) so that potential clinical effectiveness can be explored beyond the experimental study. Also, the design strategy allows for two occasions (B to A, then A to B) in showing the positive effects associated with the treatment variable. As a result, conclusions regarding the potency of its controlling effects with respect to target behaviours under observation may be enhanced.

Multiple baseline

A number of responses are identified and measured over time to provide baselines against which changes can be measured. Once baselines are established, the experimenter is then able to apply an experimental variable to one of the behaviours, producing a change in it, and maybe noting little or no change in the other baselines. The experimenter then applies the experimental variable to all identified target behaviours in a systematic fashion. The outcome of such studies is usually best summarised by use of a graph.

EVALUATING RESEARCH

The research protocol

This is the starting point for any study and communicates the framework for how a given study will be achieved. The key components are:

- investigator details (names, sites)
- sites where the research will take place
- objectives and hypothesis to be tested. An objective could be to determine how one clinical service compares to another with regard to specific parameters. A hypothesis could be that community-based staff report higher levels of job satisfaction than their hospital counterparts.
- background and reason for carrying out the study
- literature search conducted. Relevant published (and sometimes unpublished) research studies are carefully reviewed to determine the experimental context which leads to the extant research question(s).
- method/study design: includes participants (how they are to be chosen and randomised), procedure and materials to be used
- inclusion and exclusion criteria: attempts to ensure that the population(s) under scrutiny will yield the most pertinent results
- potential risks to patient/participant
- cost implications and associated funding sources
- what statistical analysis will be required (eg ANOVA), and power calculations for sample size (if relevant)
- outcome measures. Helps to clarify benefits that could be conferred for patients in receipt of a particular treatment
- implication for the service. What are the implications of the research findings for changes in clinical practice? Introducing specific recommendations for service re-design may be needed
- suggestions for future research. A given study may support a given hypothesis and provide some research answers but may raise other research questions
- dissemination of findings: specifying how this is to be achieved and to whom.

Critically appraising research (see Chapter 17)

Chapter 5

Social Sciences

Alan Butler

CONTENTS

Social Sciences

INTRODUCTION AND DEFINITIONS

Introduction

Social life is orderly and predictable. It is possible to discern patterns in the ways that people behave. Sociologists place the emphasis, when seeking to explain this, upon social conditions rather than biological, psychological, or genetic factors.

Definitions: Sociology

Sociology can be defined as:

- the science of society
- the study of human social life, groups and societies
- an attempt to understand society and the individual's part in it
- an examination of the daily way of life.

Society

Society is a system of inter-relationships which connects individuals together.

Emile Durkheim, the French sociologist and one of the 'trinity of founding thinkers' (the others being Marx and Weber), sought to explain variations in suicide rates by reference to 'social facts' related to the ways in which society was organised and operated.

Suicide, while a personal act, can be socially explained. Rapid social change may result in feelings of loss of self-worth or of cultural alienation – what he termed **anomie**.

A social fact is that insufficient social integration may help to explain personal behaviour.

Culture

Culture can be defined as

- the values held by members of a given group
- the norms (principles/rules) they follow (the do's and don'ts of social life)
- the material goods that the group creates.

SOCIALISATION

Definitions

Because sociologists put the emphasis, when trying to understand and explain behaviour, upon culture rather than biology, understanding the social rules under which we live is important.

- **Socialisation** is the process whereby the helpless infant gradually becomes a self-aware, knowledgeable person.
- Socialisation is the on-going process whereby an individual learns about the surrounding societies norms and values. The rules become internalised.
- Emile Durkheim (1858–1917) wrote about the importance of a well-ordered society and the fact that social harmony allows the individual to flourish.
- Max Weber based his analysis of society upon the meaning that individuals give to their social world and their place in it.
- This required the adoption of what he termed in German *Verstehen* – the development of an understanding and empathy with the beliefs of other people, ie trying to see the world and understand it through the eyes of another person.
- His stance sowed the seeds for much future qualitative research work and the interpretive approach adopted by such 'radical psychiatrists' as R. D. Laing.

The process of socialisation

- Most studies have been focused upon primary socialisation in the early years, usually taking place within the family.
- John Bowlby noted the importance of this when he wrote about the importance of 'maternal deprivation' as a factor explaining problems of adjustment in later life.
- However, it is now more widely appreciated that the agencies of socialisation continue throughout our life. These include our peer group, the school, and the mass media.
- Role models are an important source of influence.
- Gender-specific ways of behaving are learned.

Faulty socialisation

Children growing up in the absence of human role models lack many human characteristics, eg speech, the ability to walk upright, and the ability to maintain eye contact.

They are referred to as feral or 'wolf' children because of the belief that they were reared by animals.

Social learning may also falter if the individual lacks intellectual capacity. Somebody with a 'learning difficulty' may find it a problem to appreciate social rules and behave in an appropriate way.

Social learning may also be defective if the role models available are inadequate or a consistent view of the world is not presented. A *'folie à deux'* is such an example in mental health terms.

An obvious challenge to social science was to seek and find an explanation for grossly abhorrent behaviours, such as the rise of fascism and the holocaust. Could these be the result of child upbringing? A group of social scientists associated with the Frankfurt Institute of Social Research, became known as the Frankfurt school.

- Seeking to combine Marxism and Freudian theory, these 'critical theorists' sought to answer such questions.
- Many of them – Fromm, Marcuse, Reich – decamped to the USA to escape Fascism and developed a libertarian critique of society which attempted to explain the rise of the 'authoritarian personality'.
- Many of their ideas illuminated the critiques of psychiatry that developed in the 1960s.
- Jurgen Habermas, one of the group, continues to explore ideas that feed back into psychiatric and psychoanalytic thinking.
- One of his key beliefs is that 'I think that a certain form of unrestrained communication brings to the fore the deepest force of reason, which enables us to overcome egocentric or ethnocentric perspectives and reach an expanded … view'.

Social role

A social role is behaviour that develops as a result of the expectations of other people or of their demands upon another person.

- The analogy is the role performed by an actor given a script.
- Most of us fulfil many different roles in our lives.
- We are usually capable of maintaining a number of rolls at any one time, eg when performing the role of doctor our behaviour/use of language/tone of voice etc will be different to that when we are with a friend or member of our family.

Labelling and social deviance

Because sociologists are interested in explaining and understanding how society works it follows that they are also fascinated and challenged to comprehend what happens when things break down.

The study of crime and deviance is a major activity in the field and many of the ideas generated have spilled over into explanations for the apparently deviant behaviour of mental illness.

- Robert Merton draws upon Durkheim's concept of anomie in his '**social strain theory**'.
  - Merton believes that it is not social change at the root of the problem, rather a social structure that holds out the same goals to us all, but denies us the equal means to achieve them.
  - This lack of complementarity between what society permits us to aspire to and the equal opportunity to succeed creates a 'strain'.
  - The 'strain' created results in the breakdown of norms and subsequent deviant behaviour.

81

- **Labelling theory** developed from ideas propounded by a group of scholars based at the University of Chicago in the 1920s and 1930s known as Symbolic Interactionists.
  - Their starting point was that social structures are created and maintained during human interaction.
  - The focus was upon the role of language and symbols in the organisation of social life.
- Howard Becker, in his study of deviance *Outsiders*, neatly encapsulates the labelling perspective in this famous quote: 'Social groups create deviance by making rules whose infraction constitutes deviance and by applying those rules to particular people and labelling them as outsiders. From this point of view deviance is not a quality of the act a person commits, but rather a consequence of the application by others of rules and sanctions to an offender. The deviant is one to whom that label has been successfully applied; deviant behaviour is behaviour that people so label.'
  - **Primary deviance** – ie the initial piece of rule-breaking behaviour – may have a biological or psychological basis.
  - However, what is more important is how that behaviour is perceived and reacted to by others, thereby creating the secondary deviance.
  - Our social position or powerlessness may result in the deviant label being more successfully attached to us.
  - In part this analysis has been used to explain why certain psychiatric labels are attached to Afro-Caribbeans or migrants or the very poor more frequently than other social groups.
- The introduction of the concept of dangerous severe personality disorder (or DSPD) is also being resisted by many on the grounds that it is really a social construct. One likely to be applied as a label to certain marginal groups in society more readily than others.

KINSHIP, FAMILY AND MARRIAGE

Definitions

- **Kinship** describes the social groups to whom we are related by either marriage or blood.
- Most people, in most parts of the world, live in family groups.
- The **family** is the most basic and important social institution in society.
  - Nuclear family: parents and their non-adult children.
  - Extended family: the wider family that includes grandparents, uncles, aunts and cousins.
- **Conjugal relationship** is the relationship between husband and wife in marriage.

The changing functions of the family

Under a functionalist view of society, favoured by Talcott Parsons, it is possible to examine the function performed by various social institutions such as the family. Why do we have something called a family and how does it contribute to the smooth running of society?

- **Social status**. Our family of origin ascribes various aspects of social status to us: birth order, religion, ethnicity etc. While modern society places emphasis upon achievement as a marker of our status, whom we are and from whence we came is still very important.
- **Procreation and regulation of sexuality**. Traditionally, the family has ensured continuity and constrained sexual desire. Changing attitudes to sex and greater tolerance of different lifestyles have made this function less prominent.
- **Socialisation**. Traditionally, the family was the primary socialising agency. In recent years other agencies, such as the state, the school, and the mass media, have become influential. Sometimes this may lead to conflicts between agencies (the rows that flare up between parents, schools and the state over the appropriate way to provide sex education to young children is a common example).
- **Economic function**. In pre-industrial society the family was the unit of production. The family was self-sufficient and shared tasks. Today the family is more likely to be typified as a unit of consumption. The growth of the welfare state has also meant that we place less reliance, than we once did, upon economic support in times of need from our family.
- **Affection and emotional function**. Family relationships are seen as the emotional security and bonding that we need to be trusting and confident in life. These appear still to be important in spite of the fact that marriages break down more frequently. Most people who divorce remarry.
- **Welfare and protective function**. The family provides support and care for dependants. In spite of the growth of the welfare state the family still plays an important role in health and welfare care. Community-care policies in recent years have underlined this. With an ageing population more older people are living for longer on their own. However, for many this exercise of autonomy is a personal choice, and family ties are maintained in new and different ways. The telephone and the weekly lift to the supermarket replacing physical proximity. What has been termed 'intimacy at a distance'.
- **Recreation and leisure**. An increase in leisure time and the fact that the home now contains many vehicles of entertainment, ie video, computer games, hi-fi etc, means that many recreational activities now take place within the family.

Changes to the family

The family has undergone many changes in Britain over the past 100 years. Many of these have important implications when issues of mental health are considered.

- **Demographic**. The nuclear family is now much smaller in size. This means that women spend a much shorter period of their lives either pregnant or caring for toddlers. It also means a much smaller pool of carers in the case of dependency.
- **An ageing population**. As a society we are increasingly 'age dense'. Because of numerous factors: lower birth rates, former baby booms and increases in life span, many parts of Britain have a post-retirement population as high as 20%. This affects the pattern of mental health in those areas. What some have seen as a biological 'time bomb' also poses a challenge to our ability to maintain services for the age

group and generate sufficient resources to maintain pension levels. Increasing divorce rates, smaller families and greater geographical mobility, have all been cited as potential problems for our ageing population.

- **Mobility and urbanisation**. More of us now live in large cities and the demands of work mean that we have to be mobile. Some have suggested that city life, distance from family and the need to keep moving have resulted in high levels of anomie and increased rates of mental illness.
- **Rise in divorce rates**. About 40% of all marriages now end in divorce. This may lead to the dislocation of children from parents and grandparents with a subsequent impact upon future mental health. We are also witnessing an increase in single parenthood and what are termed 'recreated families' with adoption, fostering etc being more commonplace. Once again some researchers have sought to relate these social changes to increases in our perceived number of mental health problems.
- **Role of women**. Women now enjoy far more rights and have entered the workforce in great number. Some have seen the introduction of the contraceptive pill as marking a huge change for the role and status of women.
- **Privatisation**. Many people have noted the way in which the nuclear family has lost many of its former strong links with the extended family. The 'new' family is small and relatively isolated. Some have suggested that this enclosed 'pressure cooker' atmosphere has contributed to the rise experienced in the number of women suffering from anxiety and depression. The reliance upon the nuclear family may leave people more vulnerable and unsupported when they become distressed or ill.
- **The symmetrical family**. A development identified by Willmott and Young describing the emergence of a family with a more equal division of domestic labour between men and women. Men and women typically perform different domestic tasks but, they suggest, the load is becoming more shared.

The pathological family

Many people, from Freud onwards, have identified the family – ie the ways the children are reared, the couples relate to each other, the organisation of family life – as the seed bed for future mental health problems. It is true that most physical and sexual abuse of children takes place within the context of the family, and this has been identified as a precursor for mental health problems later in life. One consequence has been the development of a range of 'family therapies' designed to encourage family members to reflect upon their (pathological) behaviour and possibly to modify it. Something that the sociologist David Morgan has described as 'medicalising the family'.

Links between pathology and the family situation include the following:

- **Birth order**. Many studies have sought to relate birth order with subsequent mental illness. The results have been inconclusive but first-born children do tend to have an I.Q higher than siblings.
- **Divorce and remarriage**. Once again, attempts to link marital problems with subsequent mental health difficulties have produced a less than clear picture.
- **Parental style**. This has been identified as falling into one of four categories: authoritarian; indulgent–permissive; indulgent–neglectful; authoritative–reciprocal.

The last of these is thought to provide the child with the most suitable start for a life free from mental health problems.

- Three familial models of explanation for schizophrenia have been advanced:
- **Double bind**. Gregory Bateson described families where children receive conflicting parental messages about their attitudes and behaviour. The parent who expresses overwhelming love verbally but shows rejection in their body language for example. The child is thought to withdraw into a psychotic state to escape the conflicting messages.
- **Expressed emotion**. Parents or other caretakers behave with overt criticism, over-involvement and hostility towards the person with schizophrenia. A scale to measure expressed emotion has been developed. A high rate of expressed emotion is associated with relapse.
- **Schisms and skews**. Theodore Lidz described two forms of abnormal family behaviour implicated in the backgrounds of schizophrenic patients. **Marital schism** he felt occurs when one parent becomes overly close to a child of the opposite sex. **Marital skew** exists where there is a power struggle between parent and child. One partner dominates the home and may either manifest idiosyncratic or unusual beliefs about him/herself or the world. Typical families may show what he describes as a 'reversal of normal family roles'. For example, the father taking on a very expressive role and the mother being very instrumental.

SYSTEMS OF SOCIAL STRATIFICATION

Introduction

Social stratification refers to the division of a population into unequal layers or strata. Examples include, gender, age, ethnicity, religion and class.

Occupational social class

Class is a means of differentiating the strata of society by reference to inequality of wealth or income.

Karl Marx believed that a capitalist society is divided into two inevitably conflicting groups

- **Bourgeoisie**: the property-owning classes and owners of the means of production.
- **Proletariat**: the wage earners and those without property.

Occupational social class measures

Since 1911 a scale for measuring occupational social class has been used by the Office of Populations Censuses and Surveys. This is incorporated into the 10-yearly census returns.

The original scale broke society down into five categories (reproduced below). Because social class 3 has swollen over the years, as the skill level of the workforce has improved, it is usually sub-divided into two categories – manual and non-manual.

Class	Percentage of population	Title	Examples
I	5	Professional	Doctor/Lawyer
II	18	Intermediate	Manager/Teacher
III NM	12	Skilled Non-Manual	Clerical
III M	38	Skilled Manual	Carpenter/Butcher
IV	18	Semi-Skilled	Postman/Driver
V	9	Unskilled	Cleaner/Labourer

Table 5.1 Classification of occupational social class

- The scale has proved to be a powerful tool for examining health inequalities.
- The Black Report (1980) highlighted morbidity and mortality differences between the social classes, and detected a 'widening gap' between social groups.

Because of some of the social changes, indicated earlier, a more refined scale was introduced for the 2001 census, and is likely to become widely accepted in medical research. This adopts an eight-point categorisation of our society:

- 1 Higher managerial and professional occupations,
- 2 Lower managerial and professional (nurses, police etc),
- 3 Intermediate occupations (clerks, computer operatives etc),
- 4 Small employers and own account workers (publicans, taxi drivers, window cleaners),
- 5 Lower supervisory, craft and related (plumbers, train drivers etc.),
- 6 Semi-routine occupations (shop assistants, hairdressers, postal workers),
- 7 Routine occupations (waiters, cleaners etc),
- 8 Never worked/long-term unemployed.

Occupational social class and mental health

The use of occupational social class has proved to be a valuable way of exploring the epidemiology of mental illness. Studies of people suffering from schizophrenia consistently show them to be over-represented in lower social class groups. A number of explanations have been advanced to explain this.

- Schizophrenia is related to migration. Recent migrants to a new country tend to start at the bottom of the economic heap. Therefore the fact that when their illness is identified they are to be found in greater numbers in occupational social classes 4 and 5 is really a function of their migration rather than of social class per se.
- Schizophrenia is a stigmatising disorder. It has been suggested that lower class groups are less able to resist being labelled with the disease. The relationship between schizophrenia and occupational social class may therefore reflect the diagnostic practices of doctors.

- A view held particularly in the USA is that inner city life is injurious to mental health. Lower social groups tend to live in inner city areas and are exposed to many life events which are magnified by poverty and poor physical environment. This is sometimes described as a '**breeder hypothesis**'.
- In Britain that theory tends to be rejected in favour of a '**drift hypothesis**'. The early symptoms of schizophrenia lead to loss of job and exclusion from the family. When the subject is first diagnosed they have already 'drifted' down the social scale and appear to be occupying categories 4 and 5 in disproportionate numbers.
- The relationship between depression, suicidal behaviour and occupational social class has been frequently examined, but the results are less clear. Many studies have found depressed patients, particularly women, to be over-represented in lower social class groups.
- George Brown and colleagues (1978) found depression to be associated with women in lower social class groups. A constellation of other factors, such as number of young children and the availability of someone to confide in, seemed to be interwoven.

A psychosocial perspective

In 1996 Richard Wilkinson proposed a comprehensive theory to explain health differences and inequality:

- the distribution of psychological stress is an important determinant of health inequalities in modern affluent societies
- psychological stress is strongly influenced by the quality of social/interpersonal relations
- these in turn are influenced by the magnitude of society's inequalities
- he took comparative data from a number of different wealthy, industrialised countries
- the greater the inequality of wealth (a ratio between the earnings of the best paid and the lowest paid) the greater was the inequality on a range of health measures ('the health gap').

HEALTH AND ILLNESS: THE SOCIOLOGICAL PERSPECTIVE

Introduction

A central belief is that social, cultural and economic factors have a significant impact upon the patterns and distribution of health in a given population.

Lay beliefs

- **Anthropologists** (people who study pre-literate societies) highlighted the fact that individuals have complex beliefs about the meaning of health and illness.

- **Sociologists** have developed this insight to explore and explain lay belief systems in Western societies.
- Lay beliefs about mental illness may not reflect contemporary medical understanding.
- Sociologists try to discriminate between a number of terms
  - **Illness** is the subjective feeling of being unwell
  - **Disease** is the presence of a professionally validated syndrome
  - **Sickness** is the way that the individual behaves when they feel ill or have a disease.
- A patient may be ill, but not have a disease, or may have a disease but feel perfectly well.
- Many psychiatric problems fall into these grey areas and have caused a good deal of controversy. For example is ME (myalgic encephalomyelitis) a disease? What about feeling depressed following a bereavement?

The sick role

In the 1950s the American sociologist Talcott Parsons introduced the concept of 'the sick role'. Parsons was a functionalist and he was concerned to explain how social order is maintained in the modern world.

- He typified the doctor–patient relationship as a micro-social system.
- The relationship is governed by a set of rules or norms.
- Illness is potentially damaging to a society reliant upon smooth functioning and the capacity to work and compete.
- The medical system is organised in such a way that it minimises the potential disruption posed by illness.
- Patients and doctors are locked together in a relationship that has certain rights and responsibilities.
- The **doctor role** is to act in the patient's best interests.
- The **patient role** had four specific characteristics:
  - the patient gains temporary exemption from normal role responsibilities
  - the patient is not held responsible for his or her illness
  - the patient must want to get well
  - the patient should comply with legitimate medical advice.

Stigma

Erving Goffman defined a stigma as 'an attribute that is deeply discrediting'. Discrediting stigmas include things like a severe facial disfigurement or a gross deformity.

- Given that illness represents deviance from the norm it follows that some illnesses have become stigmatised.
- Historically epilepsy was discreditable – people with epilepsy were regarded as unreliable, dangerous and their behaviour as potentially disruptive.
- Many forms of mental illness have acquired the same characteristics.

- Many patients may attempt to conceal their problem from friends, family and employers.
- The general public may be fearful of the diagnosis and shun sufferers.
- These attitudes may have been amplified in the past by the way in which sufferers were incarcerated away from the public gaze.

Health care and behaviour

Three American medical sociologists have been particularly instrumental in exploring this field and providing insights into our understanding of help seeking and patterns of care in the mentally ill.

- **David Mechanic**, who spent some time at the Maudsley Hospital in London, explored the influence of non-medical factors on individuals' perception of and reaction to clinical disorders. He coined the phrase '**illness behaviour**' back in 1968 to describe, 'the way in which symptoms are perceived, evaluated and acted upon by a person who recognises some pain, discomfort, or other signs of organic malfunction'.
- The mitigating factor of 'illness behaviour' has been an influence upon the work of George Brown and his studies of depression, while Golberg and Huxley have used the concept to explore issues around psychiatric referral pathways.
- **Irving Zola** invoked the concept of 'triggers' to explain help-seeking behaviour.
- He suggests that when a patient decides to seek help the explanation may be as much social as medical.
- As a clinician you should try to become aware of potential triggers – why has this patient come to see me now?
- The five trigger areas that he identified were
  o perceived interference with vocational or physical activity
  o perceived interference with social or personal relations
  o occurrence of an interpersonal crisis
  o the time scale of symptoms
  o social sanctions from family and/or friends.
- **Kleinman** proposed a useful way of categorising health care into three overlapping sectors. The model highlights the fact that lay people theorise about their own health, and self-treat more frequently than they seek professional help.
- The three sectors – professional, popular and folk – not only overlap but frequently conflict.
- **Professional care** refers to the sort of mental health treatments currently taught in modern medical schools.
- **Popular care** is the care provided within the family, reliant upon traditional beliefs.
- **Folk care** refers to those more formalised systems of care that exist outside conventional medicine. These would include alternative and complementary medicine.
- Mental health patients will move between these three sectors, taking their own decisions and creating a unique pathway of care.

PSYCHIATRY AND SOCIAL CONTROL

As medicine, and particularly psychiatry, has developed as a discipline so a number of critics have questioned the part it plays in our life and the control it exercises over our daily life.

Medicalisation and colonisation

American sociologists such as Irving Zola and Elliot Freidson, have highlighted the fact that medicine seemed to be spreading in influence and entering areas of our lives formerly governed by the law or religion.

Medicalisation was turning 'social problems' such as alcoholism and drug addiction into a medical problem.

- The argument gathers weight when we reflect that it was not until 1980 that homosexuality was dropped as a diagnostic category from the Diagnostic and Statistical Manual of Mental Disorders (DSM).
- Thomas Szasz, an American psychiatrist and psychoanalyst, took up the theme. He wrote about what he saw as 'the myth of mental illness'; psychiatry was concerning itself too much with what he termed 'the problems of daily living' (medicalisation).
  - Genuine mental health problems, once an organic or genetic component was discovered, became re-designated as neurological problems.
  - Hence many psychiatrists were treating non-diseases and the growth and power of the profession was based upon a series of misbeliefs or fictions.
- Ivan Ilich airs some of the same ideas in his famous tract, *Medical Nemesis*.
  - He made the term 'iatrogenesis' or doctor-induced illness popular.
  - The start of his argument is fairly conventional as he outlines 'clinical iatrogenesis'. The more we treat and medicate patients the more we risk damaging them because of medical errors and the side-effects of powerful treatments.
- Claims for treatments made by doctors may not be borne out in the long run. Psychiatry has a rich history of once-vaunted treatments now consigned to the museum.
- The promise of 'wonder cure' is undermined by dependency and side-effects. Recent anti-depressive medication would seem to fit this category.
- **Social iatrogenesis** refers to the way in which we tend to convert the stresses of economic activity and industrial growth into more and more demands for therapy.
- **Cultural iatrogenesis** suggests that as we become more reliant upon technical solutions to our problems and symptoms we fail to utilise the resources inherent in our network of family and friends.
- As Illich puts it 'iatrogenic medicine reinforces a morbid society in which social control of the population by the medical system turns into a principal economic activity'.

THE DECLINE OF LARGE INSTITUTIONS

The history of psychiatry in Britain can be told by means of an examination of the ways in which the mentally ill have been contained and cared for.

- Throughout the nineteenth century the emphasis was placed upon the building of large psychiatric institutions or 'asylums' to keep the afflicted away from crowded cities, both for their protection and that of others.
- Since the mid-1950s this way of dealing with the severely mentally ill has come under sustained attack from social scientists and others. The main thrust of their various arguments is that large, relatively isolated institutions, are potentially damaging environments in which to treat people, and that rehabilitation back into normal mainstream society was made more difficult.

Foucault

The French social historian Michel Foucault, in two books, *The Birth of the Clinic* (1976) and *Madness and Civilisation* (1965) captured the critical spirit of the age:

- 'madness' was socially constructed
- punishment of rule breakers had given way to 'treatment'. But this treatment resulted in
- the need for constant surveillance in large remote hospitals
- Doctors were able to exercise more power over their patients and discipline more aspects of their behaviour and daily life.

Two English critics added to the debate

Russell Barton (1959), building upon earlier work that had identified maladaptation to long-stay, institutional life (prison stupor, psychological institutionalism) coined the phrase 'institutional neurosis'.

He felt that the 'symptoms' that he observed in the long-stay patients that he was attempting to rehabilitate, ie apathy, lack of initiative, loss of interest, submissiveness, and resignation, were not the after effects of a long illness (usually schizophrenia) but the result of spending so long in the unstimulating environment of the hospital.

Hospitals in Trouble (1985) by J. P. Martin followed a series of scandals highlighting poor conditions for patients and systematic abuse.

After reviewing the evidence he felt that various aspects of 'Isolation' were crucial. Psychiatric hospitals were geographically remote and out of the medical mainstream.

'Asylums'

Erving Goffman in a series of essays published in a book entitled *Asylums* mounted a devastating and influential critique of life in a psychiatric hospital or 'total institution' as he termed it.

- As a result of his academic background as a social anthropologist, his research technique relied upon 'participant observation'. This involves immersing oneself in a situation and becoming part of it to understand it from the inside. He worked as a hospital ward orderly in an American psychiatric hospital to gather his data.
- Many of the insights generated by Goffman appear in a popular work of fiction; *One Flew Over the Cuckoo's Nest* by Ken Kesey, and they are sharply illustrated in Milos Foreman's Oscar-winning film of the same name.
- His starting point is that 'any group of persons … develop a life of their own that becomes meaningful, reasonable and normal once you get used to it'.
- He defined the '**total institution**' as one in which all aspects of life are conducted in the same place and under the same authority. The 'total institution' was typified as one in which activities are tightly scheduled and where the 'bureaucratic organisation of whole blocks of people' takes place.
- Inmates adjust to this world in a number of ways: withdrawal; intransigence; colonisation and conversion. All these responses are illustrated in the Foreman film.
- A strict demarcation was noted between 'inmates' and staff. This resulted in the development of stereotypes. Staff are regarded by patients as harsh and authoritarian. Staff meanwhile see patients as secretive, bitter and conspiratorial.

Wing and Brown

Many of the insights generated by Goffman were to be empirically tested in a series of studies by the British sociologist George Brown and John Wing a social psychiatrist.

- They noted the social passivity and withdrawn state of patients and related this to length of stay and lack of stimulation on the ward.
- They demonstrated, by comparing different hospitals, that it was possible to bring about improvements in the patients' state by changing the nature of the hospital regime and the atmosphere on the ward.

Chapter 6

Psychopathology

Chris Fear

CONTENTS

Psychopathology

COMMON TERMS

- **Psychopathology**: The study of abnormal experiences
  - **descriptive psychopathology** describes without attributing cause
  - **dynamic psychopathology** looks for explanations for the behaviour, usually within a psychoanalytical framework.
- **Phenomenology**: The philosophical study of the experiences (normal or abnormal) described by the patients, associated with Husserl
- **Form**: The phenomenon occurring (eg hallucination, delusion, obsession)
- **Content**: The specific nature of the experience (eg persecutory, grandiose)
- **Symptom**: The patient's complaint
- **Sign**: Objective evidence on examination
- **Normal**: A term best avoided but properly used to convey statistical norm or usual state of affairs for the patient
- **Mental state examination**: A judgement about the patient's state of mind based upon observation and reported subjective experience of phenomena and psychopathology.

APPEARANCE AND BEHAVIOUR

Mental state can be inferred from appearance, response to others (manner) and movements (voluntary and involuntary), eg an unkempt, dirty and dishevelled appearance may indicate:

- alcohol or drugs
- depression
- schizophrenia (see negative symptoms)
- dementia
- physical infirmity and neglect.

Weight loss suggests:

- eating disorder
- depression
- physical illness, eg thyrotoxicosis, cancer
- chronic anxiety disorder.

Incongruous dress may suggest mania or offer a clue to a delusional system.

Scars may indicate self-harm.

Facial appearance (not exhaustive)

- Lack of facial mobility (flat affect) of depression
- 'Mask-like' facies of Parkinsonism
- Characteristic facies of myxoedema and thyrotoxicosis
- Dilated pupils of anxiety, with furrowed brow and raised eyebrows
- Constricted pupils of opiate use
- Tooth erosion caused by repeated vomiting in bulimia
- Evidence of bruising, possibly indicating violence
- Incongruence between facial appearance and behaviour/reported experiences.

Movement disorders

Disorders of **adaptive movements** include hunched depressive postures (tearfulness, unhappy facies), overactive and expansive mania, and the restless fiddling and touching of anxiety. Other adaptive movement disorders include mannerisms and certain obstructive movements in catatonic schizophrenia (see pages 101–102).

Non-adaptive movements are divided into those that are **induced**, as seen in catatonia (see pages 101–102 echopraxia, *Mitgehen* etc) and the following **spontaneous movements**:

- **akinesia**: Lack of voluntary movement (depressive stupor: retardation with muteness)
- **akathisia**: A motor restlessness, worse in the lower limbs, experienced as very unpleasant and leading to constant shifting of posture (drugs such as neuroleptics and selective serotonin re-uptake inhibitors (SSRIs))
- **athetosis**: Slow, sinuous movement of the limbs (perinatal brain injury)
- **chorea**: A continuous flow of small jerky movements from limb to limb (Huntington's disease, Sydenham's chorea, thyrotoxicosis, neuroleptics, phenytoin and oral contraceptives)
- **dystonia**: Prolonged spasms of muscle contraction (neuroleptics)
- **dyskinesia**: Choreo-athetotic movements, generalised or affecting particular muscle groups, most commonly emerging after prolonged use of neuroleptics (tardive dyskinesia); typically orofacial ('Rabbit syndrome'), trunkal and limb symptom groupings
- **hyperkinesia**: Restless overactivity (head injury, epilepsies)
- **myoclonus**: Sudden involuntary jerks of muscle groups (amitriptyline, Alzheimer's disease and Creuzfeldt–Jakob disease
- **Parkinsonism**: Triad of bradykinesia, resting tremor and rigidity
- **spasmodic torticollis**: Dystonic spasm of the neck in which the head is twisted
- **tic**: Involuntary, rapid repetitive and stereotyped twitching of small muscle groups
- **tremor**: Rhythmic and alternating movement with a number of variations and aetiologies.

There are **varieties of tremor**:

- **Essential tremor** is an autosomal dominant condition with incomplete penetrance (35% no family history); it is worsened with stress and improved by alcohol.

- **Flapping tremor** (asterixis) is associated with liver failure and comprises flapping flexion/extension movements at the wrist, worsened by outstretching arms, fatigue and stress; it is absent at rest.
- **Resting tremor** occurs when the limbs are relaxed and supported, especially in Parkinson's disease (pill-rolling).
- **Static tremor** occurs typically in the hands, head, or upper torso and is associated with drugs (lithium, neuroleptics), anxiety, thyrotoxicosis and hysteria. Essential tremor and resting tremor are varieties of this problem.
- **Syphilitic tremor** of general paresis is typically coarse and irregular and involves the face and hands.

Causes of Parkinsonism include:

- Parkinson's disease
- extra-pyramidal side-effects (EPSE) of neuroleptics, MPTP and narcotic drugs
- carbon monoxide poisoning
- diffuse Lewy body disease
- secondary to chronic minor head injury (dementia pugilistica)
- depression with psychomotor retardation.

Behaviours associated with (catatonic) schizophrenia

(These behaviours may also occur in learning disabled patients and, rarely, in dementia.)

- **advertence/aversion**: Turning towards/away from the examiner when speaking to them
- **akinesia**: A mild form of stupor in which there is paucity of movement
- **ambitendency**: Motor reflection of ambivalence
- **automatic obedience**: Carrying out of every instruction received; also called 'command automatism' (but see below)
- **'Command automatism'**: Term used synonymously with 'automatic obedience' or to describe a syndrome of echolalia, echopraxia and waxy flexibility
- **echolalia**: Repetition of the last few syllables
- **echopraxia**: Repetitive performance of every action of a nearby person
- **flat affect**: Expressionless stiffness of the face that contrasts with likely eye expression
- *flexibilitas cerea*: See 'waxy flexibility'
- **grimacing**: Abnormal facial expression, including *Schnauzkrampf* (snout spasm)
- *Haltungsverharren*: Similar to waxy flexibility but posture returns to resting state after a few seconds
- **handling**: Touching or handling of everything within reach, often associated with intertwining
- **impulsive behaviours**: Sudden outbursts of aggression or overactivity without obvious stimulus
- **intertwining**: Continuous intertwining of fingers or winding clothes/other items around hands/fingers.
- *logoclonia*: Perseveration of the final syllable of the last word
- **mannerism**: Abnormal execution of an understandable, goal-directed movement

- **Mitgehen**: Movement of body in response to light pressure until the movement is halted
- **Mitmachen**: Movement of body in response to light pressure but returns to resting state when pressure ceases
- **negativism**: Active resistance of all interventions or attempts at passive movement. Associated with Kleist
- **obstruction (blocking)**: Motor equivalent of thought block, a movement is interrupted or ceases before completion
- **opposition**: Resistance to all attempts at passive movement with exactly the same degree of pressure as that applied
- **palilalia**: Repeating a perseverated word with increasing frequency
- **parakinesia**: Continuous irregular muscle movements resulting in grimacing and twitching
- **perseveration**: Continuing a goal-directed activity beyond its necessity (may be applied to behaviour, speech, thought etc)
- **prosectic speech**: Turning towards the examiner and speaking in an undertone for as long as spoken to or encouraged non-verbally
- **psychological pillow**: Stereotyped posture in which the patient lies prone with head raised a few centimetres as if resting on an invisible pillow
- **stereotyped/manneristic posture**: Bizarre posture rigidly maintained for hours/not maintained
- **stereotypy**: Non-goal-directed movement carried out in a uniform way; may affect speech
- **stupor**: State of immobility without physical or emotional response; occasional grimacing may occur if reacting to hallucinations and the eyes are expressive
- **Vorbeireden**: Talking past the point (behaviour disorder, thought disorder or deliberate)
- **waxy flexibility**: Placed into a posture and will hold it for minutes/hours.

VOLITION

A poorly understood area, usually interpreted on the basis of individuals' subjective descriptions: encompassing urges, needs, drives, instincts and motivations.

Types of volition (Scharfetter, 1980)

These include:

- **drive**: A move to satisfy basic needs
- **instinct**: An innate pattern of behaviour to satisfy drive
- **motivation**: A clear mood leading to actions designed to satisfy needs and desires
- **need**: Work towards a goal, seen as a desire
- **will**: Planned action leading to a desired goal.

Disturbances of volition

- schizophrenic negative symptoms
- depressive retardation
- manic overactivity
- perceived external locus of control in neurosis
- passivity experiences in schizophrenia (made thoughts, made acts, made affect)
- hysterical dissociative states.

SELF-CONCEPT AND BODILY EXPERIENCES

Jasper's four aspects of self-experience

Awareness of:

- existence and activity of the self
- unity of self at a given point in time
- continuity and identity over a period of time
- boundaries of the self (ego boundaries).

Disturbances

Disturbances that can occur are:

- **depersonalisation**: Dissociative state, often with derealisation; feeling, not delusion
- **multiple personality**: The assumption of different identities in vulnerable individuals
- depressive sensation of being unable to feel emotions
- **autoscopy**: Seeing oneself and identifying with the hallucination at a somatic level (parietal lobe lesions: also **heautoscopy** or **phantom mirror image**)
- **passivity experiences**: The sensation of having thoughts, movements and emotions imposed from an external source.

They lead to disturbed:

- unity of self (multiple personality, autoscopy)
- continuity of self (schizophrenia, hysterical and dissociative states, depression)
- ego boundaries (schizophrenia, dissociative states)
- body image (dysmorphophobia, anorexia nervosa, hypochondriasis)
- use of body parts (dissociative states, non-dominant strokes).

AFFECT

Some terms used in the study of affect:

- **affect**: Short-lived feeling state, synonymous with emotion
- **feeling**: The transitory emotional reaction to an experience

- **mood**: Prevalent emotional tone at a given time
- **mood state**: As for mood but longer lasting

In describing emotional disorders, the **quality**, **appropriateness** and **constancy** should receive comment.

Abnormalities of emotion as personality traits are discussed below.

Jasper's categorisations of affect

- **object**: Eg specific phobias, love, grief, etc
- **source**: Ie as a physical feeling in a part of the body or a psychological feeling of happiness, etc
- **biological purpose**: Instinctual response to situations, evolutionary role
- **feeling**: A prevailing state
- **duration and intensity**: Eg affect is complex but brief, mood is prolonged.

Abnormal emotional reaction

All emotional reactions are normal and adaptive to some extent. Judgement of abnormality depends upon degree and context.

- **Anxiety** is a fear in the expectation, but not certainty, of an unpleasant experience. When pathological, defined as 'fear without adequate cause'. Includes physical symptoms as a result of autonomic overactivity (sweating, abdominal cramps, palpitations, dry mouth, tremor, etc). Anxiety may be free-floating, situational, or phobic.
- **Depression** is a feeling of misery, helplessness, unworthiness and hopelessness. To be clinically important, it should be accompanied by somatic symptoms of disturbed appetite, sleep and cognitive function or it may present somatically as symptoms of illness in the absence of pathology (hypochondriasis). If severe, there may be **mood congruent** delusions and/or hallucinations.
- **Euphoria/ecstasy** is unrealistic cheerfulness and elation associated with hypomania and mania. It may be accompanied by a reduced need for sleep, changes in appetite, attention and concentration, or by **mood congruent** delusions and/or hallucinations.
- **Panic attack** is the abrupt onset of intense anxiety with autonomic symptoms and a need to escape the situation, fearing death, heart attack, collapse, or madness. It usually has a duration of 10 to 20 minutes.

Abnormal expression of emotion

The emotional behaviour displayed is qualitatively different from an average response.

- **apathy**: Loss of emotional response (schizophrenia)
- **blunted affect**: Dulling of the sensitivity of the normal emotional response (schizophrenia)

- **dissociation**: Detachment from emotions, seen in hysterical states (***belle indifference***, **derealisation**, **depersonalisation**) and occasionally bereavement (denial), extreme danger
- **flattened affect**: Reduction in range of emotional response (schizophrenia)
- **incongruity**: Emotion inappropriate to the situation and not understandable to a normal observer (acute schizophrenia)
- **incontinence**: Extreme emotional lability with loss of control, seen in organic conditions (pseudobulbar palsy)
- **indifference**: Lack of expected emotional response to others or to their own antisocial behaviour (psychopathy)
- **lability**: Emotional tone may be appropriate, but excessive, and fluctuates rapidly (mania, personality disorder, organic especially brainstem lesions)
- **perplexity**: Anxious, puzzled bewilderment, seen in delusional mood (early psychosis).

SPEECH AND LANGUAGE

Problems with speech and language can be **organic**, ie aphasias/dysphasias, or **functional**, ie echolalia in schizophrenia (catatonic motor disorder, see page 101); rapid speech in mania (associated with flight of ideas, a thought disorder); slowed speech in depression; or manneristic speech in schizophrenia.

Theories of language

The psycho-physiological theory of Brain holds that concepts attached to language are refined during childhood to produce unconscious schemata for word and sentence recognition and for speech production. The key words in this theory are **word** and **sentence schemata**.

The anatomical theory of Geschwind suggests that objects stimulate the visual cortex and are named, producing associations in the auditory cortex of Wernicke's area before transfer to Broca's area (motor association cortex) for speech. The key words here are **naming**, **comprehension** and **repetition**.

Organic speech/language disorders

Detailed consideration of the various lesions that can lead to different types of aphasia or dysphasia (terms usually used interchangeably) is more properly given in a neurological text. It is worth being familiar with the following terms and their meanings:

- **acalculia**: Lack of recognition of mathematical symbols
- **agnosia**: Lack of recognition
- **agraphia**: Inability to write
- **alexia**: Inability to read with understanding
- **asymbolia**: Inability to recognise writing
- **verbigeration**: Repetition of words or syllables in aphasia.

Primary sensory dysphasia (receptive aphasia) is the inability to understand spoken speech and grammar as a result of a lesion in Wernicke's speech area (primary auditory association cortex). Hearing is normal.

- **central (syntactical) aphasia**: Inability to understand written and spoken words
- **conduction dysphasia**: Patient can understand but not repeat a message
- **nominal (amnestic) dysphasia**: Unable to name objects but can describe them/their function
- **jargon aphasia**: Fluent speech, unintelligible because of grammatical/word finding errors
- **subcortical auditory/visual dysphasia** ('pure word-deafness/-blindness'): Inability to understand the spoken word/read speech with understanding. Other aspects of language (eg speaking, writing) are unimpaired
- **intermediate aphasia**: Collective name for nominal and central dysphasias.

Primary motor dysphasia (expressive aphasia, Broca's aphasia, verbal aphasia) is the inability to choose words and construct grammar affecting both written and spoken language. Lesion in Broca's speech area also causes difficulty in understanding and carrying out complex instructions. Words are substituted or 'yes' and 'no' answers are given; patient may understand language and use swear words under stress.

- **subcortical agraphia** (may be with or without alexia)
- **subcortical verbal apraxia** ('pure word-dumbness'): Inability to say words although muscles are undamaged and understanding is unimpaired.

Functional disorders

Disorders are:

- **agrammatism**: Loss of parts of speech as a result of thought disorder
- **akataphasia**: Loss of expression of thought in speech (Kraepelin)
- **alogia**: Poverty of thought as expressed in language
- **aphonia**: Loss of the ability to vocalise; may be caused by damage to the IXth cranial nerve or in hysterical states, is common in Ear, Nose and Throat departments
- **coprolalia**: Tics of obscene verbalisations; really a movement disorder associated with Tourette syndrome
- **cryptolalia/phonia**: Use of a private spoken or written language
- **dysphonia**: A lesser form of aphonia producing hoarseness; also caused by vocal chord lesions
- **logoclonia**: Repetition on syllables associated with Parkinsonism
- **mutism**: May be elective (eg children), hysterical (aphonia), or associated with depressive (manic) or catatonic stupor
- **neologism**: New word with idiosyncratic meaning (schizophrenia)
- **paragrammatism**: Disorder of syntax leading to schizophasia
- **paralogia**: Intrusion of bizarre words because of thought disorder
- **paraphasia**: Intrusion of bizarre sounds into normal words
- **schizophasia** ('word salad', 'speech confusion'): Random words used meaninglessly so that grammar breaks down
- **stammering/stuttering**

- **Vorbereiden** ('talking past the point'): Approximate answers to questions indicating an understanding of the question but giving a deliberately false answer; characteristic of Ganser syndrome, hysterical pseudodementia, but rarely seen in young adolescent schizophrenics.

THOUGHT

Curt Schneider listed three features of healthy thinking (see below):

- **constancy**: Persistence of a completed thought
- **organisation**: Contents of a thought related to one another but separated in an organised way
- **continuity**: All thoughts, even sudden ideas, are organised in order in the whole consciousness.

Disorders of tempo

Flight of ideas is a manic form of thought in which ideas come so rapidly that the themes lack general direction and may be associated by chance or according to associations of sound (clang associations, rhyming, assonance, alliteration), external stimuli, proverbs, clichés, etc. **Prolixity** is a slowed form that occurs in hypomania and has less clang and fewer verbal associations.

Thought may be retarded or slowed; in depression it may be inhibited completely. Inhibition is seen rarely in manic stupor. Circumstantiality is a rambling, slow, convoluted but goal-directed type of thinking usually associated with obsessive personalities.

Disorders of form (formal thought disorder)

Disturbance of abstract or conceptual thinking is diagnostic of schizophrenia or organic brain disorders.

Cameron's thought disorder encompasses:

- **asyndesis**: Lack of adequate connections between thoughts causing the patient to use clusters of familiar and related words
- **metonyms**: Imprecise approximations to words or phrases
- **interpenetration**: Speech contains elements of the task in hand interspersed with a stream of fantasy thoughts
- **overinclusion**: Inability to maintain thinking within the boundaries of the problem.

Goldstein described a loss of **abstract attitude** in both schizophrenia and coarse brain disease. However, the schizophrenia patients have not lost their **fund of words**.

The five features of formal thought disorder described by Curt Schneider (NB not Karl Schneider of First Rank Symptoms) are:

- **derailment**: Thought slides onto a subsidiary thought

- **drivelling**: The constituent parts of a complex thought are broken down and intermixed
- **fusion**: Heterogeneous elements of a thought are woven together
- **omission**: Part of a thought is left out for no reason
- **substitution**: A major thought is replaced by a subsidiary one.

Disorders of possession of thought

Obsessions are unwanted (often distressing) intrusive thoughts but are recognised as coming from the patient's own mind and are resisted. **Compulsions** are the acts that arise in an attempt to neutralise the anxiety arising from the obsessions. According to Lewis there are three elements: subjective compulsion, resistance and insight. Resistance may be lost with habituation.

Thought alienation phenomena are thoughts experienced as being under the control of someone/thing else. They are not recognised as the patient's own thoughts and this distinguishes them from obsessions. They were considered, by Karl Schneider, to be first-rank symptoms of schizophrenia:

- **thought insertion**: The experience of having foreign thoughts placed in the mind by an external agency
- **thought withdrawal**: A normal stream of thoughts is suddenly removed from the mind by a foreign agency
- **thought broadcasting**: The patient's thoughts are being thought by others simultaneously.

Disorders of the content of thought

Overvalued ideas

Jasper considered overvalued ideas to be synonymous with his delusion-like ideas. They are understandable, often socially congruent, beliefs that are held with unusual force and pursued beyond the bounds of reason. Although they dominate the patient's life, they are never considered senseless.

Delusions

Delusions are defined as 'fixed false beliefs out of keeping with the individual's cultural background'. They may not be entirely false but the process by which they arise is bizarre and illogical. Jasper's ideas on delusions are pre-eminent, recognising the following forms. He divided delusions into delusion-like ideas, that are understandable (*verstandlich*) from a patient's prior experience and true delusions, which are bizarre and cannot be understood (*unverstandlich*). A variety of delusional forms are recognised:

- **primary delusion** (synonymous with autochthonous idea): A 'eureka' experience, brainwave, inspiration; the patient suddenly 'knows' what is going on, often preceded by delusional mood

- **secondary delusion**: A delusional belief that arises to explain other phenomena, eg hallucinations, passivity experiences, etc
- **delusional memory**: An event is 'remembered' but clearly delusional
- **delusional mood**: A sense of strangeness as if something peculiar is going on or something is about to happen
- **delusional perception**: A delusional belief linked to a real perception ('I saw the traffic lights change and knew the world was going to end.'); this is the only delusion that is a first-rank symptom of schizophrenia
- **religious delusions**: The distinction from true religious beliefs is difficult but in the latter, there is a possibility of doubt and a purposeful, spiritual tone whereas delusions are concrete and self-serving
- **partial delusion**: Held with less certainty/partial insight.

Folie à deux	Psychotic **principal** communicates a delusional idea to a dependent **associate** whose delusions settle on separation
Grandiose*	Special powers; mania and schizophrenia
Guilt, worthlessness	Depression
Hypochondriacal*	Illness; depression, schizophrenia
Imagined ugliness/deformity	Body dysmorphic disorder, schizophrenia, depression
Infestation	Ekbom syndrome; organic states, drug misuse
Jealousy*	Othello syndrome; associated with alcohol
Love*	De Clerambault syndrome, erotomania – the belief that another (unattainable) person is in love with the patient. Schizophrenia
Misidentification	Many subtypes. Capgras syndrome – familiar person replaced by a stranger who is an exact double; Fregoli syndrome – familiar person identified in various strangers; this may also occur for inanimate objects. Schizophrenia, paranoia and organic disorders
Nihilism	Cotard syndrome – parts of the body, the whole self, or even the world have disappeared or 'rotted away'. There may be olfactory hallucinations (decay). Depression, organic disorders, etc
Persecution*	The commonest delusion, universal in psychosis
Reference	Kretschmer's sensitive *beziehungswahn* – the belief that others/radio/TV/events are discussing or occurring for the patient. Often with grandiose/persecutory delusions.

* Subtypes of Diagnostic and Statistical Manual of Mental Disorders 4th edition (DSM-IV) delusional disorder.

Table 6.1 Some delusional types and syndromes

Conrad's four stages of **apophany** (primary delusional experience), derived from Gestalt psychology (Conrad, 1958) are:

- trema (fear and trembling): A delusional mood
- apophenia (the appearance of a phenomenon): The delusional idea
- change in world view to make sense of the delusion
- apocalypse: Breakdown of logic accompanied by thought disorder and behavioural disorders.

PERCEPTION

Normal sensory receptors, tracts and cortex are required for normal perceptions.

Sensory distortions

The intensity, size, colour, etc of a perception may become changed. In the visual range this includes macro/micropsia, dysmegalopsia (psychedelics and temporal lobe lesions) and colour (yellow or green dominance with digoxin toxicity) as well as the Lilliputian perception of normal objects as small. Hyper/hypoacusis can occur in the auditory range, abnormal perception of pain can occur in the tactile sense and affect is altered in dissociative states (eg derealisation). These changes may be associated with:

- affective disorders
- anxiety states, hysteria
- schizophrenia
- alcohol and drugs (eg LSD)
- organic conditions such as epilepsy, dementia, delirium, etc.

Illusions (Esquirol, 1838) and imagery

Illusions are false perceptions arising involuntarily from the transformation of a real object.

- **completion illusions**: Involuntarily making sense of incomplete patterns (normal due to tiredness or inattention)
- **affective illusions**: Emotion heightens perception, familiar objects are misinterpreted (normal in fear of the dark, bereavement)
- **pareidolic illusions**: Images made from shapes (may be normal)
- illusions may be abnormal if associated with psychoses, affect or organic states, eg delirium.

Imagery is the voluntary process. **Eidetic imagery** involves recreating previous perceptions as vivid mental pictures.

Pseudohallucination (Kandinsky, 1885)

Involuntary abnormal perception, which differs in quality from a normal perception and is experienced in inner space (bereavement, obsession, dissociation, borderline personalities).

Hallucination

An hallucination is a perception without a stimulus/an object. Equal in quality to a real perception and experienced in external space an hallucination may occur in any modality, commonly.

- **Auditory hallucinations** vary from sounds to voices. They can be distinguished as male/female, un/familiar, second (to)/third person (about), single/multiple, affective tone, commands/need to obey, whether reacted to, etc. They are common in schizophrenia (third person, running commentary, thought echo), affective psychosis (second person, mood congruent), and organic states (poorly formed, fleeting).
- **Visual hallucinations** vary from flashes of light to complex and panoramic images. They are more common in organic conditions such as TLE, and in the use of LSD and other drugs, also Charles Bonnet syndrome. They are rare in schizophrenia.
- **Gustatory and olfactory hallucinations** occur in schizophrenia, severe depression and TLE.
- **Tactile (haptic) hallucinations** occur in drug withdrawal (formication).
- Hallucinations may also be **kinaesthetic**, **thermic**, **hygric** and **visceral** (schizophrenia).

Extracampine hallucinations are experienced outside the sensory field (often hypnopompic and may be normal). **Hypnopompic/hypnagogic hallucinations** occur while waking/falling asleep (are usually visual or auditory and are normal). **Functional hallucinations** occur only together with an unrelated external stimulus (schizophrenia). **Reflex hallucinations** occur in one sensory modality in response to a real perception in another.

Schneider's symptoms of the first rank

Considered to be diagnostic of schizophrenia in the absence of organic disorders.

Delusion

- delusional perception (NB this is the only type of primary delusion or autochthonous idea that is included).

Auditory hallucinations

- thoughts spoken aloud
- voices arguing or discussing in the third person
- running commentary on the patient's actions.

Thought alienation phenomena

- withdrawal
- insertion
- broadcasting.

Passivity experiences

- made thoughts, acts and affect.

COGNITION

The assessment of cognition overlaps both neurological examination and psychometric testing. It is as well to be familiar with Folstein's Mini Mental State Examination, which provides a brief, but effective, assessment of orientation, attention, concentration and memory as well as visuospatial function.

Attention and concentration

Attention is the objective observation of another person, object or event and may be active or passive. It is increased in states of preoccupation (delusions, depression, etc) and reduced in dissociative states. Attention and concentration are affected by organic states and in hypomania. The following timed tests measure attention/concentration:

- serial 7s (threes)
- months of the year backwards
- digits repeated forwards and backwards
- words spelt forwards and backwards (Folstein).

Consciousness

Consciousness is defined as 'a state of awareness of self and environment'. It is tested through checking orientation in time, place and person; also by the Glasgow Coma Scale. Consciousness may be altered as:

- **clouding**: Disorientation, disturbed perception and attention, subsequent amnesia (eg delirium)
- **drowsiness**: As clouding but unconscious without stimulation, can be roused
- **stupor**: Only rousable with considerable effort; awareness of environment is maintained in functional stupor (schizophrenia, depression) but not in organic stupor
- **coma**: Little or no response to stimulus.

Memory

The registration, rehearsal, retention and retrieval of information: affected by anything that interferes with any of these processes, eg head injury, intoxication (registration/rehearsal), dementia, Korsakoff's psychosis (retention), hysterical amnesia (retrieval). Confabulation is the process by which information is made up to fill gaps in memory.

Welford's seven stages in memory comprise the following:

- adequate perception: comprehension and response to the material
- short-term storage mechanism
- formation of a durable trace
- consolidation with modification/simplification of traces by subsequent learning
- recognition that certain material needs to be recalled
- isolation of the relevant memory
- use of recalled material in new situations.

Some **tests of memory** include:

- recall of past or recent life events (that can be corroborated)
- recall of a name and address after 5 minutes
- recall of apple, table, penny after 2 and 5 minutes (Folstein)
- Babcock sentence: 'What every nation needs to become rich and great is a strong secure supply of wood'.
- general knowledge questions.

Ribot's law of memory regression: 'In dementing illnesses, memory for recent events is lost before memory for remote events'.

Intelligence

'The individual's total of abilities, those instruments of performance and purpose available to him for adaptation to life'. Intelligence requires psychometric testing (eg Wechsler Adult Intelligence Scale – WAIS) for formal testing (see Chapter 4).

Visuospatial function

This can be tested by observation or directly. The tests are mostly included in Folstein.

- copy an asymmetrical object, draw a clock face, build a star from matchsticks (constructional apraxia)
- observe right–left orientation and ability to name fingers (finger agnosia)
- observe dressing and finding way around (dressing apraxia, topographical disorientation).

INSIGHT

Insight is used to indicate the degree of correctness of patients' understanding of:

- their condition (may be lost in psychosis but usually present to some degree)
- the underlying cause of their distress (often reduced in neurosis)
- their environment (affected by delusions and hallucinations).

There is no relationship between insight and intellectual impairment, and a complex association with other psychopathology. Some patients will comply with treatment despite having no insight into its necessity. Good insight is associated with improved compliance, less readmission and better prognosis.

David's components of insight are:

- recognition of unusual mental events as pathological
- recognition, by the patients, that they suffer from a mental illness
- compliance with medication.

GENDER AND PERSONALITY

Gender is the lifelong genetically determined masculinity or femininity of an individual. **Core gender identity** is the individual's private view of their own gender, normally established by 18 months of age. **Gender role** is the public display of gender. Gender identity and sexual disorders will be covered in Chapter 14.

Personality is that, apart from physical appearance, which distinguishes an individual. It comprises different traits, expressed to a greater or lesser extent in different individuals and within the same individual in different situations. These traits are considered abnormal either as a statistical deviation from the norm or in circumstances where they interfere with others or pass beyond the bounds of social acceptability. A patient's predominant personality traits will often influence the expression or content of their psychopathology. Personality disorders per se are covered in Chapter 12.

Abnormal predisposition to emotion

This is seen as a tendency to give stereotyped emotional responses in various personalities:

- **affectless**: Emotionally cold (schizoid personalities)
- **cyclothymic**: Marked swings of mood but not sufficient for bipolar disorder (cyclothymia, emotionally unstable personality)
- **dysthymic**: Miserable (depressive)
- **hyperthymic**: Over-cheerful, unreasonably optimistic
- **irritable**: Hyper-critical, touchy individuals (paranoid personalities).

Psychogenic pain

This is associated with the following personality types (Engels):

- anxious
- depressive/cyclothymia at the depressive pole
- hysterical
- hypochondriacal
- obsessional.

Schneider's personality types

These are:

- affectionless
- asthenic
- attention-seeking
- depressive
- explosive
- fanatic
- hyperthymic
- insecure
- labile.

PSYCHODYNAMIC THEORY OF DEFENCE MECHANISMS

The inclusion of this topic in a psychopathology syllabus would appear to be an anachronism of the College examiners. It is a topic for descriptive phenomenology and is better included in the chapter on psychotherapies. However, in brief:

Theoretical frameworks and their theories of defence mechanisms

- **Attachment theory**: Patient maintains desirable relationships
- **Object-relations**: Help maintain a 'nuclear self' (authentic self-representation)
- **Psychoanalysis**: Adaptation of patient to intrapsychic conflict.

Freudian ego defence mechanisms and associated mental states

The following is not an exhaustive list.

Unconscious mental processes designed to resolve conflict between instinctive needs (id), conscientious prohibitions (superego) and reality (ego)

- **acting out**: Expression of unconscious impulse to avoid the accompanying affect
- **denial**: Refusal to accept external reality (hysteria)
- **displacement**: Directing feelings towards a less important object/person (phobia)
- **distortion**: Reshaping reality to suit internal needs
- **intellectualisation**: Thinking rather than feeling
- **isolation**: Removal of affect from an idea (obsessive–compulsive disorder; OCD)
- **magical undoing**: Using superstitious rituals to neutralise conflict (OCD)
- **projection**: Attributing own unacknowledged feelings to others (hysteria, paranoia)
- **projective identification**: Attributing unacceptable personal characteristic to others and identifying with them (hysteria)
- **reaction formation**: Behaving/feeling contrary to unacceptable instinctual impulses (OCD)

- **repression**: Basic mechanism of unconsciously inhibiting an unacceptable thought/impulse
- **splitting**: Having fantasised positive and negative parts of a relationship with different individuals (paranoia)
- **sublimation**: Indirect expression of impulses without adverse consequences
- **turning against self**: Aggression to others directed against self (depression).

Properties of defence mechanisms (Freud)

According to Freud, defence mechanisms are:

- unconscious
- help manage instincts and affects
- dynamic and reversible
- mostly adaptive, not pathological.

Inferred purposes of ego defence mechanisms

The inferred purposes are:

- to maintain bearable limits on affect during life crises
- to restore psychological 'normality' by deflecting/postponing changes in biological drives
- to create a framework for managing critical life changes
- to handle unresolved conflicts with important others.

Chapter 7
Neuroscience

Anne Lingford-Hughes & Chris Fear

CONTENTS

Neuroscience

NEUROANATOMY

Cerebral hemispheres (Figure 7.1)

- Right and left cerebral hemispheres are separated by the sagittal or longitudinal fissure.
- The central sulcus (fissure of Rolando) divides each hemisphere into frontal (anteriorly) and parietal lobes.
- The lateral sulcus (Sylvian fissure) divides these lobes from the temporal lobe inferiorly.
- The occipital lobe is posterior to the parietal and temporal lobes.
- Hemispheres communicate through short and long tracts:
  - the cingulum is a long association tract

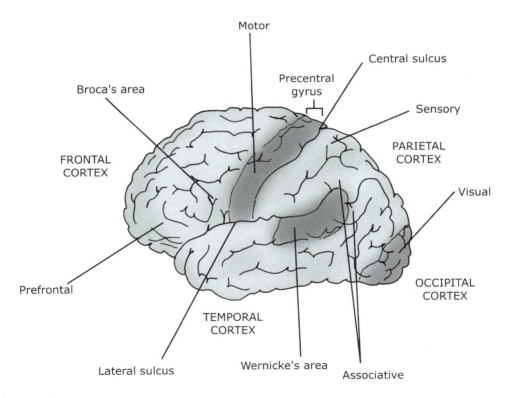

Figure 7.1

- o the commissural fibres connect homologous areas: corpus callosum (largest), anterior commissure, fornix.
- Internal capsule:
  - o is a projection tract between cortical/subcortical areas and the spinal column
  - o has the following components: anterior and posterior limbs, genu and sublentiform (retrolentiform)
  - o runs lateral to head of caudate nucleus, medial to lentiform nucleus and thalamus
  - o fans out superiorly into the corona radiata
  - o becomes the crus cerebri in the midbrain.
- Covering the brain are the meninges: pia, arachnoid and dura mater from innermost to outermost layer
  - o cerebrospinal fluid circulates in the subarachnoid space.
- In right-handed people dominance is usually contralateral to the dominant hand
  - o mediates language and speech
  - o right hemisphere is dominant in 10% of right-handed people
  - o 20% of left-handed people have right-hemisphere dominance, 64% have left-hemisphere dominance and 16% are bilaterally dominant.

Lobe functions

Frontal lobe

- **Prefrontal cortex**
  - o The dorsolateral prefrontal cortex is concerned with executive cognitive functions.
  - o Lesions impair working memory; organisation, planning and abstract thinking; and motor programming.
  - o **Dominant lobe lesions** impair verbal fluency.
  - o **Non-dominant lobe lesions** impair non-verbal fluency.
- **Primary and supplementary motor cortices, Broca's area, frontal eye fields**
- **Anterior cingulate cortex**
  - o is part of limbic system
  - o involved with attention and emotional processing.
- **Orbitofrontal cortex**
  - o is part of limbic system
  - o involves impulse control, processing reward value of stimuli and suppressing motor responses.
- Damage causes personality changes:
  - o disinhibition, decreased social awareness and control, inappropriate sexual behaviour
  - o loss of finer feelings, errors of judgement, lack of concern for others
  - o irritability, elevated mood, childish behaviour (*Witzelsucht*)
  - o lack of drive, impaired initiation, reduced abstraction, impaired concentration/attention
  - o inability to adapt
  - o perseveration of speech and movement, palilalia, decreased verbal fluency
  - o posterior lesions affect Broca's speech area (expressive dysphasia).

- Function can be tested by examining verbal fluency, proverbs and co-ordinated movements.

Occipital lobe

- Visual and visual accessory cortex
- Dominant hemisphere lesions produce:
  - alexia without agraphia
  - agnosia for colour and visual objects.
- Non-dominant hemisphere lesions produce:
  - visuospatial agnosia
  - prosopagnosia
  - image distortion (metamorphosia)
  - complex visual hallucinations.
- Occipital lobe syndrome produces:
  - contralateral homonymous hemianopia
  - scotomata
  - simultagnosia.

Parietal lobe

- This is involved in complex integration of recognition, visuospatial awareness and environmental appreciation.
- Parietal lobe syndrome presents with:
  - constructional apraxia
  - visuospatial agnosia
  - topographical disorientation (getting lost etc)
  - visual inattention
  - cortical sensory loss (items felt but not discriminated or interpreted fully).
- Dominant hemisphere lesions present with:
  - anterior – motor aphasia
  - posterior – sensory aphasia
  - agraphia with alexia, motor apraxia, bilateral tactile agnosia (plus visual agnosia if parieto-occipital area affected).
- Gerstmann's syndrome:
  - is associated with dominant parietal lobe lesions
  - produces dyscalculia, agraphia, finger agnosia, right–left disorientation.
- Non-dominant hemisphere lesions produce:
  - anosognosia
  - hemisomatognosia
  - dressing apraxia
  - prosopagnosia.

Temporal lobe

- A large and important area of the brain containing components of the limbic system. Its functions are involved with sensation, memory, personality, vision etc.

- Damage results in personality changes, visual field and sensory deficits.
- Dominant hemisphere lesions are generally more symptomatic.
- Sensory afferents
  - auditory
  - gustatory
  - olfactory
  - vestibular.
- Memory
  - bilateral medial temporal lesions result in profound amnesia
  - caused by infection, tumour, epilepsy and bilateral posterior cerebral artery occlusion
  - semantic and immediate memory preserved (digit span)
  - anterograde and retrograde memory impairment (memory for remote events may remain)
  - bilateral hippocampal lesions cause global amnesia
  - dominant lobe lesions produce problems with learning verbal material
  - non-dominant lobe lesions produce problems with learning non-verbal material.
- Personality
  - depersonalisation
  - emotional instability
  - aggression
  - antisocial behaviour
  - psychosis (eg temporal lobe epilepsy).
- Visual field
  - deep lesions of the optic radiation produce contralateral homonymous upper quadrantanopia.
- Dominant lobe lesions also produce
  - sensory aphasia
  - alexia and agraphia (posterior).
- Non-dominant lobe lesions also produce
  - hemisomatognosia
  - prosopagnosia
  - visuospatial problems.
- Wernicke's auditory association area
  - dominant superior temporal cortex
  - reduced verbal comprehension, reading and writing skills
  - receptive aphasia ('jargon aphasia').
- Kluver–Bucy syndrome
  - comprises bilateral ablation of the temporal lobes and destruction of uncus, amygdala and hippocampus
  - increased oral and sexual behaviour
  - placidity ('pet-like compliance')
  - loss of fear/anger with apathy
  - is associated with Alzheimer's and Pick's diseases, arteriosclerosis, tumours and herpes simplex encephalitis
  - is associated with visual agnosia, prosopagnosia, hypermetamorphosis (touching everything).

Limbic system

- Originally called the Papez circuit, comprising the hippocampus, anterior nucleus of thalamus, cingulate gyrus, mammillary bodies and their connections.
- Now extended to hippocampal formation, cingulate and subcallosal gyri, anterior nucleus of thalamus, amygdala, septal area and secondary olfactory areas, and nucleus accumbens.
- Controls memory and behavioural/emotional expression.
- Intralimbic and external pathways run via fimbria, alveus, fornix and mammillothalamic tracts (see Figure 7.2).
- Hippocampal formation
  - comprises the hippocampus, dentate and parahippocampal gyri, entorhinal cortex

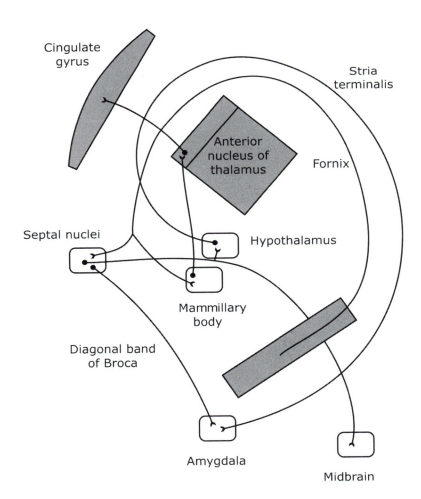

Figure 7.2

  - located in the medial wall of the temporal lobe, forming the floor of the inferior horn of the lateral ventricle
  - afferents from cingulate and dentate gyri, contralateral gyrus, septal area indusium griseum and diencephalon
  - efferent pathway via fornix (convergence of fimbria) to anterior nucleus of thalamus, then bifurcation and termination in mammillary bodies and septal nuclei; also to hypothalamus and tegmentum
  - reciprocal connections to rest of limbic system.
- Amygdala
  - contains nuclei involved in sensory and motor functions, emotional processing and associative learning
  - stimulation causes aggression, ablation causes placidity.
- Nucleus accumbens (in ventral striatum)
  - dopaminergic function
  - positive reinforcement and reward.

Basal ganglia

- Basal ganglia comprises corpus striatum (caudate nucleus and putamen), lentiform nucleus (globus pallidus and putamen), claustrum, amygdala
- afferent pathways run to caudate nucleus and putamen from all parts of the cortex projected topographically onto the globus pallidus
- efferents run to ventral nuclei of thalamus and brainstem
- reciprocal connection from thalamus to premotor cortex to monitor and modulate motor activity (Figure 7.3)
- reciprocal connection between striatum and substantia nigra (nigrostriatal and striatonigral pathways)
- dysfunction causes motor disorders: loss of automatic associated movement (gait, facial expression), rigidity, cog-wheeling, choreiform (fidgety) and athetoid (writhing) movements, hemiballismus and resting tremor, as in:
  - Huntington's chorea: Degeneration of the caudate nucleus (choreiform movements, depression, psychosis, dementia)
  - Parkinson's disease: Depleted dopamine as a result of loss of neurones in substantia nigra
  - parkinsonism: Drug-induced due to D_2 blockade in striatum
  - Wilson's disease: Copper deposition in basal ganglia (congenital, Kayser–Fleischer rings around the cornea).

Cerebellum

Cerebellum

- is involved in co-ordination of movement, maintenance of muscle tone and balance; also cognition
- comprises two hemispheres and midline vermis.

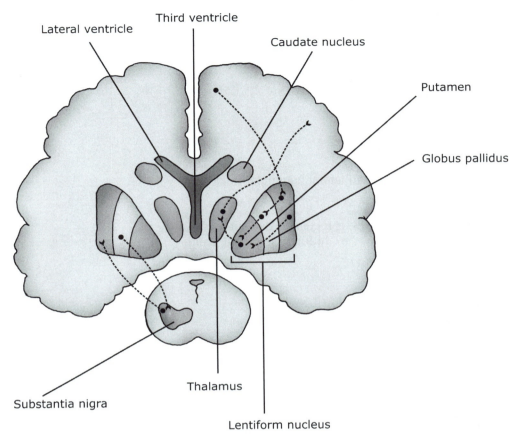

Figure 7.3 Connections of the basal ganglia

Archicerebellum	Palaeocerebellum	Neocerebellum
• interior part of the vermis • communicates with the vestibular nuclei • lesions cause broad-based gait	• anterior lobe • afferents from spinocerebellar tracts • efferents to vestibular and reticular nuclei • lesions affect extensor tone	• posterior lobe and tonsil • afferents from cortical relays in pontine nuclei • concerned with skilled voluntary movement

Table 7.1 Cerebellar components

Cerebellar dysfunction causes:

- truncal ataxia and dysequilibrium
- reduced muscle tone, fatigue and reduced reflexes

- difficulty with rapid repetitive movements (dysdiadokinesia) and finger–nose testing (dysmetria)
- intention tremor
- slurred, jerky and explosive speech
- nystagmus on fixation to object
- wide-based ataxic gait.

Diencephalon

Epithalamus

- comprises the medial and lateral habenular nuclei
- the pineal gland
- the striae medullaris
- controls melatonin synthesis regulated by light
- modulates circadian rhythm through the pineal gland.

Hypothalamus, see page 141

Thalamus

- comprises a large collection of nuclei
- is the relay for sensory and motor information.

Nucleus	Connections	Function
Anterior	Limbic system to thalamus	Part of limbic system
Dorsomedial	Hypothalamus and prefrontal cortex	Emotion (anxiety/dread)
Dorsolateral	Cingulate gyrus and parietal association cortex	
Lateral posterior	Occitipal to pariental cortex	Higher-order sensory perceptions
Ventral anterior	Basal ganglia/cerebellar nuclei	Updating and fine
Ventral lateral	to pre/motor cortex	adjustment of motor mechanisms
Ventral posterior lateral	Ascending sensory inputs	General sensory input
Ventral posterior medial	to primary sensory cortex	processing
Medial geniculate body	Relay of auditory tracts from lateral lemniscus to primary auditory area	Auditory pathways
Lateral geniculate body	Optic tract to primary visual area	Visual pathways
Pulvinar	Occipital/temporal/parietal cortex to visual cortex	Visual processing
Intralaminar	Midbrain, basal ganglia, motor, prefrontal cortex	Reticular system

Table 7.2 Thalamic relays

Brainstem

The continuation of the spinal cord above the foramen magnum, comprising medulla, pons and midbrain. It passes into the diencephalon.

	Medulla oblongata	Pons	Midbrain
Tracts	Decussation of pyramids/corticospinal Rubro/vestibulo/tecto spinal Decussation of medial lemniscus (gracilis and cuneatus to thalamus)	Corticobulbar Rubrospinal Medial longitudinal fasciculus	Medial longitudinal fasciculus Medial and lateral lemnisci Crus cerebri Inferior colliculus (auditory) Superior colliculus (visual)
Nuclei	Solitary Anterior and dorsal cochlear Medial/lateral/inferior/superior vestibular Gracilis Cuneate Inferior olivary (projects to cerebellum)	Trapezoid body Superior olivary (auditory) Lateral/superior vestibular Locus coeruleus (noradrenaline)	Substantia nigra Red nucleus (relay from cerebellum and cerebral cortex to spinal cord and cranial nerve nuclei) Raphe nuclei (serotonin)
Cranial nerve nuclei and tracts	Medial longitudinal fasciculus (III, IV, VI) – eye movements Nuclei of XII and spinal root of XI Spinal root of V Dorsal motor nucleus of X Nucleus ambiguus (motor root of IX, X, XI)	Spinal trigeminal nucleus and tract (V) Nuclei of V, VI, VII	Edinger–Westphal nucleus of III Mesencephalic of V Nucleus of VI
Other	Reticular formation Fourth ventricle Inferior cerebellar peduncle	Reticular formation Floor of fourth ventricle Middle/superior cerebellar peduncles	Reticular formation Cerebral aqueduct Periaqueductal grey matter Superior cerebellar peduncle

Numbers indicate cranial nerves.

Table 7.3 Brainstem tracts and nuclei

Major white matter pathways

- Anterior commissure
  - is part of the lamina terminalis
  - connects homologous areas of cortex
  - joins amygdala, hippocampus and parahippocampal gyrus in the two hemispheres.
- Arcuate bundle
  - association fibres connecting Broca's and Wernicke's speech areas.
- Corpus callosum
  - connects homologous cortex
  - divided into body, genu, rostrum and splenium.
- Fornix
  - main hippocampal subcortical efferent tract
  - connects the anterior hypothalamus, anterior nucleus of the thalamus, habenular nucleus, lateral preoptic area, mammillary body, septal nucleus and tegmentum.
- Papez circuit (see page 119).

Blood supply

- Arterial blood supply is from the internal carotid artery and vertebral arteries via various branches (Figure 7.4)
- The Circle of Willis is a circuit of arteries comprising the internal carotid, anterior, middle and posterior cerebral, and anterior and posterior communicating arteries. It regulates blood flow.
- Venous drainage is via the cavernous sinus in the medial cranial fossa.

Ventricular system and cerebrospinal fluid

- See Figure 7.5.
- Cerebrospinal fluid is formed in the choroid plexus of the lateral, third and fourth ventricles (about 300 ml/day).
- Non-communicating hydrocephalus
  - as a result of cerebrospinal fluid obstruction in the third or fourth ventricle or communicating pathways
  - raised intracranial pressure
  - nausea/vomiting, headache (worse on lying), bradycardia, hypertension, papilloedema.
- Communicating (normal pressure) hydrocephalus
  - cerebrospinal fluid obstruction in the subarachnoid space
  - intracranial pressure not raised
  - ataxia, urinary incontinence, nystagmus, cognitive impairment.

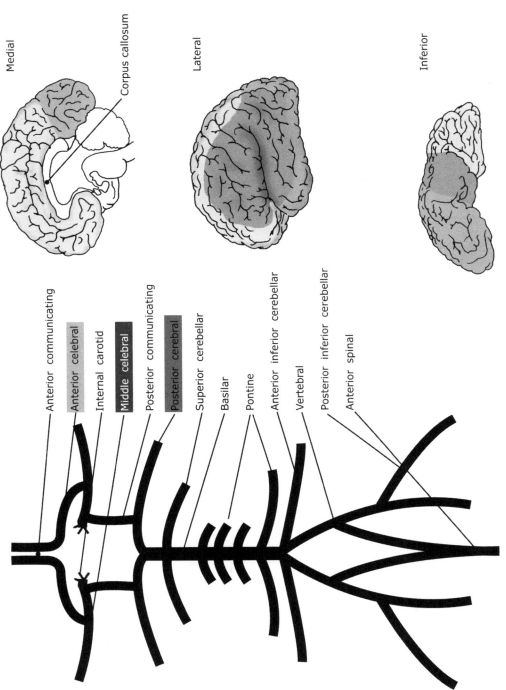

Figure 7.4

126

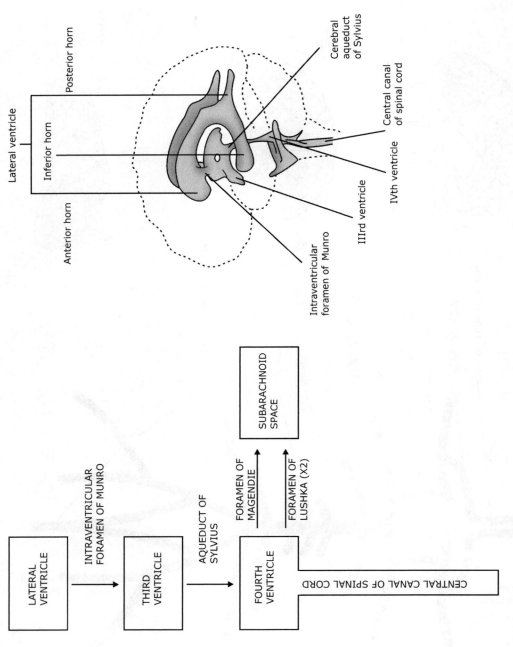

Figure 7.5

PERIPHERAL NERVOUS SYSTEM

Sensory system

- Peripheral sensory receptors comprise the following:
  - stretching, proprioception, tone: Golgi organs (tendon), annulospiral and flower-spray (muscle)
  - touch, temperature, pain: unencapsulated 'free', or Merkel's discs
  - pressure, vibration: Pacinian corpuscles
  - two-point discrimination: Meissner corpuscles.
- Myelinated fibres can be:
  - $A\beta$ (touch)
  - $A\delta$ (touch and pain).
- Unmyelinated C fibres carry temperature information.
- Signal is carried in the sensory nerve to the dorsal root ganglion and thence to nuclei specific to the modality.
- It is relayed to the thalamus.
- Projection to the post-central gyrus (parietal cortex) is organised according to area of the body (homunculus).

Motor system

- Voluntary movement is initiated in the primary motor cortex of the frontal lobe.
- Fibres from the pyramidal cells pass through the internal capsule, decussate in the midbrain and descend as the corticospinal tracts.
- Corticospinal tracts end in the anterior horn cells and interneurones.
- The signal is modulated and co-ordinated through extrapyramidal tracts to the basal ganglia (putamen) and tracts to the cerebellum.
- Upper motor neurone
  - projection is onto the anterior horn cell (ie proximal)
  - lesions cause hypertonia, spastic paralysis, hyper-reflexia and Babinski sign (eg cerebral palsy).
- Lower motor neurone
  - projection is from the anterior horn cell to the end muscle (ie distal)
  - lesions cause hypotonia, flaccid paralysis, hyporeflexia, muscle wasting, fasciculation, fibrillation (eg peripheral nerve compression).
- Corticospinal tracts tend to be excitatory and extrapyramidal tracts tend to be inhibitory of voluntary movement.

Autonomic system

- It innervates and regulates smooth and cardiac muscle and glands.
- Its actions are integrated through the central nervous system, especially hypothalamus and limbic system.
- Most of its actions are automatic.

- The sympathetic and parasympathetic systems generally act in opposition.
- It acts through two-neurone relays.
- Preganglionic fibres from the spinal cord or brainstem terminate in a peripheral ganglion.
- Postganglionic neurones innervate the end-organ.

	Sympathetic	Parasympathetic
Preganglionic neurone	Shorter	Longer
Postganglionic neurone	Longer	Shorter
Ganglia located	Close to CNS	Close to end-organ
Postganglionic neurotransmitter	Noradrenaline	Acetylcholine
Preganglionic neurotransmitter	Acetylcholine	Acetylcholine
Site of origin	Interomediolateral grey column of T1–L2	Intermediate grey matter of S2–4 Brainstem nuclei: Edinger–Westphal (III) Inferior and superior salivary (VII and IX) Dorsal motor of the vagus (X)

CNS, central nervous system; roman numerals indicate cranial nerves.

Table 7.4 Para/sympathetic neurones

The **sympathetic function** is that of 'fight or flight' and results in:

- dilated pupils
- increased cardiac and respiratory output
- peripheral vasoconstriction, sweating and piloerection
- reduced gastro-intestinal activity
- contracted sphincters
- diversion of blood from splanchnic bed.

The **sympathetic system** is divided as follows:

- Superior cervical ganglia
  - provides sympathetic innervation to the head via fibres running with the carotid arteries from the carotid plexus
  - supplies dilator muscles of the iris, lacrimal and salivary glands, levator palpebrae and erector pili muscles and small blood vessels
  - forms cardiac nerve, and sympathetic fibres with cranial nerves IX, X and XI and fibres to cardiac nerve and plexus.
- Medial cervical ganglion
  - provides innervation to thyroid, oesophagus and trachea.

- Inferior (stellate) ganglion
  - contributes to the cardiac plexus.
- Cardiac plexus
  - supplies thoracic organs
  - causes bronchial smooth muscle relaxation and inhibition of secretions.
- Mesenteric ganglia
  - supply the gut and associated organs.

The **parasympathetic system** is divided as follows:

- fibres from the Edinger–Westphal nucleus run with the IIIrd cranial nerve to the ciliary ganglion
  - these produce constriction of ciliary muscle and sphincter, causing pupillary constriction.
- innervation of the salivary glands via the pterygopalatine and submandibular ganglia
- fibres with the vagus nerve run to the heart, lungs, gut and associated organs causing:
  - reduced heart and respiratory rate and secretion
  - decreased gut motility and secretions.
- sacral component runs to the large bowel, bladder and genitalia.

Cranial nerves

There are 12 pairs of cranial nerves with both somatic and autonomic components. They are sensory, motor, or both (see Table 7.5).

	Skull foramen exited	Somatic-sensory component	Somatic-motor component	Autonomic-sensory component	Autonomic-motor component
I Olfactory	Cribriform plates of ethmoid bone	Mucous membrane of nasal cavity – olfactory bulb – hippocampus/ hypothalamus – 1°& 2° olfactory areas **Loss of sense of smell**	–	–	–
II Optic	Optic canal	Retinal ganglion cells – visual cortex via optic radiation and lateral geniculate body **Anterior to optic chiasma, loss of vision in that eye. Posterior to optic chiasma, hemianopia. Myers loop, quadrantanopia**	–	–	–
III Oculomotor	Superior orbital fissure	–	Oculomotor nuclei (midbrain) to inferior, superior and medial rectus, inferior oblique and levator palpebrae orbital muscles. Nuclei of III, IV and VI linked via medial longitudinal fasciculus. **Ptosis & deviation of eye downwards and outwards (+ dilated pupil of parasympathetic involved)**	–	Parasympathetic motor tract from Edinger-Westphal nucleus (preganglionic) – ciliary ganglion (postganglionic) – ciliary and sphincter pupillae muscles of iris (pupil constriction/ accommodation) **Argyll-Robertson pupils (neurosyphilis) – small, unequal, irregular, unreactive to light but accommodation intact***

Nerve	Exit	Motor	Sensory	Parasympathetic	Clinical
IV Trochlear	Superior orbital fissure	Superior oblique muscle of the orbit **Unable to move eye downwards and outwards**	—	—	—
V Trigeminal 1st (ophthalmic)	Superior orbital fissure		Trigeminal ganglion: Skin of head and scalp, corneal reflex (nasociliary branch)	Sympathetic and parasympathetic fibres carried in all divisions. No distinct parasympathetic nucleus.	—
2nd (maxillary)	Foramen rotundum		Skin of cheek		
3rd (mandibular)	Foramen ovale	Motor nucleus – muscles of mastication, pharynx and mouth	Skin of face, buccal cavity, external ear, lower teeth and lip **Loss of jaw jerk** Central fibres to: • Spinal trigeminal nucleus & tract (facial touch, temperature, pain) • Sensory nucleus (touch, position, two-point discrimination) • Mesencephalic nucleus of V (proprioception of muscles of mastication)		
VI Abducens	Superior orbital fissure	Lateral rectus muscle of the orbit **Cross-eyes** • commonly affected in Wernicke–Korsakoff syndrome causing Nystag	—	—	—

Table 7.5 continued overleaf

	Skull foramen exited	Somatic-sensory component	Somatic-motor component	Autonomic-sensory component	Autonomic-motor component
VII Facial	Internal auditory meatus	Geniculate ganglion – spinal trigeminal nucleus (touch pain and temperature from part of external ear)	Buccal, cervical, mandibular, temporal and zygomatic branches to muscles of facial expression, posterior belly of digastric and stylohyoid. Stapedius in ear. **Peripheral – ipsilateral paralysis or weakness (Bell's palsy)** **Central – contralateral weakness of lower face only (crossed and uncrossed fibres to forehead)**	Nucleus solitarius via petrosal nerve (taste to anterior $^{2}/_{3}$ of tongue)	Superior salivary nucleus via petrosal nerves to nasal, palatine, parotid, sublingual and sub-mandibular glands. Lacrimal nucleus to lacrimal gland.
VIII Vestibulocochlear	Internal auditory meatus	Cochlea – inferior & superior cochlear nuclei – superior olivary nucleus – lateral lemniscus – inferior colliculus. Then auditory radiation (internal capsule) to auditory cortex in Heschl's gyrus (superior temporal). Fibres cross within auditory cortex. **Peripheral nerve – unilateral deafness** **Auditory tracts – minimal deafness** Vestibular – cerebellum & nuclei of oculomotor nerves (balance)	–	–	–

	Foramen				
IX Glossopharyngeal	Jugular foramen	External auditory meatus and back of ear – spinal trigeminal nucleus	Nucleus ambiguous – stylopharyngeus and superior constrictor muscles of pharynx **Ipsilateral paralysis and difficulties swallowing**	Petrosal nerve to nucleus solitarius • Pain and poorly-localised sensation from palate tonsils and pharynx • Carotid sinus (pressure) • Carotid body (H+, CO_2 & O_2) • Taste to posterior $1/3$ of tongue	Parasympathetic from inferior salivatory nucleus to parotid gland (watery, amylase-rich secretions)
X Vagus	Jugular foramen	Exterior ear – spinal trigeminal nucleus	Nucleus ambiguous to muscles of pharynx and palate. Recurrent laryngeal nerve to laryngeal muscles. *Unilateral – partially obstructed airway & dysphonia* *Bilateral – closed vocal cords, narrowed airway*	Parasympathetic from whole GI tract, including liver, pancreas & gall bladder to cardiac, oesophageal, pharyngeal and pulmonary plexi. Superior laryngeal nerves from larynx to nucleus solitarius.	Postganglionic parasympathetic from cardiac, gastric, pulmonary and intestinal walls (smooth muscle contraction, decreased heart rate, secretion in all glands)
XI Accessory Cranial root	Jugular foramen	Nucleus ambiguous to intrinsic muscles of soft palate	–	–	–
Spinal roots	Foramen magnum & jugular foramen	Anterior horn motor neurones of C1-5/6 to sternocleidomastoid & trapezius **Head cannot be turned to affected side and ipsilateral shoulder drop**			

Table 7.5 continued overleaf

133

	Skull foramen exited	Somatic-sensory component	Somatic-motor component	Autonomic-sensory component	Autonomic-motor component
XII Hypoglossal	Hypoglossal canal	Intrinsic & extrinsic muscles of the tongue **Peripheral – ipsilateral deviation of the tongue on protrusion** **Central – contralateral deviation of the tongue on protrusion**	–	–	–

*+Horner's syndrome (cervical sympathetic lesion) – ptosis, anhydrosis, enophthalmos & constricted pupil (unopposed parasympathetic action)

Text in bold refers to the effects of damage to these nerves or parts of them.

Table 7.5 Cranial nerves: their anatomy, functions and lesions

Anoxia (chronic)

CO_2 retention

Disc infiltration

Encephalitis

Hypertension (accelerated)

Intracranial mass

Optic neuritis

Optic neuropathy

Retinal vein obstruction

Subarachnoid haemorrhage

Table 7.6 Ten causes of papilloedema

Spinal cord

The spinal cord comprises both ascending and descending tracts.

The **ascending tracts** (see Figure 7.6) carry sensory pathways from the periphery to the brain. Their functions are:

- Proprioception, tactile discrimination and vibration
  - fasciculus gracilis
  - fasciculus cuneatus
  - posterior part of cord
  - fibres lie sacral (medial) to cervical (lateral), ipsilateral to synapse with nuclei in the medulla, tracts then cross and ascend as the medial lemniscus
  - projections terminate in the thalamus (ventral posterior nucleus) and thence to parietal cortex via the internal capsule.
- Pain, temperature, light touch
  - lateral spinothalamic tract carries pain and temperature
  - anterior spinothalamic tract carries light touch
  - fibres ascend two segments of spinal cord before crossing
  - spinothalamic tracts terminate in the thalamus (ventral posterior nucleus) and project to parietal cortex.
- Brown–Sequard syndrome
  - transection of one-half of the spinal cord
  - loss of ipsilateral two-point discrimination and proprioception
  - loss of contralateral pain and temperature sensation.
- Muscle and tendon function is relayed ipsilaterally in the spinocerebellar tract.

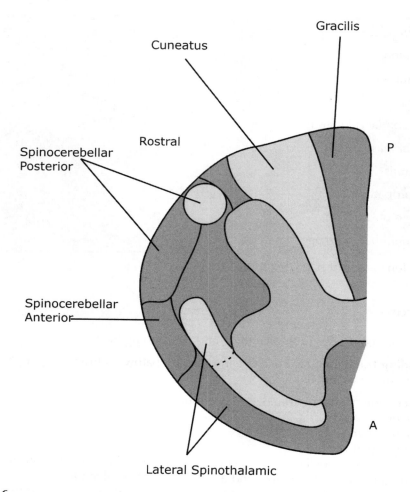

Figure 7.6

The **descending tracts** (see Figure 7.7) comprise the following:

- Pyramidal (corticospinal) tracts
  - mediation of voluntary movement
  - lateral corticospinal tract is present throughout the entire cord
  - anterior corticospinal tract is ipsilateral and terminates at the level of the thoracic vertebrae.
- Extrapyramidal tracts
  - vestibulospinal tract (vestibular nuclei) controls extensor muscles
  - rubrospinal tract (red nucleus) controls flexor muscles; it ends in the thoracic area
  - tectospinal tract (superior colliculus) visual and auditory postural reflexes.
- Reticulospinal tract (brainstem)

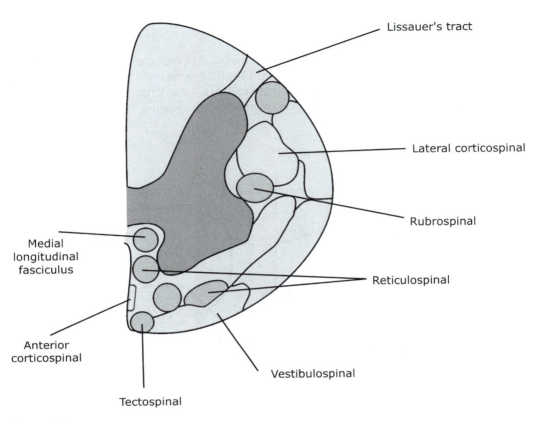

Figure 7.7

PHYSIOLOGY, EMBRYOLOGY AND HISTOLOGY

	Cerebral cortex (six layers)	Cerebellar cortex (three layers)
Surface		
I	Molecular (plexiform) layer	Molecular (basket and stellate cells)
II	External granular layer	Purkinje layer
III	External pyramidal layer	Granular layer (granule and Golgi cells)
IV	Internal granular layer	
V	Internal pyramidal layer	
VI	Polymorphic layer	
Deep		

Table 7.7 Cell layers of the cerebral cortex and cerebellum

Neurone and synapse

Two neurones meet at a **synapse**, where their surface membranes are close but do not touch, leaving a **synaptic cleft** between them. Electrical signals are transmitted across the synapse by means of **chemical neurotransmitters** (see Chapter 8). In **electrical synapses**, the membranes connect via **gap junctions**, allowing faster direct electrical transmission.

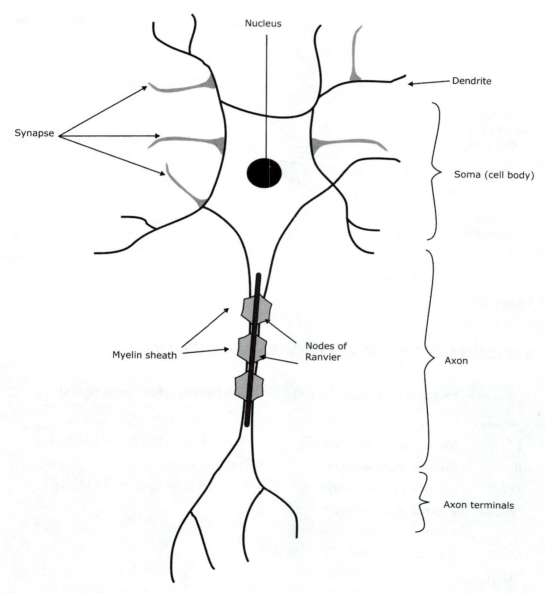

Figure 7.8 Diagrammatic representation of a neurone

At rest, the **membrane potential** is about -70 to -80 mV, maintained by the sodium pump, powered by adenosine triphosphate (ATP) to pump sodium ions out of the cell in exchange for potassium ions. The resting membrane is freely permeable to chloride ions and is relatively impermeable to organic anions.

Stimulation → **depolarisation** (membrane potential ↑) → action potential

or

Stimulation → **hyperpolarisation** (membrane potential ↓) → no action potential

The **action potential** is all-or-nothing. An influx of sodium ions and outflow of potassium ions restore the membrane potential via the sodium pump. This is followed by the **absolute refractory period** (no further action potential is possible) and then the **relative refractory period** (membrane hyperpolarised). The **saltatory motion** is the skipping from between Nodes of Ranvier in myelinated neurones.

Unmyelinated transmission is slower but increases with the diameter of the neurone.

Glia

In order of size the glial cells are:

- Astrocytes
  - are multipolar, occurring in both white and grey matter
  - provide structural, metabolic and phagocytic support to neurones
  - the 'end feet' terminations of their processes on capillaries form the blood–brain barrier
  - other process terminations form the pia–glial membrane.
- Oligodendrocytes
  - form myelin sheaths.
- Microglia
  - control phagocytosis
  - proliferate in response to injury.
- Ependyma (three types, line cavities and maintain the flow of cerebrospinal fluid)
  - choroidal epithelial cells: cover the choroid plexus
  - ependymocytes: line the ventricles and central canal of the spinal cord
  - tanycytes: line the floor of the third ventricle.

Meninges

The meninges are the three layers of connective tissue covering the brain. They can be divided into:

- Dura mater
  - is the thickest
  - lines the skull
  - forms the tentorium cerebelli through a fold between the cerebellum and occipital lobe.

- Arachnoid mater
  - is thin, middle layer
  - the subarachnoid space contains the cerebrospinal fluid.
- Pia mater
  - covers the brain surface.

Embryology

At week 4 of gestation, three vesicles form in the cranial end of the neural tube. These are:

- the **prosencephalon**
  - forms the forebrain
  - divides into the **telencephalon** and **diencephalon**
  - the telencephalon forms cerebral hemispheres, and the rhinencephalon (olfactory mucosa, tracts and bulbs) and corpus striatum.
- the **mesencephalon**
  - forms the midbrain.
- the **rhombencephalon** divides into
  - **metencephalon** (cerebellum and pons)
  - **myelencephalon** (medulla oblongata and spinal cord).

NEUROPATHOLOGICAL

Response to injury

Following damage to an axon, changes occur in the cell body (axon reaction) and the nerve fibre distally (Wallerian degeneration).

- **Axon reaction**
  - varies in different cell types and animal species (absent in spinal cord of rats and rabbits)
  - traumatic degeneration adjacent to lesion
  - gradual chromatolysis (dispersion of Nissl material)
  - cellular oedema
  - migration of nucleus.
- **Wallerian degeneration**
  - axon distal to the injury swells and breaks into fragments over five days
  - regeneration is possible through close approximation of the severed ends.
- **Simple atrophy** occurs in neurodegenerative diseases (dementia, motor neuron disease).
- **Ischaemic cell change**
  - shrinkage
  - intense eosinophilia
  - nucleus fragments
  - Nissl substance disappears.

- Transneuronal (trans-synaptic) atrophy occurs in neurons whose principle afferent fibres have been cut.

Specific disease processes

See Chapters 12, 16, 19, 22, and 23.

NEUROENDOCRINE SYSTEM

The neuroendocrine system comprises the hypothalamus and the pituitary gland.

- There are various nuclei concerned with endocrine control and neurosecretion.
- They regulate the autonomic function, body temperature, biological clock, thirst, hunger and sexual function.
- They are involved, with the limbic system, in mediating emotion, fear, anger, pleasure and reward.
- They control hormone release from the anterior pituitary.

Nuclear region	Subnuclei	Function
Arcuate		Neurosecretory fibres to anterior pituitary
Mammillary	Mammillary bodies	Integration of information from limbic system via fornix Memory (Korsakoff's psychosis)
Posterior		Sympathetic responses
Preoptic		Production of gonadotrophins
Tuberal	Ventromedial Dorsomedial	Control of hunger (stimulation produces satiation) Emotion (ablation produces rage)
Supraoptic	Anterior hypothalamic	Parasympathetic (bradycardia, gastrointestinal secretion)
	Suprachiasmatic	Secretes antidiuretic hormone (ADH)
	Supraoptic and paraventricular	Secretion of ADH and oxytocin

Table 7.8 Hypothalamic nuclei

Pituitary

A small gland situated below the cerebrum in the sella turcica. Details of its function are given in Table 7.9.

Releasing factor	Hormone	Function
Corticotrophin (CRF)	Adrenocorticotrophic hormone (ACTH)	Control of cortisol release from the adrenal cortex
Gonadotrophin-releasing factor	Follicle-stimulating hormone (FSH) Luteinising hormone (LH)	Growth of ovarian follicles; spermatogenesis Ovulation/production of corpus luteum; stimulation of interstitial cells of testis
Growth-hormone-releasing hormone (GHRH) Growth-hormone-inhibiting factor (somatostatin)	Somatotrophin, growth hormone (GH)	Growth of skeleton, muscles, connective tissue and viscera; also levels of glucose, phosphate and fatty acids
Melatonin-stimulating hormone release-inhibiting factor (MSHRIF)	Melatonin-stimulating hormone (MSH)	Stimulate release of melatonin from the pineal gland
Prolactin-releasing factor Prolactin-inhibiting factor (dopamine)	Prolactin	Stimulate progesterone secretion from corpus luteum; promote breast milk secretion
Thyrotrophin	Thyroid-stimulating hormone (TSH)	Stimulate release of thyroxine and triiodothyronine

Table 7.9 Release of hormones from the anterior pituitary

Arousal and sleep

See Chapter 16.

EEG

See Chapter 16.

NEUROCHEMISTRY

See Chapter 8.

Chapter 8

Psychopharmacology

Anne Lingford-Hughes and Jan Melichar

CONTENTS

Psychopharmacology

PHARMACOKINETICS

Pharmacokinetics describes the mechanisms involved in getting a drug to and from its site of action.

Processes determining the blood levels of a drug and explaining the variability between different people are:

- absorption
- distribution
- metabolism
- excretion.

Common	Uncommon
oral	intra-arterial
intramuscular	subcutaneous
intravenous	topical
rectal	nasal
	inhalation

Table 8.1 Routes of administration for psychotropic drugs

Simple pharmacokinetic calculations and terms

- **First-order kinetics**
  - applies to most drugs
  - rate of elimination is dependent on amount of drug present
  - amount of drug eliminated in each half-life (see below) differs, eg 100 to 50 to 25 to 12.5 etc.
- **Zero-order kinetics**
  - rate is independent of amount of drug present
  - examples are fixed intravenous infusions, absorption from depot, phenytoin when concentration saturates its metabolising enzymes
  - there is no fixed half-life.
- **Half-life ($t_{1/2}$)**
  - time taken for a drug concentration to fall to one-half of its value
  - only applies to drugs with first-order kinetics

- ○ guides dosage regimens, drugs with a $t_{1/2}$ of about 24 h need only be given once daily
- ○ 90% of drug is eliminated after four times the $t_{1/2}$
- ○ 'steady state' is achieved in approximately five times the $t_{1/2}$
- ○ drugs with $t_{1/2}$ more than 1–2 days can accumulate or only require alternate day administration (eg fluoxetine).
- **Bioavailability**
  - ○ describes the fraction of the administered drug that reaches the systemic blood without being metabolised
  - ○ low bioavailability usually means high first-pass metabolism
  - ○ bioavailability (F) =[(area under oral concentration/time curve) / (area under intravenous concentration/time curve)].
- **Steady state**
  - ○ the amount of drug eliminated from the body in a single dose interval is the same as the amount being administered
  - ○ can be reached sooner if a loading dose is given.
- **Volume of distribution** (V_d)
  - ○ $V_d = D / C$ (where D = mass of drug in body at time t, C = plasma concentration of the drug at time t)
  - ○ no anatomical or physiological representation, compartments where drug can 'go' include extracellular and intracellular water, plasma and tissue-bound
  - ○ drugs with high tissue-binding that are lipid soluble with low protein-binding have large V_d
  - ○ a low V_d is seen with high levels of protein-binding and low lipophilicity and tissue-binding
  - ○ psychotropic drugs tend to have large V_d.
- **Therapeutic index**
  - ○ relative measure of a drug's toxicity or safety
  - ○ ratio of toxic dose to therapeutic dose.
- **Monitoring plasma levels**
  - ○ monitoring is required for drugs with a therapeutic window, where higher doses can have adverse affects. Most commonly performed for lithium (12 h after last dose), due to its low therapeutic index
  - ○ most anticonvulsants require monitoring: phenytoin has an unpredictable relationship between dose and plasma concentration because of wide variability between individuals' pharmacokinetics
  - ○ many psychotropic drugs have pharmacologically active metabolites, hence measuring the parent compound's plasma levels will not be therapeutically informative
  - ○ nortriptyline is the only antidepressant which shows a relationship between plasma levels and therapeutic response
  - ○ plasma levels are also useful to assess compliance

Absorption

Orally administered drugs cross the gut wall by:

- **Passive diffusion** (down a concentration gradient): this is the most common mechanism and is dependent upon:
  - **Formulation**: the enteric coating slows down the rate of disintegration, particle size, diluents (eg lactose), binding agents (eg syrups), lubricants (eg talc), and disintegrating agents (eg starch) all have an effect.
  - **Solubility**: particle size, ambient pH (acidic stomach, alkaline small gut), and drug pK_a (derived from Henderson–Hasselbach equation: when pH $= pK_a$, then 50% of the drug is ionised) all affect solubility.
  - Most drugs are either weak acids (barbiturates) or weak bases (tricyclic antidepressants, most psychotropic drugs).
  - To be absorbed by passive diffusion, a drug must be un-ionised since it is more lipid soluble (lipophilic).
  - In the acidic pH of the stomach, basic drugs will be largely ionised and hence will not be absorbed until they reach the alkaline small bowel where they become un-ionised.
- **Active transport** (ie against a concentration gradient).
- **Pore filtration.**
- **Pinocytosis**.

Oral administration

- **Compliance**:
  - is the drug taken correctly?
  - is an alternative formulation or delivery route (eg patch, liquid) more acceptable?
- **Absorption** occurs primarily in the small bowel. Many sustained-release drugs are absorbed from the large bowel.
- **Influences** on oral administration include:
  - gastric emptying (delay by anticholinergic activity, eg tricyclic antidepressants (TCAs), monoamine oxidase inhibitors (MAOIs), opiates)
  - gastric pH
  - intestinal motility
  - food – absorption is greatest from an empty stomach, but food increases the absorption of diazepam
  - intestinal flora/wall enzymes can metabolise drugs (eg tyramine by MAO)
  - blood flow.
- All drugs absorbed from the gut (except those administered by sublingual, buccal, or rectal routes) undergo extensive metabolism in the liver, ie 'the first-pass metabolism' before passing into the systemic circulation.

Rectal administration

- overcomes swallowing problems, or 'unco-operative' patients
- has a minimal first-pass metabolism (absorbed directly into systemic circulation)

- there is no acidic gastric environment
- frequent use can be an irritant
- low acceptability in UK.

Intramuscular administration

- is useful in an emergency (eg acute disturbance, sedation, anticholinergics for acute dystonia) or for maintenance (eg depot)
- avoids first-pass metabolism
- influencing factors are:
  - **Solubility**: lipid-soluble drugs are rapidly absorbed and those with low molecular weight.
  - **Rate of absorption**: increases with increased blood flow (exercise, struggling), less with decreased blood flow (eg heart failure).
  - **Formulation**: a fatty ester added to depot slowly hydrolyses, thus releasing the active drug.
  - **Precipitation**: can crystallise (eg diazepam), onset may be slower than oral.

Intravenous administration

- Suitable for emergency as enters systemic circulation rapidly with no metabolism.
- Dose can be titrated, rapid administration can give dangerously high levels.
- Risks of injection include: sepsis, thrombosis, embolism, extra-venous injection into tissue can cause necrosis, or into an artery can cause spasm and levels that are too high.

Distribution

Distribution describes the location of a drug within the body. Some drugs are confined to body fluids, others accumulate within particular tissues.

- Blood-flow-dependent distribution:
  - Protein binding (albumin, globulins, glycoproteins) occurs.
  - Only the 'free', unbound fraction can be 'active' (ie drug can bind to receptors, pass across blood–brain barrier, be metabolised, or excreted).
  - Changes in protein binding can have profound effects on drug availability.
  - 95–99% protein-bound include diazepam, chlorpromazine, amitriptyline, imipramine.
  - 90–95% protein-bound include phenytoin, valproate, clomipramine.
  - Drugs can displace each other from protein-binding, leading to increased 'free' levels (this is an underlying mechanism of 'drug interactions'). Clinically in psychiatry, such an increase is rarely important as the volume of distribution (see above) is large for most psychotropic drugs and excess free drug is widely distributed and metabolised. Toxicity is highly unlikely.
  - Drug assays measure total (bound and free) amount of drug.
- Crossing the capillary endothelium:
  - This barrier is highly permeable.
  - Lipophilic/lipid-soluble drugs cross rapidly.

- Blood–brain barrier:
  - Not as permeable as above.
  - Lipophilic/lipid-soluble drugs cross, ie free, non-protein-bound ionised drugs (eg highly acidic or basic) cross slowly, if at all.
  - There is active transport for a few drugs such as levadopa.
  - Movement is by diffusion for small molecules such as lithium.

Metabolism

- Metabolism aims to produce increasing polar compounds for renal excretion.
- The liver is the main site, others include gut, kidney, skin and lung.
- **First-pass metabolism**: the drug is absorbed from the gut into the portal circulation and metabolised in the liver before reaching the systemic circulation.
- Metabolism can result in both inactive and active compounds.
- Differential rates account for most of the variability seen in blood drug levels and therapeutic dosage.

Phase 1	Drug metabolised by enzymes (oxidation (most common), hydroxylation, dealkylation, reduction, demethylation, acetylation, methylation). Active metabolites undergo the same processes to produce further metabolite
Phase 2	Metabolite undergoes glucuronidation or sulphation, producing a water-soluble conjugate for excretion (kidney or entero-hepatic system). Compound now inactive

Table 8.2 Hepatic transformation

Cytochrome P450 system

There are about 30 oxidative isoenzymes; they are the key enzymes involved in metabolism.

- CYP 2D6 metabolises desipramine, nortriptyline, clomipramine, risperidone, paroxetine, fluoxetine, and phenothiazine antipsychotics.
- CYP 1A2 is inhibited by fluvoxamine, induced by cigarette smoking, metabolism olanzapine and clozapine.
- CYP 2C is inhibited by fluvoxamine, fluoxetine, metabolism.
- Selective serotonin reuptake inhibitors (SSRIs) commonly inhibit: CYP 1A2 (fluvoxamine), CYP 2D6 (fluoxetine, paroxetine), CYP 2C (fluoxetine, fluvoxamine), CYP 3A4 (fluvoxamine, nefazodone).
- Sertraline and citalopram have the least effects on CYP.

The system is under genetic control, eg

- Hydroxylation (eg phenytoin metabolism)
  - there are poor and extensive metabolisers
  - inheritance is autosomal dominant
  - 8% of Whites, ethnic variability.

- Acetylation (MAOIs, eg phenelzine metabolism)
  - the enzyme involved is *N*-acetyltransferase
  - people are either fast or slow acetylators, depending on their amount of enzyme
  - fast : slow, in Europe is 40 : 60%, cf. in Japan 85 : 15%.

Enzyme induction

Enzyme induction increases the metabolism of the inducing drug and possibly of others.

There are common cause of interactions.

Inducers are carbamazepine, phenothiazines, phenytoin, which can reduce the effect of other drugs, eg oral contraceptives.

Specific drugs

- **Fluoxetine**: Active metabolite norfluoxetine ($t_{1/2}$ = 7–15 days).
- **Benzodiazepines**:
  - Oxidation (long-acting) and non-oxidative (shorter-acting).
  - Metabolites can be pharmacologically active (eg diazepam → desmethyldiazepam → oxazepam).
  - Shorter acting benzodiazepines have more abuse potential (rapid changes in plasma levels).

Drug	$t_{1/2}$ (hours)	Notes
Diazepam	14–70 (active metabolite ~200)	several days sedation possible (build-up of metabolites)
Clonazepam	20–40	
Chlordiazepoxide	5–30	
Lorazepam	8–20	no hepatic metabolism
Temazepam	6–15	
Oxazepam	6–20	no hepatic metabolism

Table 8.3 $t_{1/2}$ of benzodiazepines

- **Tricyclic antidepressants**:
  - Extensive first-pass metabolism.
  - Tertiary amines (block serotonin (5HT) uptake) → secondary amines [block noradrenaline and dopamine uptake] eg amitriptyline → nortriptyline; imipramine → desipramine; clomipramine → desmethylclomipramine.
- **Venlafaxine**: No substantial inhibition of cytochrome enzymes (including CYP 2D6, CYP 1A2, CYP 3A/4)
- **Chlorpromazine**: Metabolism in kidneys, brain, lung, gastrointestinal tract (active metabolites)
- **Ethanol**: Enzyme inducer (at least initially).

Excretion

Excretion is mostly renal; care is needed in patients with renal impairment.

Ionised state allows metabolites to diffuse passively from glomerular filtrate.

Tubular filtrate pH affects the rate of elimination of these drugs:

- Normally urine is weakly acidic, ie good for excretion of basic drugs (TCAs, amphetamines).
- Alkaline diuresis enhances elimination of aspirin or phenobarbitone, for example, in overdose.

Lithium toxicity:

- Lithium and sodium use similar reabsorption mechanisms. In sodium deficiency, increased lithium reabsorption occurs.
- Diuretics (eg frusemide, thiazide) reduce lithium excretion.

Elderly patients

Changes in pharmacokinetics are difficult to predict, $t_{1/2}$ is usually increased because of:

- Slower absorption (no change in amount absorbed).
- Decreases in weight, albumin, and % water, but increased % fat (lipophilic drugs accumulate), and increased V_d.
- Generally there is reduced metabolism and reduced kidney function.

Adverse reactions are two to three times more common than in younger adults.

Polypharmacy is common (giving increased likelihood of interactions).

There are more errors in taking the correct dosage.

Pregnancy and lactation

See Chapter 26.

PHARMACODYNAMICS

Receptor

A receptor is a protein with a recognition site and mechanisms to transmit a signal from outside to inside a cell.

Receptor type determines whether a neurotransmitter has excitatory or inhibitory effects on the cell.

There are two major superfamilies: metabotropic or ionotropic.

- **Metabotropic**:
  - ○ The binding site, G protein and enzyme (eg adenylate cyclase or phospholipase C) form a transmembrane signalling mechanism.
  - ○ Intracellular second messenger system (eg cAMP or inositol phosphates).
  - ○ Altered second messenger levels produce changes in phosphorylation of key proteins rendering them active or inactive.
  - ○ Eg Dopamine D_1 to D_5, $5HT_1$, $5HT_2$, μ-opioid.
- **Ionotropic**:
  - ○ Five subunits make up an ion channel (eg Na^+, Ca^{2+}, K^+, Cl^-).
  - ○ Eg γ-aminobutyric acid (GABA)-benzodiazepine, $5HT_3$, nicotinic, glutamatergic NMDA.

Receptors can be sited post-synaptically or pre-synaptically. Autoreceptors are pre-synaptic receptors on the same neurone that released the neurotransmitter, eg noradrenergic $\alpha 2$ receptors on noradrenergic terminals. Heteroreceptors are also pre-synaptic but are located on the terminal of a neurone containing a different neurotransmitter, eg noradrenergic $\alpha 2$ receptors on 5HT terminals.

- Autoreceptors act as a negative feedback system, stimulation reduces the release of neurotransmitter from that synapse (eg lofexidine, an agonist, at noradrenergic $\alpha 2$ receptors reduces noradrenergic activity).
- If an autoreceptor is blocked by a receptor antagonist, neurotransmitter will continue to be released (eg mirtazapine blocks noradrenergic $\alpha 2$ receptors increasing noradrenaline release).

Classification of effect

- **Agonist** activates the receptor.
- **Antagonists** block the receptor, preventing activation, but have no intrinsic activity.
- **Partial agonists** are drugs that activate the receptor but even at high dose do not induce the maximal response seen by full agonists.
- **Inverse agonists** are drugs which have the opposite effect to agonists (eg at the benzodiazepine receptor, agonists produce anxiolysis, inverse agonists are anxiogenic).
- **Chronic agonist** or endogenous neurotransmitter release can cause receptors to down-regulate or, conversely with antagonists, up-regulate. This may occur with altered numbers of receptor-binding sites available on the cell surface, or an altered response of the intracellular cascade.

Glutamate system

The glutamate system is the brain's main excitatory system: involving interneurones and some projections (cerebral cortex to basal ganglia, and in the hippocampus and cerebellum).

It is important in various disorders (eg addiction, neurodegeneration).

Glutamate is synthesised from glutamine (enzyme: glutaminase).

Glutamate **receptors** can be:

- Ionotropic: NMDA
    - in inactive state, Ca^{2+} channel is blocked by Mg^{2+} (leaves channel depolarised)
    - excessive intracellular Ca^{2+} levels are toxic, hence the role in neurodegeneration
    - antagonists include MK801, PCP, ketamine
    - glycine allosterically increases glutamate's ability to open channels (like benzodiazepines at the GABA-A receptor).
- Ionotropic
    - AMPA, kainate.
- Metabotropic
    - Group I: inositol phosphate, (Ca^{2+} linked)
    - Group II, III: reduce adenylate cyclase.

GABA system

This is the brain's main inhibitory system – with interneurones throughout the brain.

- GABA is synthesised from glutamate by the enzyme glutamic acid decarboxylase.
- Reuptake occurs, then it is recycled or metabolised by GABA transaminase (valproate inhibits, increasing GABA levels).
- GABA dysfunction is associated with anxiety, Huntington's chorea and alcoholism.

GABA **receptors** are:

- GABA-A complex is an ion channel (increased Cl^- into cell) of five subunits containing binding sites for GABA, benzodiazepine, neurosteroid, barbiturates.
    - Benzodiazepines enhance the effects of GABA.
    - Subtypes have been identified which mediate specific actions of benzodiazepines (eg $\alpha 1$, sedation; $\alpha 2$, anxiety).
    - Zolpidem and zopiclone are $\alpha 1$–selective drugs.
    - Antagonist: Flumazenil
- GABA-B receptor
    - G-protein, increases K^+ efflux
    - Agonist: baclofen.

Acetylcholine

Cell bodies (nucleus basalis of Meynert) project to the cerebral cortex, interneurones in the basal ganglia, the brainstem nucleus projects to the thalamus and midbrain.

- Acetylcholine controls memory, learning, sleep–wake rhythms.
- The nucleus basalis of Meynert degenerates in Alzheimer's disease.
- Balances dopaminergic activity in the basal ganglia.
- Synthesised by choline acetyltransferase transferring acetyl from acetyl coenzyme A to choline.
- Metabolised by acetylcholinesterase.

153

- Blocked by 'anti-dementia' drugs eg donepezi, rivastigmine to increase acetylcholine levels.

Acetylcholine **receptors** are:

- Muscarinic
  - G-protein-linked (seven types)
  - Mediates 'anticholinergic' effects of drugs (typical antipsychotics, TCAs etc)
- Nicotinic
  - ligand-gated channel.

NON-ADRENALINE (NA)

Noradrenaline (NA)

NA is a catecholamine.

- Cell bodies in the locus coeruleus (brainstem) project to the cortex, hypothalamus, limbic regions and hippocampus.
- Associated with depression, anxiety, motivation and drive, involved in maintaining cortical activity when awake and vigilance.
- **Synthesis pathway**: tyrosine to dopa through action of tyrosine hydroxylase, to dopamine and to NA through action of dopa decarboxylase.
- Metabolised by monoamine oxidase (MAO), catechol-O-methyl transferase (COMT) – main metabolite is 3–methoxy–4–hydroxyphenylglycol (MHPG).
- Reuptake mechanism for NA to be taken up into same neurone: the site of action for NA reuptake blockers (TCAs, venlafaxine (serotonin and NA reuptake inhibitor – SNRI), reboxetine (noradrenaline reuptake inhibitor – NARI).

NA **receptors** are:

- $\alpha 1$: post-synaptic
  - second messenger: Ca, inositol
  - antagonists: some psychotropic drugs (eg antipsychotics causing hypotension, sedation).
- $\alpha 2$: pre-synaptic
  - cAMP inhibition
  - agonist: lofexidine (reduces NA overactivity in opiate withdrawal)
  - antagonist: mirtazapine (increases NA release as autoreceptor and increases 5HT firing as heteroceptor).
- $\beta 1$, $\beta 2$: both post-synaptic
  - cAMP stimulation.

Dopamine

Dopamine is also a catecholamine.

- There are three main pathways:
  - **Mesocorticolimbic**: ventral tegmental area to frontal cortex, limbic system, septohippocampal area, nucleus accumbens; involved in 'emotion', reward/addiction (nucleus accumbens), affect, and goal-directed behaviour.
  - **Nigrostriatal**: substantia nigra to striatum; involved in movement and goal-directed behaviour.
  - **Tubero-infundibular**: hypothalamic arcuate nucleus to median eminence; dopamine blocks prolactin secretion.
- For **synthesis** of dopamine: see under NA.
- **Metabolism** of dopamine involves MAO, COMT to dihydroxyphenylacetic acid (DOPAC) and homovanillic acid (HVA).
- **Reuptake** mechanism for dopamine
  - Cocaine and amphetamine block uptake (increased dopamine levels are associated with 'high'; amphetamine also stimulates DA release).
  - Bupropion (drug that aids smoking cessation): dopamine and noradrenaline reuptake inhibitor.

There are five receptor subtypes, D_1 to D_5.

- D_1-like receptors: D_1 and D_5
  - D_1: post-synaptic, increases cAMP, in frontal cortex, caudate; involved in movement, role in neuropathology of schizophrenia (frontal cortex)
  - D_5: as for D_1, low levels in cortex and hippocampus.
- D_2-like: D_2, D_3, D_4
  - D_2: pre- and post-synaptic, inhibits cAMP, in basal ganglia, cerebral cortex (low), medial temporal lobe, limbic system
  - involved in movement, psychosis, prolactin secretion.
- D_3
  - as for D_2
  - in nucleus accumbens (limbic system)
  - likely role in emotion, reward, cognitive function.
- D_4
  - low concentration, found in hippocampus and amygdala.
- Dopamine receptor antagonists at D_2-like receptors
  - 'antipsychotic' activity related to D_2 receptor affinity. Some antipsychotics, eg sulpiride, amisulpride are 'pure' D_2/D_3 antagonists.
- Clozapine has a lower affinity for D_2 and a higher affinity for D_4.

Serotonin (5-hydroxytryptamine, 5-HT)

This is an indolamine.

- From the raphe nucleus (brainstem) projects to cerebral cortex, limbic system and cerebellum.

- Dysfunction is linked with depression, anxiety, impulsiveness, obsessive-compulsive disorder, eating disorders.
- **Synthesis** is via tryptophan to hydroxytryptophan (5-HTP) through action of enzyme tryptophan hydroxylase, then to 5-HT.
- Metabolised by MAO to 5-hydroxyindoleacetic acid (5-HIAA)
- Reuptake mechanism as for NA and dopamine.
- Site of action for 5-HT reuptake blockers (TCAs – preferentially clomipramine, venlafaxine (SNRI), fluoxetine, citalopram (most specific) and SSRI).
- SSRIs block 5-HT reuptake in the raphe, and will desensitise the autoreceptors, increasing 5-HT neuronal firing – this is thought to be important for SSRI efficacy.

Many 5-HT receptors exist (seven + A,B,C, etc), those most relevant to psychiatry are:

- 5-HT$_{1A}$
  - pre- and post-synaptic receptors
  - G-protein, decreases cAMP
  - pre-synaptic in raphe – stimulation decreases cell firing and release of 5-HT
  - post-synaptic in cortex, hippocampus etc
  - involved in anxiety, depression
  - partial agonist: buspirone
  - agonist: pindolol.
- 5-HT$_{2A}$/5-HT$_{2C}$
  - post-synaptic, increases Ca, inositol phosphates
  - involved in sleep, sexual function
  - agonist: LSD
  - antagonist: important to the pharmacology of some atypical antipsychotics (clozapine, risperidone) to minimise extrapyramidal side-effects and in mirtazepine (antidepressant) minimises sleep and sexual dysfunction.
- 5-HT$_3$
  - K$^+$/Na$^+$ ion channel
  - stimulation produces nausea, a common side-effect of SSRIs
  - antagonist: ondansetron.

Opioid system

These act in the periaquaductal grey matter, cerebral cortex and thalamus and include:

- Met/leu-enkephalins (derived from pro-opiomelanocortin).
- β-endorphins.

The **receptors** include:

  - μ-receptors: roles in analgesia, 'pleasure/reinforcement', respiratory depression.
  - κ-receptors: role in dysphoria.
  - δ-receptors: role in reinforcement.
- Drugs relevant to psychiatry:
  - Methadone: agonist; greatest affinity for μ-opiod receptor
  - Buprenorphine: partial agonist at æ-receptor (less respiratory depression) and antagonist at κ-receptor (less dysphoria)
  - Naloxone (short-acting), naltrexone (longer acting): non-selective antagonists.

Other peptides

- **Cholecystokinin**: a gut peptide found in the brain and implicated in anxiety and pain.
- **Substance P**: a gut peptide found in the brain and recently implicated in depression. Its receptor is neurokinin 1.
- **Neuropeptide Y**: involved in feeding behaviour and anxiety.
- **Vasopressin**: has a role in memory.

Monoamine oxidase (MAO) system

The MAO system is intracellular, in vesicles, pre- and post-synaptic.

MAO A (peripheral)	MAO A and MAO B	MAO B (central)
5-HT	tyramine	phenlyethylamine
NA	dopamine	

Table 8.4 MAO metabolises

- MAO inhibitors (ie MAOIs) are antidepressants.
  - Non-selective inhibitors: 'older' MAOIs (phenelzine, tranylcypromine) bind irreversibly. Enzyme resynthesis takes ~2 weeks.
  - MAO A inhibitor: moclobemide (RIMA) binds reversibly, allowing tyramine access to the enzyme and thus preventing build-up (there is therefore less likelihood of the 'cheese reaction').
  - MAO B inhibitor: selegiline.

Lithium

- Lithium increases the activity of Na^+-K^+-ATPase.
- It affects inositol phosphate metabolism and Ca^{2+}-dependent activities.

SPECIFIC PHARMACOTHERAPIES

Side-effects of drug treatments can be **idiosyncratic**, ie unpredictable and unpreventable, or **dose-related**, ie predictable and potentially preventable.

Hypnotics/sedatives

Benzodiazepines

- Dependence and abuse are associated with those drugs with shorter half-lives (eg nitrazepam). These should not be used long-term.
- Tolerance can develop within 14 days, efficacy can decline.
- Long-term use can result in withdrawal syndrome.
- Frequent side-effects are anxiety, insomnia, restlessness, agitation, irritability and muscle tension.
- Less frequently there can be nausea, sweating, lethargy, hyperacusis, nightmares, ataxia and blurred vision.
- Rare problems are psychosis, seizures, tinnitus and paranoid delusions.
- Management of withdrawal is achieved by switching to an equivalent dose of a benzodiazepine with longer half-life (eg diazepam). Dose should be reduced gradually (approximately 1/8 dose every two weeks).
- Side-effects are drowsiness, ataxia, reduced psychomotor performance (patients should be warned about driving, operating machinery etc), amnesia, rarely disinhibition with aggression.
- Interactions can occur; sedation is potentiated by other sedatives (alcohol, TCAs, antihistamines).

Zopiclone, zolpidem and zaleplon

These are non-benzodiazepine hypnotics that bind to the $\alpha 1$ subtype of the GABA-benzodiazepine receptor.

- Zopiclone (cyclopyrrolone) and zolpidem (imidazopyridine)
  - shorter duration of action – less risk of 'hangover'
  - chronic use is not advised – reports of dependence and withdrawal exist.
- Zaleplon (pyrazolopyrimidine)
  - half-life is ~1 hour.

Antihistamines

Promethazine (Phenergan) can be used in patients for whom benzodiazepines are not thought to be appropriate.

Chlormethiazole (Heminevrin)

- This is derived from thiamine (vitamin B_1).
- No longer recommended for outpatient alcohol detoxification (see below), because of potential fatal respiratory depression if taken with alcohol.

Chloral hydrate

This is generally used only in the elderly.

Anxiolytics

Benzodiazepines (see page 164)

Benzodiazepines are not recommended for long-term use.

- Committee on Safety of Medicines (CSM) advice: they are indicated for short-term relief (2–4 weeks only) of anxiety that is severe, disabling or subjecting the individual to unacceptable levels of distress, occurring alone or in association with insomnia or short-term psychosomatic, organic or psychotic illness. The use of benzodiazepines to treat short-term 'mild' anxiety is inappropriate and unsuitable.
- For details of dependence and withdrawal see above on page 164.

Buspirone

- An azapirone, buspirone is a partial $5-HT_{1A}$ agonist.
- When used for generalised anxiety disorder its effect evolves over 1–3 weeks.
- Advantages over benzodiazepines include no significant sedation or cognitive impairment and minimal risk of dependence/withdrawal.
- There is no potentiation of sedative effects of alcohol (not an hypnotic).
- Side-effects include nervousness, dizziness, headache and lightheadedness.

Antidepressants

All have significant anxiolytic activity, some are licensed.

Antidepressants

Tricyclic and related compounds

- **Broad pharmacology**. The inhibition of NA and 5-HT reuptake sites is important to their action. Blockade is immediate, antidepressant action takes two or more weeks to appear.
- They are the 'gold standard' for effective therapy.
- Side-effects reduce their acceptability.
- They are relatively dangerous in overdose (except lofepramine and trazodone).
- Commonly prescribed TCAs are:
  - Amitriptyline: sedative.
  - Dothiepin (prothiaden): sedative.
  - Nortriptyline (adrenergic): least sedative, less anticholinergic.
  - Imipramine: less sedative.
  - Trimipramine: most sedative, probably safest with MAOI.
  - lofepramine: less sedative, less anticholinergic and cardiotoxic, useful for elderly.
  - Mianserin ($5-HT_2$ antagonist, $\alpha2$ antagonist), maprotiline are both tetracyclics.

- Side-effects are:
  - Anticholinergic: muscarinic (M1): dry mouth, constipation, urinary retention, blurred vision. Some tolerance occurs within two weeks. Side-effects can be minimised by gradual dose increase.
  - Alpha-adrenergic: $\alpha 1$ effects, postural hypotension, dizziness, tachycardia/arrhythmias
  - Anti-histaminergic: H_1, sedation, weight gain
  - Other cardiac-related: supraventricular tachycardia, ventricular tachycardia, atrioventricular block, bundle branch block, increased PR interval, increased QRS width, increased QT interval, T wave flattening, ST depression/elevation, R-on-T phenomenon.
- Contraindications/cautions
  - Use with caution with electroconvulsive therapy (serious cardiac events), renal/hepatic/heart disease, and epilepsy (decreased seizure threshold).
  - Contraindication: prostatism, narrow angle glaucoma, post-myocardial infarction, heart block.
- Interactions
  - Potentiates alcohol, hypnotics, anxiolytics, anticholinergic drugs (eg antipsychotics), NA, adrenaline (local anaesthetics).
  - Increases plasma levels of tricyclics, tetracyclics, antipsychotics.
  - Decreases antihypertensive action of guanethidine, clonidine.
  - Interacts with MAOIs potentially causing central nervous system excitation, hyperpyrexia, coma.

Selective serotonin reuptake inhibitors (SSRIs)

- SSRIs inhibit the reuptake site for serotonin.
- They have equal efficacy to TCAs in treatment of depression.
- They have a better side-effect profile: the absence of anticholinergic activity increases patient acceptability, but initial gastrointestinal side-effects and anxiety are unacceptable for some. Lack of toxicity in overdose is a major reason why they are prescribed.
- The following SSRIs are also licensed/prescribed in:
  - Fluoxetine: obsessive-compulsive disorder and bulimia (60 mg).
  - Sertraline: obsessive-compulsive disorder, post-traumatic stress disorder.
  - Paroxetine: obsessive-compulsive disorder, generalised anxiety disorder, post-traumatic stress disorder, panic disorder and social phobia.
  - Fluvoxamine: obsessive-compulsive disorder.
  - Citalopram/escitalopram (active enantiomer): panic disorder.
- Side-effects include:
  - Nausea, diarrhoea (All SSRIs, 27%).
  - Insomnia (worse slow wave sleep) (15% with paroxetine, fluoxetine, sertraline and 5% with fluvoxamine).
  - Sedation (7% with fluoxetine and 21% with paroxetine).
  - Dry mouth (All: 5–18%).
  - Blurred vision (All: 5%).
  - Anxiety, agitation: occur in first two weeks (fluoxetine > paroxetine > sertraline).
  - Anorectic effect.

- Sexual dysfunction (delayed ejaculation, anorgasmia, rarely impotence): can be managed by a change to nefazodone or a noradrenergic antidepressant, addition of cyproheptadine (5-HT$_1$/5-HT$_2$ antagonist) may reverse sexual dysfunction.
- Serotonergic syndrome:
  - Secondary to enhanced serotonergic neurotransmission in the brainstem.
  - Inner restlessness, agitation, increased gastrointestinal motility, neuromuscular hyperactivity (tremor, myoclonus, hyper-reflexia), fever, impaired consciousness; can be fatal. Risk is enhanced with lithium or MAOI co-administration.
  - Discontinuation syndrome (dizziness, sweating and tremor) and dystonias have been reported for paroxetine – gradually decrease dose.
- Contraindications/cautions:
  - Caution should be exercised when using in epilepsy.
  - Sertraline – abnormal liver function tests.
- Interactions:
  - MAOIs (central nervous system excitation, hyperpyrexia, coma).
  - Enhances propanolol, oral anticoagulants.
  - Fluoxetine increases plasma phenytoin and carbamazepine, **but** seizure threshold is lowered (inhibition of cytochrome P450, CYP1A2).
  - Fluoxetine increases haloperidol concentration.
  - Lithium coadministration runs the risk of central nervous system toxicity.

Serotonin/noradrenaline reuptake inhibitor (SNRI): venlafaxine

- Venlafaxine is a phenethylamine bicyclic derivative.
- Similar to TCAs but fewer side-effects (low affinity for cholinergic, histaminergic (H$_1$) or α1-adrenergic receptors).
- Also blocks dopamine reuptake.
- $t_{1/2}$ is 5 hours, active metabolite 10 hours. A slow-release (once/day) preparation is available.
- It is also an effective anxiolytic used in the treatment of generalised anxiety disorder.
- Milnacipran and Duloxetine are other SNRIs which may be released in the near future.
- Side-effects:
  - As for SSRIs but lower frequency.
  - Nausea is problematic (decreases with time).
  - Hypertension (incidence is 2–4% at a dose of < 200 mg; 6–8% at > 200 mg): this should be monitored.
  - Sexual dysfunction.
  - Some fatalities have occurred in overdose with alcohol and other central nervous system drugs.
  - Seizures, increased QTc.
- Interactions:
  - Similar to SSRIs but extra caution should be used in hypertensive patients.
  - Reduce dose or avoid in hepatic/renal impairment.
  - No significant CYP2D6 inhibition (less significant interactions).
  - With MAOIs can cause serotonergic syndrome.
  - Increases effect from warfarin.
  - Increases levels of haloperidol.

Noradrenergic/specific serotonergic antidepressant (NASSA): mirtazapine

- Enhances noradrenergic and serotonergic transmission (blocks α2 auto- and hetero-receptors; see above). Blocks $5\text{-HT}_{2A}/5\text{-HT}_3$ receptors, but enhances activity at 5-HT_{1A} autoreceptors.
- Relatively high affinity for H_1 receptors (weight gain, sedation).
- Side-effects include:
  - Increased appetite, weight gain, drowsiness, sedation, dry mouth (greater at initiation).
  - Safe in overdose.
- Cautions are:
  - Risk of neutropenia/agranulocytosis, cardiac disease, hepato-renal insufficiency.
  - Potentiation of other sedatives.

Selective noradrenaline reuptake inhibitor (NARI): reboxetine

- Selectively blocks reuptake of NA.
- Side-effects are dry mouth (27%), constipation (17%), insomnia (14%), impotence and deceased libido.

Monoamine oxidase inhibitors (MAOI)

- Irreversible MAO-A inhibitors: Phenelzine, tranylcypromine, isocarboxazid.
- Mainly used in depression resistant to other antidepressants and treatment, because of dietary and drug restrictions.
- Phenelzine is used for atypical, non-biological depression with pronounced anxiety and hypochondriacal symptoms, and in phobias and panic disorder.
- Side-effects include orthostatic hypotension, hepatotoxicity (phenelzine), psychosis, weight gain, oedema, insomnia, and sexual dysfunction (less than TCAs)
- Contraindications/cautions:
  - Contraindicated in phaeochromocytoma
  - Caution should be exercised in cardiovascular disease, liver disease (except for tranylcypromine), diabetes, epilepsy, hyperthyroidism.

Food to be avoided	Drugs to be avoided
Cheese – especially mature varieties Degraded protein – chicken liver, hung game, pickled herring, smoked fish, paté, Yeast and protein extract – marmite, bovril, oxo, beer, Chianti wine Fava or broad bean pods, green banana skins, avocados	Opiates – pethidine, morphine (may be less dangerous) Sympathomimetic – these are often included in cough and cold remedies, nose drops (pseudoephedrine), and laxatives bought over the counter Cocaine SSRIs Anaesthetics containing adrenaline
These restrictions remain for at least 2 weeks after the MAOI is discontinued. Treatment of such an interaction is with the α-adrenergic blocker, phentolamine, intravenous or if not available initially, chlorpromazine 200 mg orally.	

Table 8.5 Cheese reaction

- Interactions include the 'Cheese Reaction': can block, irreversibly, MAO-A (mainly gut) and MAO-B (mainly brain) enzymes which break down NA, dopamine and 5-HT. MAO-A preferentially breaks down 5-HT and NA. Gut MAO-A breaks down tyramine in the diet. Tyramine, once in the circulation, leader to a NA-related sudden and potentially fatal rise in blood pressure as it is preferentially broken down by MAO-A leading to increased NA. Patients on MAOIs must avoid food rich in tyramine and other drug preparations containing amines. Usually patients suffer flushing and headache after ingestion of such food or drugs and this is the most important side-effect of MAOIs.

Reversible inhibitors of monoamine oxidase A (RIMA): moclobemide

- MAOI which reversibly inhibits MAO-A.
- Risk of 'cheese reaction' if high levels of tyramine are consumed (eg > 50 g of mature cheese), but in general no dietary restrictions are required.
- Efficacy probably similar to TCAs and SSRIs but not recommended as a first-line treatment.
- Side-effects include: insomnia, nausea, agitation, confusion.
- Interactions can occur with: cimetidine, pethidine, SSRIs, caution with TCAs.

Others

- Trazodone:
  - Triazolopyridine.
  - A weak inhibitor of 5-HT and NA reuptake, blocks 5-HT$_2$ receptors and anti-histamine (sedative).
  - Less anticholinergic and cardiotoxic than TCAs.
  - Used for elderly, possibly antidepressant of choice in epilepsy.
- Nefazodone (now withdrawn):
  - Weak 5-HT receptive inhibitor.
  - Also antagonises 5-HT$_{2A}$ (and 5-HT$_{2c}$) receptors and inhibits NA uptake. No sexual dysfunction, promotes slow-wave sleep.
  - Causes nausea, headache, drowsiness (as SSRIs).
  - Low seizure potential, safe in overdose.
- The dopaminergic system:
  - Nomifensine: a dopamine/NA reuptake inhibitor withdrawn because of haemolytic anaemia.
  - Buproprion: dopamine and NA reuptake inhibitor. Used as an antidepressant (not licensed in UK). Licensed as an aid to smoking cessation but can cause seizures.
- St John's Wort (*Hypericum perforatum*):
  - Used for centuries as an antidepressant.
  - Blocks 5-HT, NA and dopamine reuptake equally.
  - Receptor changes seen in animal models comparable to other antidepressants.
  - Superior to placebo in treating depression.
  - Dose (300–900 mg/tablet) but variable and mixed herbal preparations.
  - Side-effects of gastrointestinal symptoms, dizziness/confusion, tiredness/sedation.
  - Interactions: trazodone, sertraline, nefazodone (mild serotonergic syndrome), paroxetine (lethargy/incoherence), decreased theophylline concentration.
  - Potent inhibitor of some cytochrome P enzymes.

Stopping antidepressants

- Abrupt withdrawal can cause gastrointestinal disturbance, insomnia, or hypomania, especially if the treatment had been taken for > 8 weeks (symptoms usually mild and brief).
- Problems are more commonly reported with SSRIs, (paroxetine: ~85%, possibly venlafaxine and nefazodone) than TCAs and MAOIs.
- Withdraw all antidepressants over ~ 1 month, guided by the patient's tolerance.

SSRI–MAOI	Withdraw and wait ~1–2 weeks, 5 weeks for fluoxetine, before starting MAOI
MAOI–SSRI	Withdraw and wait 2 weeks
TCA–MAOI	Withdraw and wait 1–2 weeks
MAOI–TCA	Withdraw and wait 2 weeks

Table 8.6 Changing antidepressants

Augmentation of antidepressant effect

- Lithium produces a therapeutic response in 30–50% cases of antidepressant-resistant depression.
- Pindolol (a β-blocker) is antagonistic at the pre-synaptic 5-HT$_{1A}$ receptor and therefore enhances serotonergic neurotransmission. Its use is controversial as an augmentation strategy.

Antipsychotics

There are two major groupings: typical and atypical.

- Typical: Block the dopamine (primarily D$_2$) receptors but can have extrapyramidal side-effects.
- Atypicals: Multiple definitions, eg minimal extrapyramidal side-effects (a wide therapeutic ratio for anti-psychotic effects and extrapyramidal side-effects), an effective antipsychotic that does not produce catalepsy in rats.

Side-effects (primarily of typicals)

Central nervous system side-effects include:

- Acute dystonia:
  - Fixed muscle postures with spasm.
  - Young males are most at risk.
  - Early onset of extrapyramidal side-effects: Parkinsonian syndrome.
  - Days to weeks.
  - Blockade of D$_2$ receptors in the basal ganglia.
  - Treat with anti-cholinergic drugs/reduced dose/switch to atypical.

Phenothiazines:	
aliphatic side chains	chlorpromazine
piperidine	thioridazine
piperazine	trifluoperazine, fluphenazine
Thioxanthines	flupenthixol, zuclopenthixol
Butyrophenones	haloperidol, droperidol
Diphenylbutylpiperidines	pimozide
Substituted benzamides	sulpiride, amisulpiride
Dibenzodiazepines	clozapine
Thienobenzodiazepine	olanzapine
Dibenzothiazepine	quetiapine
Benzixasoles	risperidone
Imidazolidinone	sertindole
Benzisothiazole	ziprasidone
Quinolinone	aripiprazole

Table 8.7 Classification of antipsychotic drugs

- Akathisia:
  - Inner and motor, generally lower limb, restlessness.
  - Reduce dose and/or propranolol or benzodiazepine.
- Late-onset extrapyramidal side-effects: tardive dyskinesia:
  - Orofacial dyskinesia, lip smacking, tongue rotating, choreoathetoid movements of head, neck and trunk.
  - Months to years.
  - Increased risk in older patients, females and patients with organic brain damage or affective disorders.
  - 5–60% in those on chronic typicals.
  - Increasing the dose may temporarily alleviate the symptoms, reducing the dose exacerbates them.
  - Anticholinergics may increase risk.
  - Treatment: switch to clozapine, (up to 70% of patients improve); withdraw causative or exacerbating drugs (eg anticholinergics).
  - Other central nervous system sedation: $\alpha 1$ adrenergic and histaminergic H_1 blockade. Toxic confusional state – muscarinic blockade.

Autonomic system side-effects include:

- Dry mouth, difficulty urinating, constipation, blurred vision (muscarinic blockade).
- Hypersalivation can occur with clozapine – mechanism is poorly understood.
- Postural hypotension, impotence, ejaculatory failure linked to $\alpha 1$ adrenergic blockade.

Endocrine side-effects include:

- Amenorrhoea, galactorrhoea, impotence, infertility (direct effects and D_2 blockade in hypothalamic–pituitary axis produce hyperprolactinaemia).

- Poikilothermic effect – especially chlorpromazine.
- Impaired glucose tolerance.

Skin side-effects include:

- Urticaria, dermatitis, rashes.
- Photosensitivity – grey/blue/purple tinge.
- Probably an autoimmune reaction, most commonly seen with the phenothiazines.

Other

- **Eye**: conjunctival/corneolenticular/retinal pigmentation (autoimmune reaction)
- **Weight gain**: mechanism unclear
- **Blood**: agranulocytosis; neutropenia (especially clozapine)
- **Cardiovascular**: increased QT and PR intervals
- **Cholestatic jaundice** (hypersensitivity reaction).

Neuroleptic malignant syndrome presents with the following:

- hyperpyrexia, muscle rigidity, autonomic instability, tachycardia, fluctuating consciousness
- idiosyncratic reaction
- increased creatinine phosphokinase
- days to weeks
- mortality 20%, immediate medical treatment required
- Treatment of neuroleptic malignant syndrome involves:
  - stop antipsychotics
  - administer bromocriptine and dantrolene to reverse dopamine blockade and muscular rigidity, respectively
  - provide supportive treatment for dehydration
  - renal failure from rhabdomyolysis is the major cause of mortality.
- Can recur on reintroduction of neuroleptics – recommend waiting at least 2 months and introduce drug of a different class at the lowest dose.

Atypical antipsychotics

Clozapine is a broad-spectrum atypical antipsychotic.

- In the UK it is only used for schizophrenia that is unresponsive to two other neuroleptics, those with tardive dyskinesia or severe extrapyramidal symptoms, and only with blood monitoring.
- It has low affinity for the D_2 receptor (? limbic selective), higher affinity at D_4, and similar affinity at D_1 and D_3 as other antipsychotics.
- It is a 5-HT_{1A}, 5-HT_{2A}, 5-HT_{2C} and 5-HT_3 antagonist.
- Also an antagonist at muscarinic receptors, $\alpha 1$ receptors, causing sedation and hypotension.
- Balance between receptors may underlie clinical efficacy.
- Effective in 30–50% of treatment-resistant patients, may improve negative symptoms.
- Side-effects include: sedation (21%), hypotension, hypersalivation(6–20%), weight gain, tachycardia (5%), seizures (4%).

- Neutropenia (1–2%): highest risk is early in treatment; usually reversible.
- Agranulocytosis is probably the result of toxic and immunologic factors.
- Interactions:
  - Other drugs causing blood dyscrasias, eg carbamazepine, sulphonamides.
  - Other drugs that are strongly protein bound – increased levels of warfarin, digoxin.
  - Other drugs which use the cytochrome P-450 enzyme system, eg phenothiazines, antidepressants.

Olanzapine is a broad-spectrum atypical antipsychotic.

- It is similar to clozapine but with higher affinity for D_2 [? limbic selective] and 5-HT_{2A} and lower for D_1.
- No neutropenia occurs.
- Significant weight gain and sedation (H_1 and 5-HT_{2C} antagonism) can occur.
- It causes less hyperprolactinaemia than typical antipsychotics.
- It improves positive and negative symptoms.
- A short-acting intramuscular dose is available for rapid tranquillisation.
- It is licensed for use in acute mania and bipolar maintenance.

Quetiapine is a broad-spectrum atypical antipsychotic.

- It has relatively lower affinity for all receptors compared to clozapine, minimal muscarinic. [? limbic selective.]
- It can cause sedation, dry mouth, less weight gain than clozapine and olanzapine.

Risperidone is a serotonin-dopamine antagonist atypical antipsychotic.

- It is a high-affinity antagonist of 5-HT_{2A}, lower (but equal to 'typicals') affinity at D_2, and antagonist at $\alpha1$, $\alpha2$, H_1 receptors.
- It can cause extrapyramidal side-effects, but fewer than typicals (6 mg = placebo)
- Side-effects include: Hyperprolactinaemia, insomnia, anxiety, headache, weight gain (as quetiapine).

Zotepine is also a serotonin-dopamine antagonist atypical antipsychotic.

- It has high affinity for 5-HT_{2A}, 5-HT_{2C}, D_1, D_2, D_3, D_4 and it inhibits NA uptake.
- It improves positive and negative symptoms.
- There is a risk of seizure (> 300 mg/day) and of hyperprolactinaemia at higher doses.

Amisulpride is selective and equipotent for D_2 and D_3.

- It is D_2 limbic selective with negligible affinity for other receptors.
- At low doses (50–300 mg/day) it blocks autoreceptors, eg in frontal cortex, thus increasing synaptic dopamine levels – this is thought to be how it improves negative symptoms.
- Less weight gain occurs compared with risperidone or relative to olanzapine.
- Prolactinaemia occurs and there is a risk of extrapramidal side-effects at higher doses.
- **Aripiprazole**, a serotonin-dopamine partial agonist atypical antipsychotic
  - released June 2004.
  - is a partial agonist at D_2 and 5-HT_{1A} receptors, causing low weight gain.
  - commonest side-effects are insomnia, anxiety and headache.

Other atypicals include:

- **Sertindole**, a serotonin-dopamine antagonist atypical, which was withdrawn (because of cardiotoxicity concerns).
- **Ziprasidone**, also a serotonin-dopamine antagonist atypical, which is not licensed in the UK (because of cardiotoxicity concerns). It has a high $D_2/5-HT_{2A}$ blockade ratio and causes little weight gain.

Mood stabilisers

Lithium

- Lithium is the most widely used mood stabiliser:
  - It prevents relapse in bipolar affective disorder and recurrent unipolar depression.
  - It is an effective treatment in acute mania.
  - It can augment antidepressants in resistant depression.
  - Bipolar depression may need additional antidepressant (risk of precipitating mania).
- Mechanism of action is unclear: It may reduce activation of second messenger systems by neurotransmitters.
- Check urea and electrolytes and also thyroid function tests (TFTs) before commencement (if pregnant see side-effects/contraindications below).
- Plasma levels:
  - Monitor weekly after dose increase until level reaches 0.6–1 mEq/L (12 hours post dose).
  - Monitor maintenance levels, with renal function, every 2–3 months.
  - Monitor thyroid function every 6 months.
- Side-effects include:
  - Early: thirst, nausea, diarrhoea, fine tremor, polyuria; these often disappear.
  - In 30% there is weight gain, acne, oedema, T-wave flattening, tardive dyskinesia, nasal congestion.
  - Hypothyroidism (in 3–4%).
  - Diabetes insipidus: inhibition of ADH in renal tubule (polydipsia).

Plasma levels 1.5–2mEq/L:	Plasma levels > 2mEq/L:
anorexia	impaired consciousness
vomiting	nystagmus
diarrhoea	myoclonus
coarse tremor	hyperreflexia
ataxia	convulsions
dysarthria	coma and death (occur at higher levels)
confusion	
sleepiness	
Get urgent plasma level. If high, stop lithium, treat with osmotic diuresis, anticonvulsants and rehydration.	

Table 8.8 Lithium toxicity

- Interactions of lithium are often the cause of a rise in plasma levels. The following increase lithium neurotoxicity:
  - Antipsychotics (especially haloperidol if increased rapidly).
  - Non-steroidal anti-inflammatories (except aspirin, sulindac).
  - Diuretics – especially thiazides (also frusemide).
  - Cardioactive medicines – digoxin, diltiazem, verapamil, angiotensin-converting enzyme inhibitors.
  - Alcohol.
  - Salt deficiency (NaCl increases lithium excretion).
- Contraindications to lithium use are:
  - Thyroid disorders.
  - Pregnancy (can cause Ebstein's anomaly of tricuspid valve in first trimester)
  - Thyroidopathies.
  - Care in compromised renal function (elderly).

Carbamazepine

Used for the prevention of relapse in bipolar disorder but is less effective than lithium and may be less effective than other anticonvulsant drugs for acute mania, depression, 'rapid cycling' disorders.

- It is a GABA agonist and also affects calcium channels.
- It induces its own catabolic enzymes so that plasma levels fall at first and need to be monitored to establish a maintenance dose (8–12 mg/L). Blood monitoring of plasma levels and a full blood count measured fortnightly for the first 2 months of treatment are advised.
- Side-effects include:
  - Drowsiness, diplopia, ataxia, headache.
  - Nausea, rashes.
  - Haematological disturbances (warn about fever and infections), include agranulocytosis and leukopenia.
- Toxicity problems include diplopia, ataxia and sedation.
- Interactions occur with:
  - Lithium (central nervous system effects and increased risk of toxicity with 'normal' lithium plasma levels).
  - Antipsychotics (drowsiness, ataxia).
  - TCAs (decreased TCA level).
  - MAOI (two-week washout).
  - Enzyme inducer.

Sodium valproate

- Used in refractory bipolar disorder, 'rapid cyclers', mania, not clear if it is 'antidepressant'. It is the anticonvulsant of choice for clozapine-induced seizures, given as prophylaxis when clozapine doses exceed 500–600 mg per day.
- Inhibits GABA-transaminase.
- Side-effects include:
  - Common: Nausea, vomiting, diarrhoea, sedation, tremor, weight gain.

○ Dose-dependent: ataxia, dysarthria.
○ Rare: thrombocytopenia, platelet dysfunction, liver and pancreas toxicity.
- Interactions include:
  ○ Lithium (increased tremor).
  ○ Antipsychotics/other sedatives (increased sedation).
  ○ Increased plasma concentration of benzodiazepines and barbiturates.
  ○ Increased aspirin and warfarin anticoagulant effect.
  ○ Valproate level increased by amitriptyline and fluoxetine, decreased by carbamazepine.
- Contraindications: Pregnant or nursing mothers, pre-existing liver disease.

Depakote is the manufacturer's name for sodium valproate licensed for the treatment of bipolar disorder – other forms are not licensed.

Other anticonvulsants

- **Gabapentin**
- **Lamotrigine**: Stabilises sodium channels, inhibits glutamate release (causes skin rashes).
- **Clonazepam**: Benzodiazepine indicated for treatment of bipolar affective disorder unresponsive to other mood stabilisers.

Dementia

See Chapter 22.

HISTORY OF PSYCHOPHARMACOLOGY

Many drugs were found serendipitously.

- 1900s: Barbiturates.
- 1949: Mood-stabilising effects of lithium (Cade).
- 1950s:
  ○ Chlorpromazine synthesised (from antihistamines).
  ○ Iproniazid (MAOI) from isoniazid (anti-tuberculosis) found to improve mood.
  ○ Imipramine derived from chlorpromazine and tried as an antidepressant.
  ○ Haloperidol synthesised.
- 1960s:
  ○ Benzodiazepines (chlordiazepoxide).
  ○ Clozapine synthesised, though developed as antidepressant.
  ○ Sulpiride.
  ○ Depot typical antipsychotics introduced.
- 1970s:
  ○ Clozapine withdrawn (agranulocytosis).
  ○ Carbamazepine used in mania.

- 1980s:
  - Clozapine efficacious for 'treatment-resistant schizophrenia'.
  - SSRIs, NARIs, SNRIs developed
- 1990s:
  - Mirtazapine developed (based on mianserin).
  - Anticonvulsants as mood stabilisers, eg sodium valproate.

PHARMACOGENETICS

- The role of genetics/DNA in individual variation in drug response.
- The possibility exists of tailoring drug and dose to individual patients and identifying potential 'non-responders' to avoid ineffective therapies and toxicity.
- All pharmacokinetic processes (absorption, distribution, metabolism etc) and target receptors probably have genetic variants that contribute to a drug's efficacy.
  - Cytochrome P-450 family includes CYP2D6, which is involved in the metabolism of many psychotropics. Enzyme polymorphisms result in differential metabolic activity.
  - Likely to be a combination of genetic variants, not single gene.
  - Eg a polymorphism of 5-HT_{2A} receptor, His452Tyr, has a role in predicting clinical response to clozapine.

DRUG DEVELOPMENT AND TRIALS

Drug development takes between 12 and 15 years, most spent in pre-clinical models prior human testing.

Preclinical drug development involves:

- Characterisation of the drug to see if it does what is wanted.
- Use of animal models that represent the disorder being studied.
- Confirmation of drug action.
- Exploring of side-effects/toxicity.

Phase 1:	Phase 2:	Phase 3:	Phase 4:
Safety and behaviour	Carefully selected patients to assess benefit advantage over existing treatments	Investigate in clinical setting	Regulatory approval stage
• healthy volunteers • studies of bioavailability and pharmacokinetics • uncontrolled • single dosing or short regimens	• dose-ranging studies • placebo-controlled and double-blind where ethical • no. of patients is tens to hundreds • duration in months to 1–2 years	• only reached if sufficient evidence that drug is safe and clinically useful • broader range of patients included compared with phase 2 • multiple hospital settings • placebo-controlled or compared with standard comparator • double-blind trials • no. of patients is 100s to ~1000. • larger numbers make rarer side-effects and interactions more likely to be observed	• once licensed and being used in clinical practice, company is required to monitor drug and report any adverse events • in UK, 'yellow card' system for doctors to report adverse events to Committee of Safety of Medicine
Gold standard is randomised controlled trial that includes at least two arms, placebo or 'gold-standard' drug vs drug under investigation.			

Table 8.9 Clinical drug testing

ELECTROCONVULSIVE THERAPY

See Chapter 12.

NEUROIMAGING

Structural imaging

Computerised tomography (CT)

- CT scans use X-rays.
- Axial (horizontal) sections are most common – not three-dimensional.
- CT can be used to distinguish:
  - Cerebrospinal fluid (black) from brain tissue (grey).
  - Higher density areas, indicating recent haemorrhage, calcified lesions.
  - Lower density areas, indicating oedema around neoplasms, infarcts (after 24 hours), inflammations and older haemorrhage.
  - Changes in ventricular system (hydrocephalus, tumours).
  - It cannot visualise the posterior fossa (because of the radio-opacity of bone).

Magnetic resonance imaging (MRI)

- MRI depends on the magnetic properties of protons (H$^+$ nucleus) in tissues.
- A powerful cryogenic magnet produces a magnetic field of ~0.5–3 Tesla.
- The protons align in the magnetic field.
- A radiofrequency electromagnetic wave pulse disturbs the proton which relaxes (ie goes back to its original quiet state) when the pulse is switched off. Energy is given off and measured:
  - T1-weighted image: fluid appears darker than solid, grey matter has more fluid than white matter (and so appears darker).
  - T2-weighted image: fluid appears white.
- Resolution is ~1 mm.
- The superior resolution of white and grey matter and of cerebrospinal fluid allows variation to enhance differences.
- MRI can visualise the posterior fossa.
- It is easy to perform axial, sagittal and coronal images.
- Volumetric and three-dimensional analyses are possible.
- No ionising radiation is involved so multiple studies are possible.
- Disadvantages include that:
  - It is claustrophobic.
  - It is less available, being more expensive than CT.
  - It cannot image bone (which contains insufficient water).
- No adverse effects are known, but unable to scan people with metallic implants.
- Indications:
  - Head injury, neurological disease.
  - Neurological signs of unknown cause.
  - Acute confusion or gradual cognitive decline.
  - Dementia.
  - First psychosis or major personality change over 50 years old.
  - Monitor progression of chronic disorders.
  - Diagnosis of organic brain disorders.

Functional imaging

This permits visualisation of brain activity or its neurochemistry in vivo.

Functional MRI is used.

- It has a magnetic field higher than for structural MRI, eg >1.5 Tesla.
- It is based on an ability to detect differences in magnetic signal from oxygenated versus deoxygenated haemoglobin.
  - It is 'blood oxygenation level dependent' (the BOLD effect).
  - A local increase in metabolic rate as a result of increased activity of that region alters the BOLD effect.
- It is primarily a research tool but can be useful in neurosurgery to map brain function and its relationship to sites of surgery.
- It is superseding nuclear medicine neuroimaging (see below) in determining blood flow changes in health and disease.
- Pharmaco-functional MRI involves giving a drug and measuring its effects on blood flow.

Nuclear medicine neuroimaging

- Nuclear medicine neuroimaging uses radioactive tracers or radioligands.
- γ-radiation is emitted and detected by cameras around the patient.
- The involvement of radioactivity limits its use in research.
- Images of brain activity include:
  - Blood flow.
  - Glucose metabolism.
  - Receptors.
  - Uptake sites.
  - Enzymes.
  - Neurotransmitter turnover.
  - Occupancy by a drug (eg antipsychotics at dopamine D_2 receptor).
  - Release of neurotransmitter in response to a cognitive–behavioural or pharmacological challenge (eg playing a video game or using amphetamine to release dopamine that reduces radiotracer binding to dopamine D_2 receptors).

Positron emission tomography (PET)

In PET the radioligands contain a short half-life isotope (eg ^{15}O, $t_{1/2} = 2$ minutes; ^{11}C, $t_{1/2} = 20$ minutes; or ^{18}F, $t_{1/2} = 110$ minutes) and therefore require an on-site cyclotron to produce radioisotopes, restricting availability and increasing cost.

- The isotope emits a positron, which combines with an electron and 2 γ-photons are released.
- Resolution is 4–6 mm.
- Clinically it is used in oncology; for the localisation of epileptic foci; but in psychiatry it is used almost entirely for research.

- Tracers available
  - Blood flow: $H_2^{15}O$ is used to obtain maps of regional cerebral blood flow at rest and when performing tasks.
  - Glucose metabolism: ^{18}F-2-fluoro-2–deoxy-D-glucose is used.

Dopamine system	
D_1	^{11}C-SCH 23390
D_2	^{11}C-raclopride
Extra-striatal D_2	^{11}C-fallypride
DA turnover	^{11}C-FLB 457
	^{11}C-dopa
Serotonin system	
5-HT1A	^{11}C-WAY100 633
5-HT2A	^{11}C-MDL100 907
GABA-benzodiazepine receptor	^{11}C-flumazenil
Opioid system	
μ	^{11}C-carfentanil
Non-selective	^{11}C-diprenorphine

Table 8.10 Commonly used PET neurotransmitter tracers

Single photon emission computed tomography (SPECT)

- The radioligands contain ^{99}Technetium ($t_{\frac{1}{2}}$ = 6 hours) or ^{123}Iodide ($t_{\frac{1}{2}}$ = 13 hours).
- These have longer half-lives and are therefore commercially available.
- Resolution is 7–10 mm.
- SPECT is regarded as inferior to PET because of its lower resolution and sensitivity, however newer machines have improved resolution.
- It is more widely available and cheaper.
- It is used for localisation of epileptic foci and to assess brain perfusion where there is cognitive impairment and a normal structural scan (hypoperfusion is seen before structural changes).
- Tracers available include ^{99}Tc-HMPAO for measuring blood flow/perfusion.

Dopamine	
D_2	^{123}I-IBZM
extra-striatal D_2	^{123}I-epidepride
reuptake site/transporter	^{123}I-β-CIT
	^{123}I-FP-CIT
5-HT transporter	^{123}I-β-CIT (non-selective)
GABA-benzodiazepine receptor	^{123}I-iomazenil

Table 8.11 Commonly used SPECT neurotransmitter tracers

Chapter 9

Genetics

Nicholas J. Bray and Michael J. Owen

CONTENTS

Genetics

BASIC GENETICS

DNA

Genetic information is stored as **deoxyribonucleic acid** (DNA).

The basic repeat unit of DNA is the nucleotide, comprising:

- a deoxyribose sugar
- a phosphate group
- a nitrogenous base (either guanine (G), adenine (A), thymine (T) or cytosine (C)).

The order of the associated nitrogenous bases is referred to as the **DNA sequence**.

Chromosomes

DNA is principally stored in the cell nucleus, packaged into chromosomes.

The normal complement of chromosomes (**karyotype**) in humans is 23 pairs:

- 22 homologous pairs of **autosomes**
- one pair of sex chromosomes (XX = female, XY = male).

One chromosome from pair is derived from each parent.

Cell division

There are two basic types of cell division.

Mitosis is the principal form of cell division in human tissues, whereby the daughter cells acquire an identical set of chromosomes to that of their parent cell (possessing both copies of each autosome as well as both sex chromosomes, and therefore described as **diploid**).

Meiosis occurs in the formation of gametes (sperm and ova), whereby the chromosome pairs in the parent cell separate (**segregate**) to form cells that possess only one of each pair (which are therefore described as **haploid**). The union of gametes at fertilisation usually restores the diploid state.

Genomic structure

The **genome** is the full complement of DNA in a cell or organism.

The human genome is estimated to contain approximately 30,000–40,000 **genes**, often separated by long nucleotide sequences of no known function. Genes are stretches of DNA sequence that give rise to an RNA product, which may then encode a polypeptide.

Each gene is located at a specific site (**locus**) on a chromosome. Genes typically consist of:

- **Exons**: sequences that are expressed as messenger ribonucleic acid (mRNA)
- **Introns**: intervening sequences that are transcribed (see below), but removed when mRNA is formed
- **Promoter/regulatory elements**: sequences that drive or modulate RNA expression.

Transcription and translation

Transcription is the process by which DNA is copied (**transcribed**) into RNA.

Translation is the process of protein synthesis whereby the amino acid sequence is specified by the mRNA code.

Allelic variation

The DNA sequence can vary between individuals of a species, which can potentially influence the observable characteristics, or **phenotype**, of an organism.

DNA variants that are sufficiently common in the general population (a frequency of at least 1%) are known as **polymorphisms**.

Different forms of a given variation in DNA sequence are called **alleles**. Since each individual has two copies of each autosomal gene (derived from each parental chromosome) they also possess two alleles at a given locus, the combination of which is the **genotype**.

Individuals in whom the two alleles are the same are **homozygous**, whereas those who possess two different alleles are **heterozygous**.

PATTERNS OF INHERITANCE

Mendelian inheritance

Genetic traits of which the presence or absence depends on the genotype at a single locus are known as **Mendelian**. Such traits are said to be **dominant** if they are manifest in heterozygotes and **recessive** if they are only seen in homozygotes for a given allele.

There are five basic Mendelian patterns of inheritance:

- **Autosomal dominant**: parents are usually an affected heterozygote and an unaffected homozygote. In this case, the average ratio of unaffected to affected offspring is usually 1 : 1.

- **Autosomal recessive**: both parents are usually unaffected heterozygotes. In this case the average ratio of unaffected to affected offspring is 3 : 1.
- **X-linked recessive**: the mother is usually an unaffected heterozygote, or **carrier**, and the father is unaffected. In this case, 50% of sons will be affected (as males possess only one copy of the X chromosome), and 50% of daughters will be carriers. Father-to-son transmission does not take place.
- **X-linked dominant**: where the mother is an affected heterozygote and the father is unaffected, the average ratio of unaffected to affected offspring is 1 : 1, irrespective of their sex. Where the father is affected but the mother is unaffected, 100% of daughters, but no sons, will be affected.
- **Y-linked**: traits inherited only from the father. These are transmitted to 100% of sons, but to no daughters.

Non-Mendelian inheritance

Most psychiatric disorders show patterns of inheritance that are complex and non-Mendelian. Complex **multifactorial** disorders, such as schizophrenia, are assumed to reflect the involvement of multiple genes, in addition to environmental factors. They may be:

- **Oligogenic**: where susceptibility alleles at relatively few genetic loci increase the risk of the disorder, but are individually insufficient to cause disease (eg the ε4 allele of the *ApoE* gene in late-onset Alzheimer's disease)
- **Polygenic**: where disease risk depends upon the combined action of many susceptibility loci, each of small effect.

Complications to pedigree patterns

Various factors may complicate patterns of inheritance.

- **Locus heterogeneity** is where mutations in several different genes result in the same clinical phenotype.
- **Non-penetrance** describes where conditions that usually display a dominant inheritance pattern skip a generation, as a result of environmental or additional genetic factors.
- **Mitochondrial inheritance**: because the mitochondrial genome is almost always maternally derived, diseases resulting from mutations in the mitochondrial genome show a maternal transmission pattern.
- **Genomic imprinting** describes cases where there is differential expression of genes depending on whether the chromosome is maternally or paternally derived.
- **Dynamic mutation** is where an unstable DNA sequence (eg repeat sequence) mutates when transmitted from one generation to another. This can be associated with the phenomenon of **anticipation**, whereby disease severity increases and/or age of onset decreases in successive generations.

QUANTITATIVE GENETIC TECHNIQUES

Genetic epidemiological studies make use of a number of natural designs to explore the contribution of genetic factors to a trait or illness.

The three principal study designs are:

- family studies
- twin studies
- adoption studies.

Family studies

Family studies investigate the degree of family clustering of a trait or illness.

The frequency of the illness in relatives of affected **index cases** (or **probands**) is compared with the prevalence in the general population or in the relatives of a demographically matched control sample.

- **Family history method**: where information on the diagnostic status of family members is obtained from the proband or a relative
- **Family study method**: where the diagnostic status of the proband and all available relatives is directly assessed by personal interview.

Potential confounds in family studies include ascertainment bias and misdiagnosis when an illness has a delayed onset (eg Alzheimer's disease).

While family studies indicate the extent to which diseases aggregate in families, they cannot distinguish between genetic and shared-environment effects.

Twin studies

Twin studies explore the contribution of genetic factors to a disease by investigating whether monozygotic (MZ) twins are more similar (**concordant**) for a trait than dizygotic (DZ) twins. MZ twins inherit all their genes in common, whereas DZ twins share, on average, 50% of their genes. Based on the assumption that both MZ and DZ twins share environmental risk factors to an approximately equal extent, higher concordance rates in MZ twins indicate a genetic contribution to the illness.

The concordance rate (CR) can be calculated from two perspectives:

- **Pairwise CR** = Number of twin pairs in which both are affected/Total number of twin pairs
- **Probandwise CR** = Number of affected co-twins/Total number of co-twins.

Potential confounds in twin studies are ascertainment bias, mis-specification of zygosity and sex-discordance in DZ twins. Other methodological problems are that MZ twinning is itself an error in development, associated with increased risk of several defects (eg congenital heart disease), and that MZ twins may be treated more similarly and share their microenvironment to a greater extent than DZ twins.

Adoption studies

Adoption studies provide a means of disentangling genetic factors from the shared family environment. There are three common study designs:

- **Adoptee strategy**: the risk of illness in the adopted away offspring of affected parents is compared to the risk in adopted offspring of unaffected biological parents.
- **Adoptee's family strategy**: the risk of the illness is compared between the biological and adoptive relatives of affected adoptees, and in the biological and adoptive relatives of unaffected adoptees.
- **Cross-fostering design**: the risk of the illness is compared in adoptees where the biological parents are affected but the adoptive parents are unaffected, and in adoptees where the biological parents are unaffected but the adoptive parents are affected.

In each case, a genetic contribution is suggested when the risk of the illness is higher in the biological relatives of probands than in the associated control groups.

Potential confounds in adoption studies include ascertainment bias and non-random adoptive placement.

MOLECULAR GENETIC TECHNIQUES

DNA cloning and amplification

Many molecular genetic techniques require initial amplification of target DNA sequence (eg specific gene sequence) from a complex source (eg whole genomic DNA).

Cell-based DNA amplification: In cell-based **DNA cloning**, the target DNA sequence is attached to a sequence that is capable of independent replication. The hybrid DNA is then transferred into host cells (usually bacterial or yeast cells), which are propagated and the amplified DNA is harvested.

Polymerase chain reaction (PCR) is the principal method of DNA amplification in modern molecular genetic laboratories. DNA sequence is exponentially amplified in an enzymatic, *in vitro* reaction using synthetic DNA **primers** that are specific to the DNA sequence of interest.

Molecular hybridisation

Molecular hybridisation uses labelled nucleic acid **probes** (either DNA or RNA) to detect the presence of closely related nucleotide sequences from a complex target source.

Southern blotting: Target DNA is digested using **restriction endonucleases** (see page 190) and the resulting fragments are separated by size using gel electrophoresis. DNA fragments are denatured, transferred onto a synthetic membrane and allowed to associate with the single-stranded probe DNA.

Northern blotting is a variation on the Southern blotting method that uses RNA instead of DNA as the target source. Northern blotting is commonly used to investigate the expression pattern of genes. A gene probe is hybridised against RNA derived from different tissues. The level of hybridisation observed for each tissue sample indicates where, and to what extent, a gene is expressed.

Genotyping methods

Several methods are available to determine which alleles are possessed by an individual at a given locus:

Short tandem repeat polymorphism (STRP) genotyping: STRPs (or **microsatellites**) are short sequences (usually between one and four nucleotides long) that are repeated in tandem a variable number of times within the population. The fundamental difference between alleles is the number of repeats and therefore the size of the target molecule. Genotyping is based on measuring the size of the amplified sequence, which is usually achieved by labelling one of the PCR amplification primers and separating the variable-sized PCR products by electrophoresis.

Restriction fragment-length polymorphism (RFLP) genotyping: Specific stretches of DNA sequence are recognised and cleaved by enzymes called **restriction endonucle-ases**. Some DNA variants, such as the relatively common **single nucleotide polymorphism (SNP)**, can alter the sequence that is usually recognised by these enzymes, so that one allele will be cut and the other will not. When subject to electrophoresis, PCR products that have been digested using a restriction endonuclease will show differences in fragment size depending on which alleles are present. Differences in restriction fragment size resulting from DNA variation are called **RFLP**s.

Primer extension genotyping is a relatively new technique for genotyping SNPs, whereby a third primer is used in a further extension reaction of PCR products. The extension primer anneals to the sequence that is directly adjacent to the polymorphism and extends by one nucleotide base (that which is complementary to the variable base). Several methods are available to detect the incorporated base, and therefore genotype for the polymorphism.

Mutation detection

Numerous techniques are available with which to identify unknown variants in a defined stretch of DNA.

Methods for screening sequences for the presence of a DNA variant include **single-strand conformation analysis (SSCA)** and **heteroduplex analysis (HA)**.

Having identified a DNA fragment that contains a variant, **DNA sequencing** may be used to identify the polymorphism.

CHROMOSOMAL ABNORMALITIES

Chromosomal abnormalities fall into three main categories:

- abnormal chromosome number
- structural chromosome abnormalities
- abnormalities of parental origin.

Abnormalities in chromosome number

Trisomy is the possession of an extra copy of a single chromosome, resulting from a failure of segregation during meiosis.

Monosomy is the loss of one copy of a chromosome. Monosomy is lethal except in cases of Turner syndrome (see below).

Structural chromosomal abnormalities

Structural abnormalities result from chromosome breakage and include:

- **Inversions**, where a chromosomal segment is reattached in the opposite orientation.
- **Translocations**, where a portion of one chromosome becomes attached to another (non-homologous) chromosome. Translocations that result in a net gain of chromosomal material are described as **unbalanced**.
- **Deletions/duplications**, where a chromosomal segment is lost or duplicated.

Abnormalities of parental origin

Occasionally, both homologous chromosomes originate from the same parent. Phenotypic consequences may arise when genes on the abnormal chromosome are subject to parental imprinting.

In **uniparental heterodisomy** both copies of the chromosome are different (ie they represent the simultaneous transmission of both homologous chromosomes carried by one parent).

In **uniparental idiodisomy** two identical copies of a single parental chromosome are inherited.

Conditions caused by chromosomal abnormalities

Down syndrome is the most common form of mental retardation resulting from a chromosomal abnormality. It usually reflects **trisomy 21** (ie an additional copy of chromosome 21). A small proportion ($\sim$ 5%) of cases result from translocations of a portion of chromosome 21.

Velocardiofacial syndrome (VCFS) is characterised by facial dysmorphology, palatal abnormalities and heart defects and is associated with high rates of psychosis. Patients usually have deletions within the long arm of chromosome 22, encompassing several genes.

Sex chromosome aneuploidies include, **Turner syndrome** in females, which is caused by the complete or partial absence of one X chromosome, and **Klinefelter syndrome** in males, in which there is an additional X chromosome. These abnormalities are indicated by examination of the **Barr body** number in cells from a buccal smear.

INHERITED CONDITIONS RELEVANT TO PSYCHIATRY

Mendelian disorders with a neuropsychiatric phenotype

Certain conditions encountered in psychiatric practice follow basic Mendelian patterns of inheritance. Examples of Mendelian disorders relevant to psychiatry are shown in Table 9.1.

Inheritance pattern	Condition
Autosomal dominant	Huntington's disease Familial Alzheimer's disease Acute intermittent porphyria Neurofibromatosis Tuberous sclerosis
Autosomal recessive	Wilson's disease Galactosaemia Tay–Sachs disease
X-linked recessive	X-linked mental retardation Lesch–Nyhan syndrome Hunter's disease

Table 9.1 Examples of Mendelian disorders relevant to psychiatry

Disease genes have been identified for many of these conditions, resulting in major advances in our understanding of pathogenesis. Examples include:

- **Huntington's disease**: clinical features include a progressive generalised chorea and intellectual deterioration. It is caused by expansion of a trinucleotide repeat encoding a polyglutamine tract in the *huntingtin* protein.
- **Familial Alzheimer's disease** is a rare form of Alzheimer's disease with an unusually early onset. It can be caused by missense mutations in the genes for amyloid precursor protein (*APP*), presenilin-1 (*PS-1*), or presenilin-2 (*PS-2*).
- **Fragile-X syndrome** is the commonest known inherited cause of mental retardation. It usually reflects the expansion of the trinucleotide repeat sequence at a fragile site on the X chromosome, leading to loss of expression of the *FMR1* gene.

Complex psychiatric disorders

The majority of psychiatric disorders are complex **multifactorial** diseases.

Quantitative genetic studies have indicated a significant genetic component to many psychiatric disorders, although the genes involved are largely unidentified.

Estimates of the **heritability** (the proportion of variance attributable to genetic effects) are shown in Table 9.2 for common psychiatric conditions.

Disorder	Heritability estimate
Schizophrenia	0.80
Bipolar disorder	0.60–0.70
Major depression	0.25–0.40
Panic disorder	0.50–0.60
Autism	0.90

Table 9.2 Estimates of heritability of common psychiatric conditions

As indicated on page 187, these conditions are likely to be **polygenic** or **oligogenic**. Risk alleles will be present in unaffected individuals (**non-penetrant**) and different risk alleles may be present in individuals with the same diagnosis (**locus heterogeneity**).

A massive international research effort has been invested in the identification of genes that promote susceptibility to complex psychiatric disorders.

IDENTIFYING DISEASE GENES

There are three principal methods used to identify disease genes:

- linkage studies
- cytogenetic approaches
- association studies.

Linkage studies

- Linkage studies examine the segregation of a disorder with alleles of polymorphic genetic markers (eg microsatellites) in multiply affected families.
- Alleles at loci that are close together on a chromosome tend to be inherited together, as they are less likely to be separated by **recombination** (cross-over of portions of homologous chromosomes during meiosis).
- Co-segregation of the disorder with a particular marker allele in a family is therefore suggestive of **genetic linkage** to a disease locus.

- The **lod score** (logarithm of the odds) is a measure of the likelihood of genetic linkage between loci.
- Linkage approaches are principally suited for Mendelian disorders involving genes of major effect.

Cytogenetic approaches

- Chromosomal abnormalities in affected individuals may be investigated as a potential clue to the location of general susceptibility genes.
- Cytogenetic abnormalities (eg deletions or translocations) may implicate a gene or region by disrupting a gene directly or by showing genetic linkage with a susceptibility variant.

Association studies

- Allelic association is where an allele at a particular locus co-occurs with disease at a level above that expected by chance.
- The simplest design to test for genetic association is the **case–control study**, where allele or genotype frequencies are compared between unrelated affected and unaffected individuals drawn from the same population.
- Association may occur when there is a direct effect of the variant itself on disease susceptibility or where the true susceptibility allele is in close enough proximity that co-occurrence of the two alleles is maintained over many generations (**linkage disequilibrium**).
- Spurious associations may result from chance or where samples are unequally matched as a result of **population stratification**.
- Association studies are able to detect genes of small effect, and are therefore suited to test individual candidate genes in complex diseases. Such genes may be **positional** candidates (located within a linkage or otherwise implicated chromosomal region) or **functional** candidates (where involvement is inferred from known pathophysiology).

PRENATAL IDENTIFICATION AND GENETIC COUNSELLING

Prenatal diagnosis is generally suitable only for single-gene disorders and chromosomal abnormalities. It requires specialised genetic counselling. Testing and counselling are organised by local medical genetics services. Such services are usually offered for severe disorders causing learning disability (which can be associated with mutations in single genes or chromosomal abnormalities) and autosomal dominant dementias (eg Huntington's disease).

Some genetics services offer counselling for common psychiatric disorders where there is evidence of familial recurrence, though here genetic testing is not appropriate unless there is evidence for co-existence of single-gene or chromosomal disorders.

Chapter 10

Ethics and the Law

Trevor Hicks

CONTENTS

Section 135
Section 136
Mental Health Act Review Tribunal
Mental Health Act Commission

Ethics and the Law

ETHICS

The dictionary defines ethics as 'the science of morals, that branch of philosophy which is concerned with human character and conduct; a system of morals, rules of behaviour; a treatise on morals'.

Codes

Codes provide a framework for good practice. They protect and promote the profession by setting out members' obligations to one another and supporting the resistance of doctors to abusive practices under oppressive regimes. There are various codes relevant to medical practice.

- **The Hippocratic Oath**. Hippocrates was born in 460 BC and is known as the 'Father of Medicine'. This was the first ethical code of conduct for doctors, probably devised by Hippocrates' students. It is the basis for codes governing early Islamic and Christian medicine. It promotes medical teaching, acting in the best interests of patients, abstention from any deleterious or mischievous action, and patient confidentiality.
- **Caraka Samhita** was an Indian physician in the first century AD. He proposed confidentiality, considerateness towards patients, and keeping abreast of medical knowledge.
- **Code of Institutes and Percepts** was defined by the English physician, Thomas Percival (1803) who was responsible for the foundation of the British Medical Association's early codes.
- **Helsinki and Geneva declarations** were made after World War II, following the Nuremberg War Trials. They were introduced because Nazi doctors had conducted experiments on Jews, homosexuals and disabled people (among others).
- **Medical school promise/oath** is taken on graduation by newly qualified doctors. It is based on the Hippocratic Oath, modified by later declarations.

Rights

The *Human Rights Act 1998* enshrined basic human rights into statutory English law. To have a right there is a corresponding duty on others to ensure that the right is not infringed.

Article 2: Right to life.

Article 3: No one shall be subjected to torture or to inhuman or degrading treatment or punishment.

Article 8: Right to respect for private and family life.

Casuistry

Casuistry tackles ethical problems by considering particular cases from the ground up. Particular circumstances can be varied in imagined situations where a course of action becomes more obvious, or by considering related cases where the ethical outcomes are clearer.

1 Autonomy: respecting patients' wishes and freedom of choice (ie people should be allowed to make their own decisions about what happens to them).
2 Beneficence: acting in the patients' best interests.
3 Non-maleficence: 'above all do no harm'.

4 Justice: ensuring that people are treated fairly and equally.
        principles considered pertinent to any medical ethical problem.
        principles' reasoning is top-down (cf casuistry), applying widely held values to specific cases.

Table 10.1 The four principles of bioethics (USA: Beauchamp & Childress, UK: Gillon)

Paternalism

The doctor acts as the patient's 'parent', telling them what to do and making choices on their behalf (cf autonomy).

Utilitarianism/consequentialism

John Stuart Mill (in the nineteenth century) described a principle of the 'greatest good for the greater number'. This depends on calculating outcomes and predicted benefits for the individual compared to society in general.

Kantianism/deontology

Immanuel Kant, an eighteenth century Prussian philosopher, argued against utilitarianism in that some things were either just 'right' or 'wrong'. He stated that people should not be considered as a means to an end but as an 'end in themselves'. No person should be subject to anything that was not 'right' even if it may have resulted in greater benefit to others.

Narrative ethics

This type of ethics rejects rules and principles. It considers the lives of individuals in context when determining ethical correctness.

THE LAW

The dictionary defines the law as: 'a rule of action established by authority; a statute; the rules of the community or state'.

It is also the formal mechanism for the creation and maintenance of social order.

British Judicial System

- **Statute law** is made by Parliament via its legislative process.
- **Common law** ('Case law') considers similar previous cases that have been tested in Court. Subsequent judgements made in these cases become part of the Common Law.
- **Criminal law** deals with acts which are forbidden or an omission to perform an act which is commanded by the Common Law, by statute or by regulations made by a subordinate authority; the remedy for which is the punishment of the offender.
- **Civil law** deals with non-criminal activity and is a form of private law involving the relationships between individual citizens. An action causing injury to another can be pursued as a criminal and/or a civil (tort) case. A 'tort' is a wrong that has caused damage to someone, eg assault, battery, or negligence. Negligence usually provides a remedy in the form of compensation to the injured party.

Court hierarchy	
European Courts	Most binding
House of Lords	
Court of Appeal	
High Court	
Crown Court	
Magistrates Court	Least binding

Table 10.2 Doctrine of precedence where the decision of a higher court is binding on a lower court

Consent

All adults are assumed to be competent to consent to or refuse medical treatment unless shown otherwise. Consent can be expressed or implied.

For minor procedures, eg blood pressure measurement, co-operation may be taken as legally valid implied consent. Expressed consent is needed for more complicated or invasive medical procedures. Verbal and written consent are equally valid. Failure to obtain valid consent can lead to the criminal charge of assault or the civil action of negligence.

Capacity is established in **Re C** and based on:

- ability to understand and retain treatment information
- ability to believe in it
- ability to weigh it in the balance
- ability to arrive at an informed choice.

The level of capacity needed for more complex procedures is higher than for simpler ones.

Patients can lack capacity to give consent because they are too young (under the age of 16), or because of physical illness or mental disorder.

Gillick competence. Medical treatment for children under the age of 16 generally requires consent from one person with parental responsibility. However, some children under the age of 16 have been deemed, by the Courts, to possess the legal capacity to consent if they are of sufficient maturity and intelligence to understand the nature of the proposed treatment. Such children are termed **Gillick competent** and can give consent despite parental objections. Paradoxically those with parental responsibilities can override the wishes of a 'Gillick-competent' child by consenting to treatment that the child is refusing!

Emergency treatment. English Common Law allows doctors to give emergency or life-saving treatment to patients if it is necessary and in their best interests and the necessary consent cannot be obtained, eg the patient is unconscious.

Advocacy

An advocate enters into a relationship with the patient to speak on their behalf, represent their wishes and stand up for their rights. An advocate has no legal status.

Appointeeship

- An appointee is authorised by the Department for Work and Pensions (DWP) to receive and administer benefits on behalf of someone who is unable to manage their own affairs.
- The appointee can only administer monies from the DWP but not other income/assets.
- Application to the Public Trust Office or Court of Protection may be needed to access accumulated funds.

Powers of attorney

One person (the **donor**) gives legal authority to another person (the **attorney**) to manage their affairs. The donor has sole responsibility for the decision provided they fully under-stand the implications of what they are undertaking.

Ordinary power of attorney allows the attorney to manage the donor's financial affairs generally or can be limited to specific matters. Such powers are revoked by law if the donor loses mental capacity to manage their own affairs.

Enduring power of attorney was introduced in 1985 to allow a donor to decide who should manage their affairs if they later become mentally incapacitated. Such powers continue after the donor has lost mental capacity providing it is registered with the Public Trust Office. The attorney then applies to the Public Trust Office for registration of the **Enduring Power of Attorney** to allow the attorney continuing authority to act on behalf of the donor. This procedure is useful where the donor suffers from a progressive illness (dementia) and anticipates loss of mental capacity.

Court of Protection

The Court of Protection exists to protect the property and affairs of persons incapable of managing their own financial affairs as a result of mental disorder. Once application is made, the Court of Protection acts to appoint a **receiver** to manage the patient's affairs on their behalf. Receivers are often family members, friends or solicitors and must keep accounts, only spending the patient's money on items that will be of benefit to them. Permission is needed from the Court of Protection to dispose of capital assets (property).

Testamentary capacity

A person must be of **sound disposing mind** to make a will. They must:

- understand to whom they are giving their property
- understand and recollect the extent of their property
- understand the nature and extent of the claims upon them, both of those included and those excluded from the will.

A valid will is not invalidated by the subsequent impairment of testamentary capacity.

Driving

The Driver Vehicle Licensing Authority (DVLA) is responsible for granting permission to drive by issuing licences.

- Drivers have the duty to inform the DVLA of any condition that may impair their ability to drive.
- Doctors are responsible for advising patients to inform the DVLA if they develop a condition that is likely to make driving dangerous.
- If the driver fails to heed this advice then General Medical Council guidelines advise breaking confidentiality and informing the DVLA directly (see www.gmc-uk.org)
- Before resuming driving, a driver must satisfy the standards of fitness for driving and be free from any effects of medication which will affect driving adversely.

The DVLA publishes a regular updated guide for doctors concerning various medical and psychiatric conditions that affect driving that is available at www.dvla.gov.uk.

Table 10.3 summarises current (2004) advice on fitness to drive in patients with psychiatric disorders:

Psychiatric illness	Group 1 entitlement	Group 2 entitlement
ANXIETY OR DEPRESSION	**DVLA need not be notified** and driving may continue.	Very minor short-lived illnesses need not be notified to DVLA.
MORE SEVERE ANXIETY STATES OR DEPRESSIVE ILLNESSES	Driving ceases pending medical enquiry. Period of stability required before driving resumed. Particularly dangerous are those who may attempt suicide at the wheel.	Driving permitted when well and stable for 6 months or if anxiety/depression long-standing but symptom-free on medications that do not impair. Medication must not cause side-effects which interfere with alertness or concentration. DVLA may require psychiatric reports.
ACUTE PSYCHOTIC DISORDERS OF ANY TYPE	**Driving must cease** during the acute illness. Re-licensing can be considered when patient: a. has remained well and stable for at least 3 months. b. is compliant with treatment. c. is free from adverse effects of medication which would impair driving *and* d. Subject to a favourable specialist report. Drivers with history of instability and/or poor compliance require a longer period off driving.	**Driving should cease** pending the outcome of medical enquiry. Must be well and stable for 3 years with insight before driving can be resumed. DVLA requires a consultant examination. Medication at minimum effective dosage, not interfering with alertness, concentration or impairing driving performance. No significant likelihood or recurrence.
HYPOMANIA/MANIA	**Driving must cease** during the acute illness. Following an isolated episode, re-licensing can be reconsidered when all the following conditions can be satisfied: a–d. above plus e. Has regained insight. **REPEATED CHANGES OF MOOD**: When there have been four or more episodes of mood swing within the previous 12 months, at least 6 months stability will be required under condition (a), in addition to satisfying conditions (b) to (e).	As acute psychotic disorders.
CHRONIC SCHIZOPHRENIA & Other Chronic Psychoses	**Driver must satisfy**: a. stable behaviour for at least 3 months. b., c. and. d. above. **Continuing symptoms** do not necessarily preclude licensing.	**Driving must cease** pending the outcome of medical enquiry. The person must be well and stable for a minimum of 3 years with insight into their condition before driving can be resumed. At that time, DVLA will usually require a consultant

DEMENTIA OR ANY ORGANIC BRAIN SYNDROME	Symptoms should be unlikely to cause significant concentration problems, memory impairment or distraction whilst driving. Particularly dangerous, are those drivers whose psychotic symptoms relate to other road users. **Assessment extremely difficult**. If poor short-term memory, disorientation, lack of insight/judgement, then not fit to drive. Medical reports needed. **Early dementia**, sufficient skills retained, progression slow, licence issued subject to annual review. Formal driving assessment may be necessary.	examination. Any psychotropic medication should be of minimum effective dosage and not interfere with alertness, concentration or in any other way impair driving performance. There should be no significant likelihood of recurrence. Refuse or revoke licence.
LEARNING DISABILITY	Severe LD not compatible with driving; licence application must be refused. In milder forms, with no other relevant problems, may be possible to hold a licence, but necessary to show adequate function at the wheel.	Permanent refusal/revocation if severe. Minor degrees of learning disability when the condition is stable with no medical or psychiatric complications may be compatible with the holding of a licence.
PERSISTENT BEHAVIOUR DISORDER (eg. post head injury syndrome, psychopathic disorders, non-epileptic seizure disorder).	If seriously disturbed e.g. violent behaviour or alcohol abuse and likely to be a source of danger at the wheel, licence would be revoked or the application refused. Licence will be issued after medical reports confirm that behavioural disturbances have been satisfactorily controlled.	Recommended refusal or revocation if associated with serious behaviour disturbance likely to make the individual a source of danger at the wheel. If the person matures and psychiatric reports confirm stability then consideration would be given to restoration of the licence but Consultant Psychiatrist report would be required.

Group 1 entitlement: cars and motorcycles.

Group 2 entitlement: lorry and bus standards (more stringent because of size and greater time spent at the wheel).

Table 10.3 Summary of fitness to drive regulations

MENTAL HEALTH ACT 1983

The *Mental Health Act 1983* applies to England and Wales. Scotland has its own *Mental Health Act 1984* and Northern Ireland has its *Mental Health Bill 1986*.

Section 1

Section 1 explains what the Act is about and who it is intended to deal with. It attempts to provide a legal (rather than medical) definition of the types of mental health problems the Mental Health Act is intended to cover.

- **Mental disorder**: mental illness, arrested or incomplete development of mind, psychopathic disorder and any other disorder or disability of mind. The four categories are:
  - **severe mental impairment**: a state of arrested or incomplete development of mind which includes severe impairment of intelligence and social functioning and is associated with abnormally aggressive or seriously irresponsible conduct on the part of the person concerned.
  - **mental impairment**: a state of arrested or incomplete development of mind (not amounting to severe mental impairment) which includes significant impairment of intelligence and social functioning and is associated with abnormally aggressive or seriously irresponsible conduct on the part of the person concerned.
  - **psychopathic disorder**: a persistent disorder or disability of mind (whether or not including significant impairment of intelligence) which results in abnormally aggressive or seriously irresponsible conduct on the part of the person concerned.
  - **mental illness**: not defined; a matter of clinical judgement. The Act states that a person may not be dealt with under the Act 'by reason of promiscuity or other immoral conduct, sexual deviancy or dependence on alcohol or drugs'.
- **Patient**: a person suffering from, or appearing to suffer from, mental disorder.
- **Medical treatment**: includes nursing, and rehabilitation under medical supervision.
- **Responsible Medical Officer (RMO)**: the registered medical practitioner in charge of the treatment of the patient.
- **Approved doctor**: a registered medical practitioner approved under Section 12 of the Act by the Secretary of State (with authority being delegated to the Regional Health Authority) as having special experience in the diagnosis and treatment of mental disorder.
- **Approved Social Worker (ASW)**: an officer of the local social services authority with appropriate training who may make applications for compulsory admission.
- **Nearest relative**: the first surviving member of the following list, with full-blood relatives taking precedence over half-blood relatives, and the elder of two relatives of the same description or level of kinship taking preference. Preference is also given to a relative with whom the patient ordinarily lives or by whom they are cared for:
  - husband or wife
  - son or daughter
  - father or mother
  - brother or sister

- ○ grandparent
- ○ grandchild
- ○ uncle or aunt
- ○ nephew or niece.

Section 2 (Assessment Order)

Section 2 provides authority for detention in hospital for up to 28 days for assessment.

- Application by the ASW is based on two medical recommendations.
- Grounds for the application are that the person is suffering from mental disorder of a nature or degree which warrants the detention of the patient in a hospital for assessment (or for assessment followed by medical treatment) for at least a limited period and that they ought to be so detained in the interests of their own health or safety or with a view to the protection of other persons.

Section 3 (Treatment Order)

Section 3 provides the authority for someone to be detained in hospital for up to six months for treatment.

- Application by the ASW which is based on two medical recommendations.
- The order may be renewed for a further six months and then for a year at a time.
- Grounds for the application are that the person is suffering from mental illness, severe mental impairment, psychopathic disorder or mental impairment and that their mental disorder is of a nature or degree which makes it appropriate for them to receive medical treatment in a hospital.
- Also, in the case of psychopathic disorder or mental impairment, such treatment is likely to alleviate or prevent a deterioration of the condition.
- It is also necessary for the health or safety of the patient or for the protection of other persons that they should receive such treatment and it cannot be provided unless they are detained under this Section.

Section 3 cannot normally be imposed if the Nearest Relative objects.

Section 4

Section 4 is intended for emergency admissions where, if it were not for the extreme urgency, a Section 2 would be appropriate:

- requires one medical recommendation
- lasts up to 72 hours
- during that time, if a second Medical Recommendation is made, the Section 4 converts into a Section 2
- grounds for the application as for Section 2
- must be stated that it is of urgent necessity for the patient to be admitted and that compliance with the usual Section 2 requirements would involve 'undesirable delay'.

Section 5(2) (Doctor's Holding Power)

A voluntary patient in hospital can be legally detained there for up to 72 hours if a registered medical practitioner provides the Mental Health Act Managers with an appropriate report.

- There is no provision to extend.
- The Section ends when an assessment has been completed as to whether admission under another Section is required.

Section 5(4) (Nurse's Holding Power)

A voluntary patient in hospital can be legally detained for up to six hours if it appears to a suitably qualified nurse that the patient is suffering from mental disorder to such a degree that it is necessary for his health or safety or for the protection of others for them to be immediately restrained from leaving the hospital and that it is not practicable to secure the immediate attendance of a medical practitioner for the purpose of furnishing a report under Section 5(2).

- The nurse records in writing that the conditions are met and the written record has to be conveyed to the Mental Health Act Managers as soon as possible.
- There is no provision for extension.
- Section ends when a doctor who is entitled to impose a Section 5(2) arrives.
- The 72-hour period of the Section 5(2) starts from the time of the original Section 5(4) report by the nurse.

Section 35

Magistrates or the Crown Court can send a person to hospital for 28 days, renewable at 28-day intervals for up to a maximum of 12 weeks, for a report to be prepared on his/her mental condition, instead of remanding the person to prison.

- Court satisfied that the accused person may have at least one of the four types of mental disorder.
- Evidence supplied by one approved doctor.
- Specific hospital is willing and able to admit within 7 days.

Section 36

Crown Court sends a person to hospital for 28 days renewable at 28-day intervals for up to a maximum of 12 weeks for treatment, instead of remanding the person to prison.

- Court satisfied that the accused person has a mental illness or severe mental impairment.
- Evidence supplied by two doctors (at least one approved).
- Specific hospital willing and able to admit within seven days.

Section 37 (Hospital Order)

Magistrates or Crown Court can send a person to hospital for 6 months, renewable for a further 6 months and then annually, for treatment, when otherwise the outcome might have been a prison sentence.

- Court satisfied that they have a specified type of mental disorder.
- Evidence supplied by two doctors agreeing on at least one of the types of mental disorder.
- Other conditions as Section 3.
- Specific hospital willing and able to admit within 28 days.

Section 38 (Interim Hospital Order)

This Section can be made prior to deciding whether to make a Hospital Order under Section 37 or whether to deal with an offender in some other way.

- Prisoner must have been convicted of an offence (other than murder) for which imprisonment is a possible penalty.
- Court satisfied that one of the four forms of mental disorder applies and there is reason to suppose that Section 37 may be appropriate and a specific hospital will admit within 28 days.
- Up to 12 weeks initially, renewed by the Court for periods of 28 days, up to a maximum of 12 months in total.

Section 41 (Restriction Order)

Crown Court making a Section 37 can impose restrictions on the patient's discharge. Leave granted only with the agreement of the Secretary of State (Home Office). The Home Office, in addition to the RMO, can recall the person from leave.

Section 47

Home Office, using powers given to the Secretary of State, can make a **Transfer Direction**, to transfer a prisoner to hospital for treatment:

- prisoner has at least one type of mental disorder
- reports from two doctors (one approved)
- mental disorder stipulations as for Section 3
- Home Office must be of the opinion that a transfer is expedient in the circumstances, having regard to the public interest.

Section 48

People remanded in custody by a magistrates' court or suspected of being illegal immigrants. Must have a mental illness or severe mental impairment and be in urgent need of the treatment which is to be provided.

Section 49 (Restriction Direction)

This prevents discharge in the same way that Section 41 restricts the discharge of someone detained under Section 37. Can be used with Section 47 or Section 48 where the person has been remanded in custody by a court.

Section 57 (Treatment requiring consent AND a second opinion)

Any surgical operation for destroying brain tissue, its functioning, or the surgical implantation of hormones for the purposes of reducing the male sex drive.

- Three people (doctor and two non-doctors, appointed by Mental Health Act Commission) certify that the patient is capable of understanding the nature, purpose and likely effects of the treatment and has consented to it.

Section 58 (Treatment requiring consent OR a second opinion)

This includes medication for the person's mental disorder three months after they first had the treatment during their current period of detention.

In the first three months the treatment can be given without consent or Section 58 (the three months start when medication is first given and the 'clock keeps running' even if there is a break in the medication, the Section is renewed or the type of medication changes). This Section also covers electroconvulsive therapy (ECT).

Section 62 (Urgent Treatment)

Treatment immediately necessary to save the patient's life and to prevent a serious deterioration in the patient's condition can be given urgently and Section 57 or Section 58 arrangements made later.

Section 117

Statutory authorities (eg social services) have a duty to make arrangements for a person's continuing support and care.

- Applies to detention under Sections 3, 37, 47, or 48.
- Steps have been taken to improve aftercare planning, for example, by the appointment of a Key Worker under the **Care Programme Approach**.
- The *Mental Health (Patients in the Community) Act 1995*, created **Supervised Discharge** (S25A) whereby a person can be legally required to reside at a certain place and attend for treatment.
- Neither the 1983 Act nor the 1995 Act include any legal power to treat someone in the community against their will.

Section 135

An ASW can seek a warrant from a Justice of the Peace to allow a police officer to enter premises (by force if necessary) to search for someone with mental health problems and take them to a **Place of Safety** (hospital, police station etc). Detention lasts up to 72 hours from the time the person first arrives at the Place of Safety. There is no provision for renewal or extension.

Section 136

This enables a police officer to remove someone from a public place and take them to a Place of Safety to enable examination by a doctor and interview by an ASW and to make necessary arrangements for treatment or care. Lasts up to 72 hours from the time of arrival at the Place of Safety. No provision for this time to be renewed or extended.

Mental Health Act Review Tribunal

The Mental Health Act Review Tribunal was established under the 1959 Mental Health Act as an independent body to review the need for continued detention of those held under the Act.

- Three members: legal chair (must be a judge for restricted patients), medical and lay members.
- Have powers of immediate or delayed discharge of Sections.

Patients discharged from Section by a Tribunal can only be sectioned again if circumstances have significantly changed from those considered by the Tribunal.

S2	Within 14 days.
S3	Within first 6 months, second 6 months if renewed, then annually. Compulsory every 3 years.
S4, S5(2), S5(4) S35, S36	None.
S37 and S41	During second 6 months, then annually. Compulsory every 3 years.
S47, S48 (and S49)	Once in first 6 months, once in second 6 months, then annually.

Table 10.4 Tribunal appeals

Mental Health Act Commission

The Commission was set up under the 1983 Mental Health Act and responsible to the Secretary of State to:

- visit and inspect hospitals, interviewing patients to oversee the use of their detention
- provide second opinion doctors for Sections 57 and 58
- maintain and amend the *Code of Practice*
- investigate complaints
- advise Government
- publish a report biennially.

Further reading

Mental Health Act Code of Practice. Published by the DoH and available in all hospitals.

Chapter 11

Epidemiology

Keith Lloyd

CONTENTS

Epidemiology

Epidemiology is 'the study of the distribution and determinants of health-related states or events in specified populations and the application of this study to control of health problems' (Last, 1988). It focuses on populations rather than individuals and links strongly to the population-based approaches of public health medicine.

The main applications of epidemiology have been:

- the causes, distribution, spread and control of communicable diseases
- the aetiology, distribution, course and outcome of diseases in populations
- the description of population health status
- the evaluation of preventive and treatment interventions and health services
- genetic epidemiology.

POPULATIONS AND SAMPLES

Samples

In every study you will ever see (except for a full decennial census) data presented are based on a **sample** selected from a much larger group called a **population**, eg a random controlled trial of case management for schizophrenia was based on a sample of 700 drawn from the population of all people in the UK with schizophrenia. Because of chance, different samples give different results (**sampling variation**).

Observations

On each of the 700 subjects in the above example, a number of **observations** are made (demographics, severity of illness, service utilisation, adverse incidents, clinical and social outcomes etc).

Variables

Any aspect of an individual that is measured (eg age, sex, diagnosis) is called a **variable**. A variable can be:

- **qualitative**: Either **binary** (male/female) or **categorical** (White, Black African, Black Caribbean, etc)
- **quantitative**: Either **discrete** (number of service contacts) or **continuous** (height, weight, age).

Summarising data

The first step of an analysis is to summarise the data. Qualitative and quantitative data, frequencies, proportions and descriptive statistics are covered in Chapters 4 and 17.

STUDY DESIGN

Choice of study design

- **Define objectives** (what's the question?). There are three main types of study objective:
  - **estimation** of certain feature of the population (what percentage of the population have anorexia nervosa?)
  - investigation of an **association** between a factor of interest (eg snowboarding) and a particular outcome (eg death)
  - **evaluation** of a drug therapy or intervention.
- **Vital statistics**: Occasionally it is possible to answer objectives using vital statistics or other routinely collected health data.
- The choice of study design follows on from the type of question and objectives.

Type of question	Type of study	Type of statistics for binary outcome variable
Diagnosis or diagnostic test	Cross-sectional	Sensitivity/Specificity, predictive value
Prevalence	Cross-sectional survey	Prevalence rate, risk ratio
Aetiology	Case–control study (retrospective)	Odds ratio
Aetiology or prognosis	Cohort study (prospective)	Risk ratio, rate ratio, odds ratio
Therapy or harm	Randomised controlled trials	Numbers needed to treat
Synthesis of evidence	Systematic review or meta-analysis	Pooled effect, odds ratios or relative risks

Table 11.1 Study types and statistics

OBSERVATIONAL STUDIES

Ecological study: correlational study

- **Unit of analysis**: Populations or groups of people, not individuals.
- Example: Demonstrate an **association** between high average sales of cannabis and the occurrence of an unusually high level of psychosis.
- **Problems**: Socio-economic confounding.

Cross-sectional studies

Cross-sectional studies can be surveys or screening studies.

Surveys

- **Uses**: Discovering prevalence to plan services; comparisons with other services/countries, screening, diagnostic tests.
- Associations are often reported as percentages or risk ratios.
- The Epidemiological Catchment Area Study in the USA and the National Surveys of Psychiatric Morbidity are good examples of large surveys yielding useful data about prevalence of disorders.
- **Prevalence**: The total number of cases in the population or the proportion of persons with a particular disease within a given population at a given time.
- **Incidence**: The number of new cases per unit time or the number of new cases of illness commencing, or of persons falling ill, during a specified time period in a given population.

Screening/diagnostic studies

- The development of screening or diagnostic tests involves comparing a new measure against a 'Gold Standard' (a method, procedure, or measurement that is widely accepted as being the best available).
- **Sensitivity**: The proportion of truly diseased persons, as measured by the gold standard, who are identified as diseased by the test under study.
- **Specificity**: The proportion of truly non-diseased persons, as measured by the gold standard, who are so identified by the diagnostic test under study.
- **Predictive value**: The probability that a person with a positive test is a true positive (ie really does have the disease), or that a person with a negative test truly does not have the disease. The predictive value of a screening test is determined by the sensitivity and specificity of the test, and by the prevalence of the condition for which the test is used.
- **Likelihood ratio**: The ratio of the probability that a given diagnostic test result will be expected for a patient with the target disorder rather than for a patient without the disorder.
- **Choosing cut-offs**: This is done by plotting sensitivity against (1 − specificity) using a receiver operating characteristic curve (or ROC curve) when binary outcomes are

derived from a numerical value. In other words, this technique lets you estimate the best cut-off on your scale for determining whether or not someone is a case of, for example, depression.

Screening for a disease in a population

- **Targeted screening**: Is applied to specific groups at risk (eg screening for depression in postnatal mothers).
- **Mass screening**: The whole population is screened (eg neonates for phenylketonuria).
- **Opportunistic screening**: Is the application of a screening test to someone who has consulted for some other reason.

Criteria for a screening programme

- **Disease**:
  - seriousness, prevalence, or severity merits screening
  - course is understood
  - window exists for intervention between detection and overt disease.
- **Diagnostic test**: Should be sensitive, specific, simple, cheap, safe, acceptable and reliable.
- **Diagnosis and treatment**: An effective, acceptable and safe treatment should be available and deliverable.
- **Health economics**: A screening programme for diseases that occur infrequently benefits few individuals but might prevent some deaths. While preventing even one death is important, given limited resources a more cost-effective programme for diseases that are more common should be given a higher priority, because it will help more people.

Case–control study

- Case-control studies can be unmatched or matched.
- The most famous case-control study in medicine is that of thalidomide.
- **Retrospective** comparison of exposures of persons with disease (cases) with those of persons without the disease (controls).
- Associations between exposure and disease outcome are usually reported as odds ratios with confidence intervals.
- The study starts with people who already have a disease, compares them with a group of people similar in all other respects except that they do not have the disease and then looks back in time to see what happened differently to them that might be associated with contracting the disease.

Cohort study

- People without a disease but with differing environmental exposure are tracked over time to see who gets a disease.

- There is follow-up of environmentally exposed and non-exposed defined groups, with a comparison of disease rates during the time covered.
- The most famous example in medicine is Richard Doll's study of smoking in doctors (exposure) with follow-up to see who developed lung cancer (disease).
- **Prospective** study design where one or more groups (cohorts) of individuals who have not yet had the outcome event in question are monitored for the number of such events which occur over time.

	Ecological	Cross-sectional	Case–control	Cohort
Investigation of rare disease	++++		+++++	
Investigation of rare cause	++			+++++
Testing multiple effects of cause	+	++	++++	+++
Measurement of time relationships	++		+	+++++
Direct measure of incidence			+	+++++

Table 11.2 Merits of different observational study designs

Measures of association in case–control and cohort studies
(see Chapter 17)

- **Association**: Statistical dependence between two or more events, characteristics, or other variables. An association may be fortuitous or may be produced by various other circumstances; the presence of an association does not necessarily imply a causal relationship.
- **Odds**: A proportion in which the numerator contains the number of times an event occurs and the denominator includes the number of times the event does not occur.
- **Odds ratio** (OR; also called cross-product ratio or relative odds): A measure of the degree of association. For example, the odds of exposure among the cases compared with the odds of exposure among the controls.
- **Risk ratio** or **Relative risk** (RR): The ratio of the probability of developing, in a specified period of time, an outcome among those receiving the treatment of interest or exposed to a risk factor, compared with the probability of developing the outcome if the risk factor or intervention is not present.

Interpreting odds and risk ratios:

- For a randomised trial, there is strong association if RR or OR > 1.
- For a cohort study, there is strong association if RR > 3 or OR > 4.
- Accept a lower strength of association if there is a serious consequence/outcome to exposure.

- Require a higher strength of association if there is a more trivial consequence/outcome to exposure.
- When outcomes or events are rare, the estimates of RR are similar to those of OR. As the outcomes become more common, this approximation no longer holds.

Probability of:	Ecological	Cross-sectional	Case–control	Cohort
selection bias		medium	high	low
recall bias			low	high
loss to follow-up	high	medium	medium	low
confounding	high	medium	medium	low
time required	low	medium	medium	high
cost	low	medium	medium	high

Table 11.3 Weaknesses of different types of observational study

EXPERIMENTAL STUDY DESIGNS

Randomised controlled trial

A study in which a sample of people drawn from a population are randomly allocated into groups to either receive or not an intervention to answer a research question. Outcomes between the two groups are then measured and compared. Results should contain a calculation of number needed to treat (NNT) and/or number needed to harm (NNH). The **consort** statement gives clear criteria against which to assess a randomised controlled trial.

Effectiveness

A measure of the benefit resulting from an intervention for a given health problem under usual conditions of clinical care for a particular group. This form of evaluation considers both the efficacy of an intervention and its acceptance by those to whom it is offered, answering the question, 'Does the practice do more good than harm to people to whom it is offered?'

Efficacy

A measure of the benefit resulting from an intervention for a given health problem under the ideal conditions of an investigation; it answers the question, 'Does the practice do more good than harm to people who fully comply with the recommendations?'

NEEDS ASSESSMENT

- **Need**: What is beneficial.
- **Supply**: What is available.
- **Demand**: What is asked for.
- **Utilisation**: What is used.
- **Mortality, morbidity, incidence** and **prevalence**: When assessing population health-care needs, an epidemiological approach can establish **incidence** (number of new cases per unit time); **prevalence** (total number of cases in the population); **morbidity** and **mortality**.
- **Actuarial statistics**: Birth rates, death rates, life expectancy, census data can all inform a population-based needs assessment.
- **Deprivation indices** and the above measures are useful in assessing social inclusion or exclusion.

Pathways to care

The concept of **levels** and **filters** is helpful (Goldberg & Huxley, 1992) and should inform the provision of services.

- Level 1: Mental disorder in the community.
- Filter 1: The decision to consult.
- Level 2: Primary-care attenders.
- Filter 2: Detection of mental disorder.
- Level 3: Identified mental disorder.
- Filter 4: Referral to specialist services.
- Level 4: Contact with specialist services.
- Filter 5: The decision to admit.
- Level 5: Inpatient care.

Each filter is harder to pass through than the one before. Ninety-five per cent of all treated mental disorders are managed in primary-care settings. Only 1 in 20 persons in whom a mental disorder is diagnosed is referred to secondary care.

Access to care: a number of factors influence access to care such as: age, sex, gender, ethnicity, socio-economic status and availability of services. A full assessment of these factors is central to the provision of equitable accessible services.

Population-based needs assessment

This process should be central to planning a psychiatric service.

- National, regional, or local.
- Thornicroft & Tansella (2000) set out a process for service planning that should include:
  - establishment of principles based on autonomy, continuity, effectiveness, accessibility, comprehensiveness, equity, accountability, co-ordination, efficiency, user-carer involvement

- clearly defined boundaries
- assessment of current provision
- assessment of need
- a strategic plan to get from current to new provision
- implementation of strategy
- monitoring and reviewing of services.

Individual needs assessment

The individual needs assessment should:

- be systematic
- be standardised, eg Camberwell Assessment of Need, Needs for Care Assessment and Cardinal Needs Assessment
- have broadly similar range of domains that can be summarised as **shares**:
  - symptoms
  - housing
  - activities of daily living
  - recreation, training and occupation
  - employment
  - significant others.

When conducting a needs assessment each of these domains should be covered as part of a multidisciplinary assessment and formulation.

Comprehensive psychiatric service

A comprehensive psychiatric service should comprise the following:

- **Primary care**
  - Close working with primary-care team who manage 95% of psychiatric morbidity.
  - Focus of work is on severe mental illness but needs to address explicitly strategies and responsibilities for common mental disorders.
- **Secondary care**
  - Acute versus recovery/ongoing care.
  - Home-based.
  - Day-based.
  - Residential.
  - In each domain a range of provision is required.
  - Outpatient and community services.
  - Day services.
  - Inpatient services.
  - Other residential services.
  - Services for special groups.
  - Social and welfare support.
  - Liaison with other agencies.
- **Tertiary care**
  - Access to a range of specialist services on a regional basis.

QUESTIONNAIRE DESIGN

Questionnaires can be structured, semi-structured, or open-ended, self-report or interviewer-rated, face-to-face, or telephone- or web-administered.

Structured questionnaire

- Fixed standardised questions.
- Batteries of questions.
- No variation in wording or layout.
- An example is the General Health Questionnaire.
- Unambiguous, easy to count.
- May miss key information and force a choice.
- Administered in a set order.

Semi-structured

- Mainly fixed responses.
- Not always administered in a set order.
- Less reliance on response codes.
- Scope to record open-ended responses.

Psychometric validation

The process of assessing an instrument for reliability and validity.
Reliability: Test–retest, inter-rater, internal consistency, multiple form, split half.
Validity: Face, content, criterion, construct, precision.

UNSTRUCTURED (OPEN-ENDED) INTERVIEWING

This is an important tool in qualitative research. Its purpose is to determine the meaning individuals assign to events and the complexities of behaviour, beliefs, attitudes and experience in a social context.

- Use **main questions** (to guide interview), **probes** and **follow-ups**.
- Content of interview is largely determined by respondent not interviewer.
- Data usually taped, transcribed and coded using an explicit set of coding rules.

SOME CLASSIC PAPERS IN PSYCHIATRIC EPIDEMIOLOGY

Brown, G. W. & Harris, T. O. 1973. 'Life-events and psychiatric disorders. 1. Some methodological issues.' *Psychological Medicine*, 3, 74–87.

Faris, R. E. & Dunham, H. W. 1939. *Mental disorders in urban areas*. Chicago: Chicago University Press.

Frank, E., Kupfer, D. J., Perel, J. M. *et al*. 1990. 'Three year outcomes of maintenance therapies in recurrent depression.' *Archives of General Psychiatry*, 47, 1093–1099.

Geddes, J., Freemantle, N., Harrison, P. & Bebbington, P. 2000. 'Atypical antipsychotics in the treatment of schizophrenia: systematic review and meta-regression analysis.' *British Medical Journal*, 321, 1371–1376.

Goldberg, D. & Huxley, P. 1992. *Common mental disorders: A bio-psychosocial model*. London: Routledge.

Harrison, G., Owens, D., Holton, A., *et al*. 1988. 'A prospective study of severe mental illness among Afro-Caribbeans.' *Psychological Medicine*, 18, 643–657.

Kendler, K. S., Thornton, L. M. & Gardner, C. O. 2001. 'Genetic risk, number of previous depressive episodes, and stressful life events in predicting onset of major depression.' *American Journal of Psychiatry*, 158(4), 582–586.

Kessler, R. C., McGonagle, K. A., Zhao, S., Nelson, C. B., Hughes, M., Eshleman, S. & Wittchen, H. U. 1994. 'Lifetime and 12–month prevalence of DSM-III-R psychiatric disorders in the United States. Results from the National Co-morbidity Survey.' *Archives of General Psychiatry*, 51(1), 8–19.

Kessler, R. C., Berglund, P., Demler, O. *et al*. 2003. 'The epidemiology of major depressive disorder results from the National Co-morbidity Survey Replication (NCS-R).' *JAMA*, 289, 3095–3105.

Last, J. M., 1988. *A Dictionary of Epidemiology, 2nd ed*, World Health Organisation. New York: Oxford University Press.

Lewis, G., Hawton, K. & Jones, P. 1997. 'Strategies for preventing suicide.' *British Journal of Psychiatry*, 171, 351–354.

Marder, S. R. & Meibach, R. C. 1994. 'Risperidone in the treatment of schizophrenia.' *American Journal of Psychiatry*, 151, 825

Mcguffin, P., Katz, R., Watkins, S. & Rutherford, J. 1996. 'A hospital based twin register of the heritability of DSM-IV uniploar depression.' *Archives of General Psychiatry*, 53, 129–136.

Odegaard, O. 1932. 'Emigration and insanity.' *Acta Psychiatrica Scandanavica*, Suppl. 4.

Parkes, C. M. 1970. 'The first year of bereavement. A longitudinal study of the reaction of London widows to the death of their husbands.' *Psychiatry*, 33, 444–467.

Robins, L. N. 1978. 'Sturdy childhood predictors of adult antisocial behaviour: Replications from longitudinal studies.' *Psychological Medicine*, 8(4):611–622.

Rutter, M., Tizard, J., Yule, W. *et al*. 1976. 'Isle Of Wight Studies' 1964–1974. *Psychological Medicine*, 6, 313–332.

The Cochrane Library, Issue 4, 2003. Chichester: John Wiley & Sons, Ltd.

Thornicroft, G. & Sartorius, N. 1993. 'The course and outcome of depression in different cultures: 10–year follow-up of the WHO Collaborative Study on the Assessment of Depressive Disorders.' *Psychological Medicine*, 23, 1023–1032.

Thornicroft, G. & Tansella, M. 1999. *The mental health matrix: A manual to improve services*, Cambridge: Cambridge University Press.

Vaughn, C. E. & Leff, J. P. 1976. 'The influence of family and social factors on the course of psychiatric illness.' *British Journal of Psychiatry*, 129, 125–137.

Weissman, M. M., Bland, R. C., Canino, G. J. et al. 1996. 'Cross national epidemiology of major depression and bipolar disorder.' *JAMA*, 276, 293–299.

Chapter 12

Psychiatric Disorders

Chris Fear

CONTENTS

Psychiatric Disorders

CLASSIFICATION AND DIAGNOSIS

Diagnoses are constructs used to describe common aggregations of symptoms and are essential in understanding course, prognosis and treatment. Before operationalized diagnostic criteria (1960s), diagnoses lacked reliability. For example, the US/UK study (1972) and International Pilot Study of Schizophrenia (WHO, 1973) showed that the different prevalence of schizophrenia in the USA, UK and USSR was the result of different diagnostic criteria.

Classification can be by categories (these are familiar, easy to understand/remember/use, relate diagnosis to management, and are clear-cut) or dimensions (these are more informative, flexible, and have no artificial boundaries). Various diagnostic systems have culminated in two current systems. Both are **categorical** and **multiaxial**:

- **International Classification of Disease** (ICD-10: WHO 1992)
  - International, covering all recognised diseases.
  - Alphanumeric system: letter F denotes psychiatric disease, numbers indicate narrower diagnostic groups, course over time or characteristic features.
  - The letter X, Y or Z is added to denote additional circumstances or symptoms.
- **Diagnostic and Statistical Manual of Mental Disorders** (DSM-IV: American Psychiatric Association, 1994)
  - National (USA), only mental disorders.
  - Numeric system with additional numbers clarifying and narrowing diagnostic criteria.

Dimension	ICD-10	DSM-IV
Psychiatric clinical disorders	Axis I	Axis I
Personality disorders and learning disability	Axis I	Axis II
General medical conditions	Axis I	Axis III
Psychosocial and environmental problems	Axis III	Axis IV
Disability (Global Assessment of Functioning)	Axis II	Axis V

Table 12.1 Dimensions of classification systems

SCHIZOPHRENIA

Chronic disorders characterised by distortions of thinking, perception, affect and cognition and affecting the most basic aspects of personality and social functioning.

History of ideas

1850	Morel	Démence précocé
1868	Kahlbaum	Catatonia
1871	Hecker	Hebeprenia
1896	Kraepelin	Dementia praecox
1911	Bleuler	Schizophrenia, 'splitting of mental functions', 'primary symptoms' of ambivalence, association, affect and autism
1913	Jaspers	Un-understandability of mental processes
1939	Langfeldt	Process schizophrenia, schizophreniform illness
1959	Kurt Schneider	Symptoms of the First Rank
1960s	Rosenhan, Scheff	Social labelling theory
	Szasz, Laing	Antipsychiatry movement
	USA, USSR	Clinical and political abuse of the diagnosis

Standardising diagnosis

1972	Feigner	St Louis diagnostic criteria
1975	Spitzer	Research Diagnostic Criteria
1980	American Psychiatric Association	DSM-III

Classification

ICD-10	DSM-IV		
F20.0	Paranoid schizophrenia	295.30	Schizophrenia: Paranoid type
F20.1	Hebephrenic	295.10	Disorganised type
F20.2	Catatonic	295.20	Catatonic type
F20.3	Undifferentiated	295.90	Undifferentiated type
F20.4	Post-schizophrenic depression		
F20.5	Residual	295.60	Residual type
F20.6	Simple schizophrenia		
F20.8	Other schizophrenia	295.40	Schizophreniform disorder
F21.0	Schizotypal disorder		
F22.0	Persistent delusional disorder	297.1	Delusional disorder
F23.x	Acute and transient polymorphic psychotic disorder ...	298.8	Brief psychotic disorder
F24	Induced delusional disorder	297.3	Shared psychotic disorder
F25.0	Schizoaffective disorder, manic type	295.70	Schizoaffective disorder: Bipolar type
F25.1	depressive	295.71	Depressive type
F25.2	mixed type		

Table 12.2 Classification of schizophrenia

Crow's (1980) classification:

- Theoretical notion of underlying pathology
  - ○ Type I: positive symptoms, good response to neuroleptics, related to dopamine receptor hyperactivity
  - ○ Type II: negative symptoms (may be positive at presentation), poor response to treatment, related to neurological damage.

Liddle's (1987) three syndromes of schizophrenia:

- **Disorganisation**: formal thought disorder, inappropriate affect, bizarre behaviour
- **Psychomotor poverty** (negative syndrome): poverty of speech, blunted affect, reduced motor activity
- **Reality distortion**: delusions and hallucinations.

Clinical picture

Positive symptoms include delusions, hallucinations and thought alienation phenomena deriving from abnormal mental processes. Negative symptoms are a reduction or loss of mental process.

Typical presentation is at age 20–24 years with a history of withdrawal or bizarre behaviour reflecting the psychopathology, often following a prodromal period. There is commonly co-morbid substance use or a recent life-event.

ICD-10	DSM-IV
One month or more	One month or more
At least one of:	Bizarre delusions or third person
Thought alienation and thought echo	hallucinations/running
	commentary
Delusions of control, passivity	or
experiences, or delusional perception	Two or more of:
Auditory hallucinations discussing the	Delusions
patient, coming from another part of the	Hallucinations
body or giving a running commentary	Disorganised speech
Persistent delusions that are 'culturally	Grossly disorganised or
inappropriate and completely impossible'	catatonic behaviour
or	Negative symptoms
Symptoms from two of:	
Persistent hallucinations in another	
modality with non-affective fleeting	
delusions/over-valued ideas or every	
day for 'weeks or months on end'	
Thought disorder with incoherence, irrelevant	
speech or neologisms	
Catatonic behaviour	
Negative symptoms	

Table 12.3 Criteria for schizophrenia

Epidemiology

- **Prevalence**: 1.4–4.6/1000 population at risk.
  - high in north Sweden, Finland, Croatia, western Ireland (high migration away)
  - low in Hutterites (a religious sect in South Dakota) and Pacific islanders.
- **Annual incidence**: 0.16–0.42/1000 population at risk: usually cited as 15–30/100,000. Higher in men to age 35 years and women over age 40.
- **Morbid risk**: about 1%.
- **Onset**: peak in men is 20–24 years, later in women; median: men 28 years, women 32 years; there is a small peak in the 40–50-year-olds.
- **Comorbidities**:
  - substance misuse
  - cigarette-smoking (two- to three-fold)
  - 46–80% inpatient, 20–43% outpatient medical conditions (7% life-threatening)
  - diabetes, coeliac disease, porphyria, epilepsy
  - ischaemic heart disease, arteriosclerosis
  - genetic abnormalities
  - reduced rate of rheumatoid arthritis.

Aetiology

Physical aetiology

- **Genetic linkage** is the most significant risk factor.
  - Monozygotic twin – 46%.
  - Two affected parents – 48%.
  - Sibling/dizygotic twin – 9–12%.
  - Second degree relative – 3–5%.
  - Theories are (i) multiple genes (polygenic model) but a small number (oligogenic), (ii) a single gene with variable penetrance (monogenic), (iii) heterogeneous disorders with their own aetiologies.
  - Loci on chromosomes 1, 6, 8, 10, 13, 15, and 22 have been reported.
  - Twin studies (Gottesman & Shields, 1972) have shown 46% concordance in monozygotic twins, 14% in dizygotic twins.
  - Adoption studies (Heston & Denny, 1968; Kety et al, 1994) have shown that adopted-away children of schizophrenics have higher rates of illness compared with control adoptees. Based on 'schizophrenia spectrum disorder'.
- **Dopamine (DA) hypothesis** – overactivity in mesolimbic pathways
  - **For**: amphetamine and disulfiram psychosis (increase DA), action of antipsychotics (decrease DA), post-mortem findings of increased DA receptors, postsynaptic supersensitivity, increased DA levels in nucleus accumbens.
  - **Against**: decreased homovanillic acid (HVA, a metabolite of DA) in cerebrospinal fluid, antipsychotics increase HVA, L-dopa reduces negative symptoms, apomorphine (which increases DA) can improve chronic schizophrenia.
  - Other findings: increased striatal D_2 and D_4 receptors, increased cortical D_1 and D_3, dimerization of D_2, altered DA receptor/G-protein coupling.

- **Serotonin (5-HT) hypothesis** – over-/underactivity
  - **For**: LSD psychosis, efficacy of some neuroleptics mediated through 5-HT.
  - **Against**: no post-mortem evidence.
  - Other findings: increased cortical 5-HT_{1A} and decreased cortical 5-HT_{2A} receptors, relationship of cerebrospinal fluid 5-hydroxy indole acetic acid (metabolite) to negative symptoms.
- Other biochemical theories
  - Noradrenalin under-/overactivity.
  - Glutamate dysfunction: phencyclidine psychosis, altered concentration of metabolites.
  - Gamma aminobutyric acid (GABA), second messengers and neuropeptides.
  - Transmethylation, abnormal melatonin, histamine.
- Other physical factors
  - Larger lateral ventricles, cerebral asymmetry, delayed P300 potentials in schizophrenics and relatives.
  - Hippocampal neurones smaller; fewer synaptic and dendritic markers.
  - Loss of temporal and thalamic volume and hippocampal neurones.

Environmental aetiologies

- Higher incidence of pre/perinatal complications, winter/spring births, second-trimester exposure to influenza/rubella, poorer maternal nutrition
- 25–50% of offspring of schizophrenic mothers show soft signs in childhood (hypotonia, delayed milestones, poor co-ordination/attention/information-processing)
- 'Social drift hypothesis' (Goldberg & Morrison, 1963): schizophrenics gravitate to deprived urban areas
- Urban birth, low socio-economic status families/fathers ('breeder hypothesis': Faris & Dunham, 1939)
- Life events
  - excess in three weeks preceding onset
  - more important in women than men
  - 'high expressed emotion'.
- Immigration (Odegaard, 1932)
  - selective migration
  - stress
  - low social class
  - Surinamese in Holland, Afro-Caribbeans in UK (also high in second generation).
- Marriage – later onset, less severe disorder
- Substance misuse
  - 20–60% co-morbid substance misuse: more than controls
  - causal relationship controversial (eg. Swedish conscript study, Andreason *et al.* 1987)
  - self-medication versus social affiliation.
  - cannabis exposure under age 15 increases risk (Dunedin study).

Psychological aetiologies

- Schizophrenogenic mother (Fromm-Reichmann)
- Cognitive and linguistic deficits
- Concrete thinking (Goldstein)
- Personal constructs invalidated (Bannister, Kelly)
- Defective filter/sensory bombardment (Broadbent)
- Double bind (Bateson)
- Marital skew and schism (Lidz)
- Overarousal as a reaction to stress (Venables)
- Over-inclusive thinking (Cameron).

Differential diagnosis

- Schizophreniform psychosis – less than six months duration
- Schizoaffective disorder
- Delusional disorder
- Affective disorders – mood congruence
- Organic disorders
    - epilepsy (TLE), presenile dementias, neurosyphilis, AIDS, tumour, metabolic (thyroid, hypercalcaemia, Wilson's disease, porphyria)
    - history, physical examination and investigations.
- Substance intoxication
- Alcoholic hallucinosis, amphetamine psychosis, psychosis due to phencyclidine, cocaine, LSD, ecstasy, cannabis
    - Suspicion, history, physical examination & investigations
- Prescribed medication (steroids, dopamine agonists).

Clinical course

Most patients have a lifelong relapsing, remitting pattern of illness but there are no reliable ways of predicting this at onset unless they fall into the 1–4% with a catastrophic illness that progresses rapidly to a defect state. Negative symptoms increase with episodes and chronicity. WHO patterns are:

- 1 Single psychotic episode with complete remission
- 2 Single psychotic episode with incomplete remission
- 3 Two or more episodes with complete remission between
- 4 Two or more episodes with incomplete remission between
- 5 Continuous illness.

There are three stages:

- Early deteriorating (5–10 years)
- Stabilisation
- Gradual improvement.

Prognosis

The prognosis for schizophrenia is as follows:

- 20–26% complete recovery
- 14–24% chronic negative picture
- 50–75% relapsing, remitting course, clinically stable after five years
- 1–4% catastrophic deterioration to negative state
- Suicide: 14–22% over 20 years.

Presentation	Sociodemographic factors	Rehabilitative factors
later onset abrupt onset precipitating life event paranoid schizophrenia (hebephrenia = poor prognosis) affective symptoms	female higher IQ higher social class normal premorbid personality marriage, social integration no family history low expressed emotion	availability and utilisation of family and social support personal skills intelligence good response to medication insight and compliance

Table 12.4 Indicators of good prognosis

Hebephrenic	Catatonic	Simple
Onset age 15–25 Prominent affective symptoms, silliness and inappropriate behaviour Fleeting delusions and hallucinations Mannerisms, grimacing, solitary aloofness Rapid deterioration to negative symptoms Poor prognosis	Marked psychomotor disturbance (waxy flexibility, negativism, bizarre postures etc) May be dream-like oneiroid state, echolalia, echopraxia, stupor Exclude organic disease	Uncertain status Gradual onset of odd behaviour and social withdrawal Develops increasing negative symptoms without ever having delusions or hallucinations

Table 12.5 Subtypes of schizophrenia

Schizoaffective disorder

A disorder in which both schizophrenic and affective features occur. Symptoms are insufficiently severe for diagnosis of one disorder.

- Theories:
    - is schizophrenia or an affective disorder
    - is a unique aetiology

- ○ is a point on a continuum of psychopathology between schizophrenia and affective psychosis ('unitary psychosis')
- ○ is a mixture of disorders including all of the above.
- Must meet criteria for schizophrenia and major affective disorder concurrently
- Sudden onset may lead to initial confusion and perplexity (oneirophrenia)
- Prevalence: it is less common than schizophrenia, but data are lacking
- Annual incidence: 1.7/100,000 (schizomania), 4/100,000 (schizodepression)
- Relatives of patients with schizoaffective disorder are more likely to develop affective disorders and equally likely to develop schizophrenia
- Morbid risk in first-degree relatives: 1.8–6.1%
- Associated with better premorbid functioning than schizophrenia
- Precipitating life event is common
- Outcome is better than for schizophrenia but worse than for affective disorders.

Management

Candidates should be familiar with the NICE guidance on the treatment of schizophrenia and on atypical neuroleptics (www.nice.org.uk). There is also a Cochrane library review of atypical neuroleptics (www.cochrane.org).

Physical management

Neuroleptics are the mainstay of treatment. Better outcomes are associated with good compliance and early commencement. Early intervention services are considered a national priority, covering the age range 15–35 years.

Drugs that block dopamine D_2 receptors are effective in treating positive symptoms but negative symptoms appear to benefit from the modulation of the meso-cortical dopaminergic pathway through serotonin agonism by atypical neuroleptics. Although there is no evidence that atypical neuroleptics are more effective treatments, they have better side-effect profiles and a survey by Rethink (previously National Schizophrenia Fellowship) indicated that patients prefer them.

Adherence (compliance) is a major issue, up to 80% are incompletely adherent

- 10–30% of fully-adherent patients relapse within two years
- 60–70% who stop treatment relapse within one year and 85% within two years
- adherence is increased through the use of depot neuroleptics but only one atypical neuroleptic (risperidone) is available in this form.

Up to 30% of patients are **treatment resistant**, a state that is usually defined as failure to respond to adequate treatment with three neuroleptics. NICE recommendations changed this in 2002 to failure to respond to an 8-week treatment with two different atypical neuroleptics. For these patients, clozapine is recommended and benefits about 30% but has a significant incidence of side-effects including neutropenia, for which regular blood monitoring is required. Other treatments for resistant patients include combinations of neuroleptics, eg clozapine + amilsulpride, or adjunctive treatment with anticonvulsants or lithium, especially if there is a schizoaffective component.

Electroconvulsive therapy (ECT) has been used for schizophrenia, especially catatonic, but is not recommended and benzodiazepines are now first-line for Catatonia.

Psychological management

Psychological management techniques include:

- Cognitive behavioural therapy, which is effective for residual symptoms, especially delusions, hallucinations and a variety of behavioural disturbances
- Voice-hearers' groups
- Family work on expressed emotion
- Social skills training
- Specific work on cognitive deficits.

Social management

- The milieu affects development and expression of negative symptoms.
- Hospitalisation (under Mental Health Act) may be necessary in acute episodes.
- Risk assessment and management.
- Day hospital provision can provide stimulation and reduce negative symptoms.
- No deterioration after five years with properly resourced community care and supported accommodation (TAPS study).
- Assertive community treatment (or assertive outreach) services are a national priority, providing intensive services to the most disabled and difficult to engage.

PARANOID PSYCHOSES (DELUSIONAL DISORDERS)

The term 'paranoid psychosis' is outmoded and now found only in the MRCPsych curriculum, having been dropped from ICD, DSM and all modern texts in favour of 'delusional disorder'.

Classification

Both classificatory systems place it with schizophrenic spectrum disorders. ICD-10 (F22.0) gives examples of delusional content but not classification by subtype. DSM-IV classification is by subtype: erotomanic, grandiose, jealous, persecutory, somatic, mixed and unspecified type. The validity of this is unclear.

The primary feature is a persistent delusional system of 1-month (DSM) or 3-month (ICD) duration. The criteria for schizophrenia are not fulfilled and any schizophrenic symptoms (especially hallucinations) are absent, 'transitory' or 'not prominent'. There must be no significant affective or physical factors. DSM specifies that the delusions are 'non-bizarre' although this is entirely subjective and is used to distinguish them from schizophrenic hallucinations.

Clinical picture

An egocentric view of the world is evidenced by a longstanding delusional system in which strange and inexplicable things are happening to the patient. These may be everyday, but are distressing and there is no objective evidence to support them. The patient has deep emotional investment in the delusion and is preoccupied to the exclusion of other things, constantly searching for evidence to support their world view and bending real experiences to do so. They may act on the delusion and although violence is generally rare it is more common with delusional jealousy. A characteristic feature is that the delusions are encapsulated and the patient is able to function perfectly well in other areas, they only respond when the situation touches on their delusions. It is therefore difficult to estimate the prevalence but this is considered to be a rare disorder.

Erotomanic	Jealous	Somatic	Misidentification
• De Clerambault syndrome • Delusion of being loved by someone uattainable • Often make no effort to contact them but can act out if 'spurned' • May be tactile hallucinations of lovemaking 'incubus syndrome' • May lead to harassment and stalking behaviour, especially in men	• Othello syndrome • Continuum, normal-morbid-delusional jealousy • Heterosexual or homosexual • Emotional abuse, interrogation and following may lead to domestic violence • Homicide/suicide recognised • Alcohol associated • Prognosis poor and may be dangerous to victim	• Monosymptomatic delusional hypochondriasis • Parasitosis (Ekbom syndrome) skin irritation, search for parasites, excoriation of skin differentiate from OCD • Delusional form of body dysmorphic disorder (underlying delusional disorder in some anorexia nervosa) • Delusion of smell with/without hallucination	• Close relative or friend replaced by a double (Capgras) • Strangers have changed appearance to familiar person so as to deceive/persecute (Fregoli) • Doubles of self exist (subjective doubles) • People exchange identities (intermetamorphosis) • Variant described involving inanimate objects • Shared delusional disorder (folie à deux) • Probably represents organic condition with pathology in the right parieto-temporal area • Occasional violence

OCD, obsessive-compulsive disorder.

Table 12.6 Subtypes & eponymous syndromes

Epidemiology

- **Prevalence**: estimated to occur in 0.03% of the population, makes up 1–2% of psychiatric admissions
- **Lifetime risk**: 0.05–0.1%
- **Onset**: middle to late life
- Persecutory is commonest form.

Aetiology

- No apparent genetic link to schizophrenic spectrum disorders
- Familial tendency to avoidant/paranoid/schizoid personality traits
- Organic brain disease can be a cause:
  - head injury
  - dementia
  - amphetamine, cocaine, L-dopa, α-methyldopa.
- Dopamine overactivity in limbic and temporal areas
- Affective disorder
- Psychodynamic theories
  - regression from homosexual phase to primary narcissistic phase (Freud)
  - fixation at paranoid–schizoid position (Klein).
- Cognitive theory of defence against depression.

Differential diagnosis

- schizophrenia
- substance misuse/withdrawal
- obsessive-compulsive disorder (OCD)
- somatoform disorders, hypochondriasis, body dysmorphic disorder
- affective disorder
- organic psychosis.

Management and prognosis

This disorder may be short-lived but is usually chronic with varying degrees of intensity. It is difficult to treat even when help is sought. Neuroleptics are often ineffective (pimozide was recommended for monosymptomatic delusional hypochondriasis but evidence is poor). Cognitive therapy for delusions is partially effective in < 50% and only if initial uncertainty in delusions.

AFFECTIVE/MOOD DISORDERS

Classification

The classification in **ICD-10** (F30–39) is as follows:

- **Depressive**
  - episode vs disorder
  - mild, moderate or severe
  - with/without somatic syndrome.
- **Bipolar**
  - hypomania vs mania
  - hypomanic/manic episode vs bipolar disorder
  - presence or absence of psychotic symptoms
  - depressive, manic, or mixed
  - severity and with/without somatic syndrome.

The classification in **DSM-IV** (296.xx) is as follows:

- Major depressive disorder (episode or recurrent)
- **Bipolar I disorder**
  - manic depressive illness
  - single manic episode
  - most recent episode depressive, hypomanic, manic or mixed.
- **Bipolar II disorder** (296.89)
  - major depression with episodes of hypomania
  - current episode hypomanic or depressed.
- For depression of bipolar I – mild/moderate/severe, with/without psychotic features, full/partial remission.

Clinical picture

Depression

- Triad of emotional/psychomotor/negative belief symptoms
- Depressed mood for most of most days
- Anhedonia (loss of interest/pleasure)
- Loss of energy/fatigue
- Poor concentration/memory
- Loss of confidence/self-esteem
- Sleep disturbance with insomnia (early morning waking) or hypersomnia
- Appetite disturbance with weight change, food tastes odd
- Inappropriate guilt, worthlessness (delusional)
- Nihilistic thoughts
- Thoughts of death or suicide, passive to active planning and behaviour
- Psychotic features (mood congruent delusions, second-person hallucinations)
- Physical complaints (pain, weight loss, insomnia etc).

Hypomania

- Triad of emotional/psychomotor/expansiveness
- Unusual feeling of well-being for at least 4 days
- Restlessness, mildly pressured speech
- Impairment in social/occupational functioning
- Louder, more extrovert.

Mania

- Extension of hypomania
- Elevated/irritable mood
- Grandiosity, pressure of speech and flight of ideas
- Less need for sleep
- Distractibility
- Increase in projects/ideas/social activities
- Psychomotor agitation
- May be aggression, hostility and violence
- Risk-taking behaviour across the range of activities, may jeopardise finances, relationships, work, etc
- Psychotic features include mood congruent (grandiose, expansive) delusions and hallucinations (second person).

Epidemiology

This disorder is increased in classes I, II and V.

Bipolar

- **Prevalence**: lifetime 0.3–1.5%, annual similar due to chronicity
- **Onset**: in teens, range 17–27 years (bipolar I younger)
- Gender distribution is equal
- Co-morbidity common with bipolar I – substance misuse, anxiety and conduct disorders
- Excess of manic episodes late spring and summer
- Disruption of circadian rhythms is a risk factor (shift work, jet-lag).

Depression

- **Prevalence**: lifetime 10–20%, annual 2–5%
- Female : male = 2 : 1
- 50% have features of bipolar spectrum disorders
- 85% have recurrent episodes
- Heritability estimated at 40–70%
- Neuroticism risk for later onset
- Chronic physical illness
- Spring peak for suicide (10–20 times more likely), small peak in October
- May be a seasonal component to episodes (winter).

233

Aetiology

Current theories favour a gene–environment interaction.

Physical aetiology

- Genetic factors are strongly involved as shown by twin and adoption studies
  - incidence in first-degree relatives is 15–20% for bipolar, 10–15% for unipolar
  - 'depression spectrum disorder' (alcoholism and antisocial personality in family)
  - adoption studies link depression in women to an alcoholic genetic diathesis when an adoptive parent is mentally ill, excess substance abuse in biological mothers and alcoholism in relatives
  - twin studies: ratio of incidence in monzygotic to dizygotic twins is 68 : 20%, bipolar 79 : 19%, unipolar 54 : 20% (Bertelsen 1977)
  - interest has been shown in chromosomes 4, 5, 11, 12, 18, 21 and X in bipolar disorder
  - serotonin transporter and tryptophan hydroxlase gene on chromosome 17 have been linked.
- Neurobiological vulnerability programmed into genes by early stressors such as cingulate cortex and amygdale
- Abnormal thyrotropin response
- Weak slow-wave sleep processes
- Monoamine theory of depression
  - reserpine depletes presynaptic amines associated with depression
  - amphetamine causes amine release and euphoria
  - antidepressants increase monoamine transmission
  - evidence is inconclusive, however
  - 5-HT turnover decreases in some depressives (suicide)
  - noradrenaline turnover decreases in depression but increases in mania
  - DA turnover decreases in retarded depression
  - this is supported by typtophan depletion studies
  - it is not supported by cerebrospinal fluid/urine metabolite studies.
- Disordered cortisol regulation – cortisol improves mood and cortisol-releasing hormone antagonists act as antidepressants
- Secondary to physical illness (endocrine, post-infective, neurological, drugs/alcohol)
- Secondary to prescribed medications (steroids, L-dopa, reserpine etc).

Environmental aetiology

- Parental style of critical disapproval, overprotection, control through guilt; but recall may be distorted in retrospect
- Impaired social, family and marital relationships in depression
- Socio-economic stress, low education
- Environmental stress precedes first admission for depression or mania in 80%, and is 50% for subsequent admissions
- Life events – more than in controls over preceding six months

- Depression in women associated with life events, unsupportive husband, unemployment, loss of mother before age 11, 3+ children under 15 at home (Camberwell Study: Brown & Harris).

Psychological aetiology

- Mainly apply to depression, mania seen as 'manic defence'
- Maternal deprivation (Bowlby)
- Learned helplessness (Seligman)
- 'Negative cognitive schemata' and 'cognitive triad' (Beck)
- Loss of love object leading to regression and attack by superego (Freud)
- Dysfunctional attributional style (internal, global, stable for negative events) but cause or consequence of depression?
- 'Response style theory' – women are more likely to be depressed because more ruminative response style. Women are more likely to admit distress while men are more likely to resort to alcohol.

Differential diagnosis

Depressive and manic presentations are generally easy to recognise but milder degrees of depression and hypomania may be more problematic. Consider

- adjustment disorder/acute stress reaction
- physical illness (hypothyroidism, Addison's disease)
- schizophrenia, schizoaffective disorder
- anxiety disorders (OCD, co-morbid anxiety)
- dissociative states
- chronic fatigue syndrome
- organic disorders – substances, dementia.

Course and prognosis

- Most episodes are short but they may last two years untreated
- Typically relapsing and remitting
- Time from first to second episode is longer than that from second to third and shortens until individual cycle is established
- Bipolar patients experience twice as many episodes as unipolar patients over a lifetime
- Chronic residual symptoms (mood, anxiety, somatic) occur in 30% and there is increased risk of recurrence in 25% to 75%
- Long-term definitive recovery is 25% in depression, 16% in bipolar
- Risk of suicide in severe depression 12–19%
- Standardised mortality ratio (risk of death compared with normal population) for suicide:
  - normal population 1.0
  - bipolar disorder 15

- o major depression 20
- o dysthymia 12
- Increasing evidence of cognitive deficits associated with chronicity in bipolar disorder.

Rapid cycling

This specifier can be applied to either bipolar disorder in DSM-IV to indicate four or more distinct episodes occurring in a 12-month period. Prevalence is 5–15% of bipolar disorders, 70–90% are women but it is not linked to the menstrual cycle. Association with hypothyroidism, multiple sclerosis, learning disability, head injury and antidepressant treatment. It has a poorer prognosis. It is not recognised in the ICD-10.

Management

Physical

- **Unipolar depression**
  - o give antidepressant (eg selective serotonin re-uptake inhibitors (SSRI)) at adequate dose for at least eight weeks, continuing with response until remission (return to premorbid self)
  - o if an inadequate response: increase dose (side-effects permitting)
  - o if no response: use an antidepressant from a different group
  - o venlafaxine above 150 mg has been shown to be marginally more effective
  - o response rate 60% (placebo 30%)
  - o can use augmentation strategies with lithium, antidepressant combinations, tryptophan (eosinophilia myalgia syndrome), liothyronine
  - o ECT (see below) is used for severe, life-threatening depression and non-response to drugs where there are physical symptoms. It is more effective in the elderly
  - o 'atypical' disease is said to respond better to monoamine oxidase inhibitors (MAOIs)
  - o continue antidepressants until recovery (4–6 months in uncomplicated first episode in younger person); may need to continue much longer if disease is complicated or resistant. If several episodes, consider life-long prophylaxis.
- **Bipolar depression**
  - o can treat as unipolar but the risk of a switch to hypomania is significant
  - o if switch occurs with one medication, risk of switch with another is 50%
  - o mood stabilisers can be effective, valproate and lamotrigine as adjunctive treatments are more effective than lithium
  - o evidence for olanzapine ('OFC' combination with fluoxetine better and licensed in USA) and quetiapine to be effective.
- **(Hypo)mania**
  - o it is imperative that the acute episode is managed, this usually requires admission as compliance is likely to be poor
  - o neuroleptics or mood stabilisers are first-line treatment
  - o atypical neuroleptics, such as olanzapine and quetiapine, are also mood-stabilising

○ valproate (Depakote) is effective for acute treatment
○ benzodiazepines may be useful as adjuncts
○ mood stabilisation with lithium, valproate, olanzapine (or carbamazepine) should be considered after the first severe episode and continued for three years initially
○ risk of relapse is 80% if treatment is discontinued abruptly within three years (it is better not to start if this is likely)
○ adherence is poorer in younger patients, patients who enjoy being slightly 'high' and patients who feel it dampens their spontaneity or creativeness.

Psychological

- Cognitive therapy was developed for depression and is now also used for mania
- Interpersonal and behaviour therapy are also used
- Compliance therapy may help with medication
- Psycho-education can be aimed at early signs of relapse (prodrome) and 'rainy day plans' in the event of relapse
- Education (anxiety management, support) or counselling sometimes used in primary care for mild 'depressions'.

Social

- Education of families and involvement in prodromal work.
- May benefit from open access to admission, day hospital and assertive community treatment work.

Electroconvulsive therapy (ECT)

Electricity was first used to induce seizures in schizophrenia by Cerletti and Bini (in Rome, 1938). Prior to this, Meduna had used parenteral camphor to induce a seizure in a catatonic patient who then recovered. ECT has since been used for a variety of psychiatric disorders but is only recommended for use in major depression (see Table 12.7). It is occasionally used for intractable mania that is unresponsive to medication and for catatonic schizophrenia (see above). Use for maintenance treatment of depression is not now recommended (see NICE guidance) although this is a controversial area.

Stupor
Nihilistic or paranoid delusions
Marked retardation
Continuing moderate to severe depressive symptoms despite an adequate trial of antidepressants (number of drugs and dosage is arbitrary)
Life-threatening depression due to refusal of food/fluids or severe suicidality
Severe puerperal depression or severe depression during pregnancy
Inability to tolerate drug treatment

Table 12.7 Indicators of positive response to ECT in depression

237

Method of administration

Most trainees will have experience of administering ECT. Patients have a standard anaesthetic and muscle relaxant such as suxamethonium. Seizure duration is monitored using an electroencephalogram (EEG) recording. ECT is usually given bilaterally but if memory disturbances occur it may be given unilaterally to the non-dominant hemisphere. There are various methods of determining stimulus dose, with formulae based upon patient characteristics to give a low initial stimulus following which the dose can be increased to be just supra-threshold. Another method involves estimating the stimulus by taking half the patient's age as percentage of 500 mC. Most machines deliver 25–500 mC in increments of 5 mC. As seizure threshold rises with each fit, the stimulus dose is usually titrated up during a course.

The usual seizure duration is 30–120 seconds. A very short fit (< 15 seconds) is likely to be ineffective, while prolonged seizures (> 180 seconds) may need to be halted with diazepam. Treatments are usually continued until the patient is judged clinically well, initially as twice-weekly treatments but weekly towards the end of the course. An average course is six to eight treatments, rarely fewer than three or more than 12.

Mode of action

The mode of action is uncertain, however, the following have been suggested:

- changing neuroendocrine function through haemodynamic changes
- release of hypothalamic and pituitary hormones
- increasing seizure threshold and thus 'stabilising' the brain in a manner akin to anticonvulsants
- inducing amnesia for early life experiences (psychodynamic)
- interseizure EEG changes.

Contraindications and adverse effects

ECT is a very safe treatment with few absolute contraindications. Patients have to be fit for anaesthesia and should not have raised intracranial pressure, recent brain or cardiac lesion, uncontrolled arrhythmias, or severe hypertension.

Adverse effects are few and usually restricted to headache, muscle pains as a result of the suxamethonium, perioperative confusion and limited amnesia for the treatment and personal events that occurred during the illness. Severity of confusion is proportional to the haemodynamic changes during treatment and is more profound with increasing stimulus. Some patients have difficulty with anterograde memory that wears off over a week or two following treatment. Much has been made of patients claiming to suffer gaps in memory for past events or biographical information. The effects of the illness are likely to have had a bearing on this and most hark back to days when large stimuli were used to induce seizures. There is no evidence that ECT causes severe, permanent memory disturbance.

Other affective disorders

Cyclothymia

Cyclothymia is a disorder of subsyndromal fluctuating mood swings that occur frequently and never reach the severity for depression or hypomania. About 30% of sufferers develop bipolar disorder. It may be prodromal or personality variable. Onset is in early life, and it is more common in the relatives of bipolar patients. Mood stabilisers (eg lithium) and/or cognitive therapy are sometimes effective but prognosis is poor.

Dysthymia

Chronic depression of mood that does not fit the criteria for major depression (although there may be periods of clinical depression). There are periods of feeling well but otherwise chronically brooding, tired, sleep-disturbed and insecure. Onset is in the teens, and it has a chronic course. Lifetime prevalence is 6%, being more common in the relatives of major depressives (may be personality variable). Prognosis is poor but antidepressants, cognitive and individual psychotherapies can be tried.

Seasonal affective disorder

This disorder is popular with some patients and clinicians to explain seasonality in depression, however, it is of low diagnostic validity.

ORGANIC PSYCHOSES

Occur in any condition interfering with cerebral functioning, especially the diencephalon and temporal lobes. Schizophrenia is mimicked in insidious onset conditions (syphilis, AIDS, cerebral abscess, tumour, dementia, thyroid, sarcoidosis, Wilson's disease, epilepsy) but acute presentations are easier to diagnose (substance abuse/withdrawal, acute infection, head injury, epilepsy). Symptoms are typically fleeting and unsystematised with reduced orientation.

See Chapters 16, 20, 22, and 23.

NEUROSES

First coined by the Edinburgh physician William Cullen in 1785 to mean an organic brain disorder (eg epilepsy), the term 'neurosis' has changed to mean a disorder of psychological functioning in which an individual's perceived relationship to the world is normal.

Adjustment disorder

- A reaction to a psychological stressor that bridges normal experience and mental illness. The symptoms are more than those seen in normal reactions; they impair social functioning but do not meet the criteria for a major psychiatric diagnosis.

- Classified by associated symptoms and duration – anxiety, depression (brief or prolonged), conduct, emotion
- No quantification of the stressor; any personally relevant domain or severity
- Accounts for 5–20% of psychiatric outpatients
- In adults the prognosis is good but adolescents are likely to go on to mental illness
- No specific treatment
- Risk of suicide/deliberate self-harm.

Acute stress reaction

- Transient reaction to exceptional physical or mental stress
- Duration up to three days but DSM-IV suggests predisposition to post-traumatic stress disorder (PTSD)
- Initial daze and disorientation followed by anxiety, anger, or depressive symptoms
- May experience brief PTSD symptoms, numbness, detachment, dissociative symptoms
- PTSD diagnosed if symptoms persist
- Level of stress/severity of symptoms less in ICD-10 than DSM-IV
- Differential diagnosis from PTSD, adjustment disorder, head injury, dissociative disorder, brief psychosis
- Incidence 13–17% in road traffic accident survivors, 19% after assault, 33% in witnesses of mass shootings
- Aetiology
  - process of adjustment of self schema to trauma
  - pathological memory network, easily triggered by stress
  - process of 'working through' trauma memory impaired by avoidance
  - dissociative restriction of emotional reaction
  - effect of extreme stress on neurone function.
- Spontaneous remission in 50%
- Specific treatment rarely needed but short-term (days) benzodiazepines most effective (no RCT)
  - occasionally admitted due to bizarreness of presentation
  - observe while drug-free, administer benzodiazepines if indicated.
- Psychological treatments include debriefing and cognitive behaviour therapy
- May progress to PTSD.

Post-traumatic stress disorder

Term coined for Vietnam war veterans, previously 'shell shock', 'survivor syndrome', 'combat neurosis' etc. The characteristic symptoms occur in response to a major stressor. The definition of that stressor is broad in ICD-10 but narrow in DSM-IV (threat to life or physical integrity).

Clinical picture (re-experiencing)

- Nightmares
- Flashbacks – act/feel/witness the trauma in the mind's eye

- Intrusive sensations/images
- May be provoked by similar circumstances/TV representations
- Avoidance of reminders
- Excessive rumination
- Range of emotional symptoms
- Hyperarousal/hypervigilance.

Epidemiology

- Risk after traumatic stressor: 8.1% men, 20.4% women
- Lifetime prevalence: 7.8% (women > men)
- Greater risk in women, Blacks and Hispanics, in those with a family history of mental illness, in those with previous traumatic stressor, in prolonged/repeated trauma, trauma with children involved, higher perceived risk to life/loss of control/threat to autonomy and causal attribution
- Co-morbidity with affective and anxiety disorders, somatisation and substance misuse (secondary); increased prevalence of these plus sociopathy in relatives
- Increased monozygotic v dizygotic twin concordance.

Aetiology

- Classical conditioning to fear
- Other psychological theories as for acute stress (see page 246)
- Thought suppression/avoidance maintains symptoms
- Abnormal hypothalamo–pituitary–adrenal axis
- Dysregulation of noradrenergic/α_2-adrenergic system; sensitisation of 5-HT; endogenous opiate release; increased corticotrophin-releasing factor; DA and GABA also implicated
- Dysfunction of thyroid or amygdala
- Massive stress-induced release of neurotransmitters leads to powerful encoding of memories.

Differential diagnosis

- Adjustment and acute stress reactions, anxiety, depression, OCD, psychosis, substance-induced state.
- Repeated severe trauma may lead to a syndrome of somatisation, dissociation, affective symptoms, impulsive self-destruction and pathological relationships in ICD-10 as F62.0: Enduring personality change after catastrophic experience ('complex PTSD').

Treatment

- Psychological treatment should not be started too early and immediate debriefing may be harmful.
- Cognitive behavioural therapy is most effective with limited evidence for psychodynamic or hypnotherapy. The approach involves anxiety and anger management, cognitive restructuring of negative schemata, education and self-monitoring of symptoms.

- Eye-movement desensitization reprocessing is controversial.
- Evidence for MAOIs and tricyclic antidepressants but SSRIs show most promise (paroxetine and sertraline are licensed in the UK).
- There is some evidence for carbamazepine, propranolol and clonidine.
- Benzodiazepines are ineffective.

Course and prognosis

- 50% recover during the first year.
- 33% are still symptomatic six years later.
- Recovery is helped by social support and positive attitude, ability to discuss and recognise the nature of symptoms.

Generalised anxiety disorder

This covers the remainder of non-specific anxiety states that do not fit into any of the more specific categories.

Clinical picture

- Psychological symptoms of anxiety and worry relating, but out of proportion, to the everyday circumstances of work, family etc.
- Somatic symptoms of tension headaches, urinary frequency, dry mouth, stomach cramps, fatigue, sweating, exaggerated startle etc (sympathetic nervous system).
- Association with atypical chest pain, irritable bowel syndrome.

Epidemiology

- **Prevalence**: 12 months 3–4%; lifetime 5–9%
- Mean age of onset 21 years
- Occurs more in women than men
- Causes increased presentation to GP with physical complaints
- Co-morbidity with other anxiety disorders – 74% have one or more additional lifetime diagnoses.

Aetiology

- 20% first-degree relatives have generalized anxiety disorder, genetics unclear
- 70% environmental factors
- Psychosocial factors
  - traumatic life events
  - disrupted attachment in childhood
  - critical unsupportive early parenting
  - excessive parental control.
- Neurobiology – dysfunctional
  - hypothalamo–pituitary–adrenal axis (cortisol response)
  - autonomic nervous system (noradrenaline)
  - amygdala (threat detection)

- o anxiety mediation through 'behavioural inhibition system' (septohippocampal)
- o GABA$_A$ receptor sensitivity
- o 5-HT regulation and cholecystokinin.

Differential diagnosis

- Normal worry/anxiety
- Physical illness – cardiac arrhythmias, thyrotoxicosis, hypoglycaemia, hyperparathyroidism, TLE, respiratory disease, phaeochromocytoma etc
- Drugs, alcohol, caffeine, prescribed medication – side-effect or withdrawal
- Other anxiety disorders
- Depression.

Management

- Psycho-educational approach
- Cognitive behaviour therapy
- Antidepressants at low dose to start and increasing; begin taper six months from recovery (eg imipramine, venlafaxine)
- Short-term benzodiazepines as an adjunct to psychological treatment
- Buspirone.

Course and prognosis

- Chronic and disabling
- Higher rates of unemployment and marital dysfunction
- Remission 15% at 1 year, 27% at 3 years with treatment
- Remission with co-morbid mental illness 8% and 17% at 1 year and 3 years, respectively.

Panic disorder (and agoraphobia)

Clinical picture

Panic attacks are periods of intense anxiety symptoms beginning abruptly and usually reaching a peak over about 10 minutes before subsiding within minutes. They involve all the autonomic and somatic features of severe anxiety and are so severe that the patient feels they are going to die, have a heart attack, or go mad. They often try to flee the situation or seek help through emergency services. The attack is followed by worry and ruminations about recurrence and the possibility of dying during a further attack. Variants include **nocturnal panic attacks** that occur during, and wake a patient from, sleep. **Non-fearful panic attacks** comprise the physical symptoms without the anxiety/fear and often present with cardiac symptoms.

Epidemiology

- **Prevalence** of panic attacks is 7–9%
- **Panic disorder**: lifetime occurrence is 1.5–2.5%, annual occurrence is 1%

- Ratio of women to men is 3 : 1.5
- **Peak of onset**: 15–24 and 45–54 years, rare over 60
- Associated with separation (any cause) and living alone, early parental loss and abuse, poor education, urban living.

Aetiology

- Up to 40% in first-degree relatives, increased concordance in monozygotic twins
- Childhood loss/trauma, continuity with childhood anxiety
- Precipitating life events
- Dependent personality traits.
- Dysfunctional GABA, 5-HT, noradrenaline, cholecystokinin systems

Differential diagnosis

- OCD, specific phobias, agoraphobia, generalised anxiety disorder (occurs with excessive worry)
- Medical illness – cardiac, respiratory, epilepsy, endocrine (thyroid, phaeochromocytoma, carcinoid syndrome, diabetes)
- Prescribed and illicit drugs (amphetamine, caffeine, steroids, alcohol withdrawal)
- Psychological relationship to phobias.

Treatment

- Tricyclics, MAOIs, SSRIs and benzodiazepines are all effective (75%)
  - citalopram and paroxetine are licensed in the UK
  - alprazolam has RCT evidence but problems of benzodiazepines.
- Behavioural and cognitive behavioural therapies are useful first-line treatments or as adjuncts to drugs
- No evidence for psychodynamic therapy.

Course and prognosis

- Often becomes chronic and stable with phobic aspect from circumstances in which panic first occurs
- 10–30% recover over five years, 50% become chronic, mild, stable
- Longer duration but less severe (less co-morbid depression, agoraphobia in men).

Agoraphobia (see Table 12.8)

This classification reflects the American view that panic is primary and that agoraphobia occurs with it as a consequence of where the first panic attack happened. DSM-IV sees the condition of agoraphobia without a history of panic as representing a milder form in which the panic disorder criteria are not satisfied. This condition is a phobic disorder in ICD-10. There is little work on agoraphobia without panic and, as most research on panic disorder uses DSM-IV, it could be said not to exist as a researched entity.

For agoraphobia see panic disorder (see page 249).

ICD-10	DSM-IV
In F40 Phobic anxiety disorders: F40.00 Agoraphobia without panic disorder F40.01 Agoraphobia with panic disorder In F41 Other anxiety disorders F41.0 Panic disorder [episodic paroxysmal anxiety]	In Anxiety disorders: 300.22 Agoraphobia without history of panic disorder 300.21 Panic disorder with agoraphobia 300.20 Panic disorder without agoraphobia

Table 12.8 Classification of agoraphobia

Social phobia

Clinical picture

Incapacitating levels of psychological and somatic anxiety in social situations or where they may be evaluated by others. Perfectionistic, exacting personal style leading to anxiety reinforced by a performance that cannot meet the standard.

Epidemiology

- **Prevalence**: 2.4–13.3% (lifetime), 7.9% (annual)
- **Onset** peaks before 5 years and 11–15 years, presentation around 30 years
- Occurs in more women than men but equal numbers present for treatment
- Lifetime co-morbidity with one or more psychiatric disorder 81% (anxiety disorder, depression, substance abuse).

Aetiology

- Genetic and environmental
- 16% in first-degree relatives
- Twin concordance: monozygotic 25%, dizygotic 15%
- Psychosocial conditioning.

Differential diagnosis

- Normal social anxiety
- Other anxiety disorders
- Avoidant personality disorder
- Self-consciousness over appearance/dysmorphophobia.

Treatment

There is evidence that SSRIs and MAOIs, also benzodiazepines, buspirone and β-blockers, give symptomatic relief. Exposure (with cognitive restructuring), cognitive behavioural therapy, social skills training and relaxation strategies are effective psychological treatments.

Course and prognosis

It is probably chronic and lifelong, leading to impairment in social, educational and occupational achievements.

Specific phobias

- Psychological and somatic symptoms of anxiety in the presence of a phobic object or stimulus, which is avoided wherever possible. DSM-IV has five categories: animals, natural environment, blood/infection/injury, situational, other.
- **Prevalence**: lifetime 11.3%, annual 8.8% (environmental > animal > blood/infection/injury)
- **Age of onset**: animal, 7 years; blood, 9 years; dental, 12 years; claustrophobia, 20 years;
- Occurs more in women than men
- Co-morbidity with affective, anxiety, substance misuse 83%
- First-degree relatives 31%, concordance in twins is monozygotice 26%, dizygotic 11%
- Theories on causes are: unconscious Oedipal fears (Freud – 'Little Hans') versus classical conditioning (associate negative experience with object), evolutionary advantage to avoid harm
- Differential diagnosis from other anxiety disorders, OCD, dysmorphophobia
- Chronic course but usually adapt; seek help when aspects of life are threatened (eg air travel)
- Treatment as social phobia but mainly psychological.

Obsessive-compulsive disorder

Clinical picture

Obsessions are intrusive, repetitive, ego-dystonic thoughts that are unpleasant and produce anxiety but are recognised as the product of a person's own mind (unlike schizophrenic thought alienation). Compulsions are repetitive, eg dystonic, goal-driven behaviours that have to be performed to prevent anxiety. Both are experienced as irrational and resisted, although resistance diminishes with chronicity. As resistance diminishes, obsessions may appear increasingly as overvalued or delusional ideas.

Epidemiology

- **Prevalence**: lifetime 2.5%, annual 1.5–2.1%
- **Age of onset**: 6–15 years in men, 20–29 years in women
- Ratio of men to women is 1 : 1.

Obsession	Compulsion
Dirt, germs, contamination, sticky substances, urine, faeces	Washing/avoiding
Causing an accident through omission	Checking
'Just-rightness', magical protection	Ordering, arranging, eating, dressing, hoarding
Causing a disaster through thought	Magical thinking, prayer rituals, mantras
Intrusive distressing thoughts of harming others, abusing children, sexual or aggressive acts	Obsessive thought rituals, resistance, neutralising thoughts

Table 12.9 Obsessive-compulsive disorder

Aetiology

- 35% of first-degree relatives are affected, higher monozygotic twin concordance
- Principal biochemical theory involves dysregulation of 5-HT and/or DA
  - therapeutic response to serotonergic drugs (eg SSRIs, fenfluramine, clonidine)
  - symptoms worsened by 5-HT antagonists
  - improvement with treatment correlates with pretreatment platelet serotonin levels
  - inconsistent findings of increased 5-hydroxyindoleacetic acid in cerebrospinal fluid
  - benefit of adding dopaminergic drugs in some OCD
  - obsessive symptoms in DA-mediated disorders (post-encephalitic parkinsonism).
- Other biological theories include:
  - autoimmune condition affecting basal ganglia (OC symptoms in 70% of Sydenham's chorea as a result of rheumatic fever)
  - smaller caudate nucleus
  - dysfunction of frontal/limbic/basal ganglia/thalamic circuit.
- Psychological theories include:
  - conditioned stimulus in which compulsive behaviours serve to reduce anxiety
  - regression from oral to anal phase with ambivalence and associated ego defence mechanisms of magical undoing, isolation and reaction formation.

Differential diagnosis

- OCD symptoms are common in other conditions, eg depression, postnatal depression, other anxiety disorders, schizophrenia, Tourette syndrome, autism and organic brain disease. The primary pathology must be identified.
- Distinguished from schizophrenia as obsessive thoughts are ego-dystonic, owned and resisted. Delusions are ego-syntonic and derived from external experience.
- 15% of schizophrenics satisfy the diagnostic criteria for OCD but psychosis trumps neurosis and the presence of OCD symptoms indicates poorer prognosis
- Distinguish from normal worries and superstitions

- OCD spectrum disorders include dysmorphophobia, hypochondriasis, trichotillomania, morbid jealousy
- Anancastic and schizotypal personality disorder.

Treatment

- Drug treatments:
  - SSRI or clomipramine at high-dose for 12 weeks
  - different SSRI or clomipramine as above
  - combination with neuroleptic, SSRI + clomipramine, or addition of lithium, trazodone, buspirone or tryptophan
  - atypical neuroleptics, thyroxine, clonidine, MAOI, intravenous clomipramine, clonazepam.
- Behavioural and/or cognitive therapy essential
- ECT or neurosurgery in resistant cases (failure of adequate drug treatment and 16+ hours of cognitive behavioural therapy).

Course and prognosis

- A chronic disorder, arising suddenly in early adult life (occasionally childhood) but presenting 10+ years after onset
- 20–30% show significant improvement, 40–50% a moderate improvement, 20–40% become chronic
- Poor prognosis indicated by childhood onset, poor social adjustment, precipitating life event, episodic symptoms, personality disorder, failure to resist symptoms, and co-morbid depression.

DISSOCIATIVE AND SOMATOFORM DISORDERS

Classification (see Table 12.10)

Emphasis in DSM-IV is on the difference between dissociation as a disruption of consciousness and conversion, in which physical symptoms are manifested (somatoform).

Aetiology

- Increased incidence in first-degree relatives; no twin studies
- Personality
  - hysterical and extroversion in dissociation
  - neuroticism and negativity in hypochondriasis.
- Psychological theories
  - conversion of emotional energy to physical symptoms, avoidance of 'direct coping', unresolved oedipal conflicts (Freud – hysteria), repression of instinctual wishes and drives
  - 'sick role' (Parsons), 'illness behaviour' (Mechanic), primary and secondary gain, non-verbal communication (Pilowsky) especially in alexothymia
  - life events.

ICD-10	DSM-IV
F45 Somatoform disorders	**Somatoform disorders**
F45.1 Somatization disorder	300.81 Somatization disorder
F44 Dissociative [conversion] disorders	
F44.4 Dissociative motor disorders	F300.11 Conversion disorder with motor symptoms or deficit
F44.0 Dissociative convulsions	– with seizures or convulsions
F44.6 Dissociative anaesthesia and sensory loss	– with sensory symptoms or deficit
F44.7 Mixed dissociative [conversion] disorders	with mixed presentation
F45 Somatoform disorders	
F45.4 Persistent somatoform pain disorder	307.80 Pain disorder associated with psychological factors
(F54 Psychological or behavioural factors associated with disorders or diseases classified elsewhere)	307.81 Pain disorder associated with both psychological factors and a general medical condition
F45.2 Hypochondriacal disorder	300.7 Hypochondriasis
F45.2 Hypochondriacal disorder	300.7 Body dysmorphic disorder
F44 Dissociative [conversion] disorders	**Dissociative disorders**
F44.1 Dissociative amnesia	300.12 Dissociative amnesia
F44.0 Dissociative fugue	300.13 Dissociative fugue
F44.8 Other dissociative [conversion] disorders (Ganser, multiple personality etc)	300.14 Dissociative identity disorder
F44.2 Dissociative stupor	300.15 Dissociative disorder NOS
F44.3 Trance and possession disorders	300.15 Dissociative disorder NOS
F48 Other neurotic disorders	
F48.1 Depersonalization–derealization syndrome	300.6 Depersonalization disorder

NOS, not otherwise specified.

Table 12.10 Classification of dissociative and somatoform disorders

- Childhood exposure to disabling illness
- Pursuit of physical illness by doctors
- Neurobiological theories
  - patients with dissociative amnesia show reduced peripheral receptor sensitivity and there may be a central mechanism of sensory inhibition
  - deficit of attention in somatisation (arising from limbic system).

Differential diagnosis

- Reasonable attempts must be made to exclude physical illness: the onset of multiple symptoms over age 40 in previously well person is almost certainly physical
- Hypochondriasis (cognitive) versus somatisation (physical symptoms)
- Epilepsy and other organic conditions
- Dissociative disorder, other anxiety disorders, depression, psychosis, OCD, PTSD, substance withdrawal/intoxication
- Factitious disorder, malingering.

Dissociative and conversion disorders

Clinical picture

- To establish a diagnosis there must be:
  - the symptoms should be inconsistent with the nature or extent of the pathology
  - evidence that the patient can do the thing that they deny being able to do
  - psychological trauma proportionate to the condition.
- The classical dissociative state is a fugue, in which an individual travels away from their usual haunts and is found without knowledge of personal details or preceding events. Amnesia and stupor can also occur.
- Conversion symptoms can mimic any motor (tremor, paralysis, seizure, hyperventilation, tics, posturing), or sensory (blindness, deafness, sensory loss, hallucinations) symptoms.
- Globus hystericus is a sense of having something stuck in the throat and being unable to swallow. It usually disappears during eating/drinking. A physical abnormality is present in 80%.
- Astasia–abasia involves unsteady gait and difficulty in standing despite normal leg movements.
- There is a classical 'belle indifference' of unconcern.
- In multiple personality disorder/dissociative identity disorder, the person is apparently taken control of by other identities and is unable to recall information about themselves. The nosological validity is questioned and it may be iatrogenic as such individuals often find themselves the subject of attention.
- ICD-10 recognises trance and possession and these may be included in DSM in the future.

Epidemiology

- Occurs more commonly in women than men (but this has been claimed as observer bias)
- Make up 3–4% of psychiatric consultations
- **Prevalence**: 0.2% (fugue).

Course and prognosis

- Acute onset resolves in 70%.

- Good prognosis for monosymptomatic.
- Chronic with co-morbidity resolves in 30% of cases.

Cultural variations

- *Pibloktoq* (Inuit), *grisi siknis* (Honduras/Nicaragua), *amok* (Western Pacific) are all examples of fugue.
- Dissociative identity disorder in the USA.

Ganser syndrome

Condition of 'approximate answers' (*Vorbereiden*) and confusion, described in prisoners ('prison psychosis').

Depersonalization/derealization

- Depersonalization is experienced by 50% of the normal population and 80% of psychiatric patients.
- It is a dream-like sense of being an outsider 'looking in' on one's activities, or of an alteration in the quality of the surroundings. Occurs in clear consciousness.
- Associated with significant stress, it probably represents an adaptive response.
- Association with organic brain disease suggests a biological basis, possibly in the limbic and parietotemporal cortex.

Somatisation disorder

Clinical picture

Physical symptoms are experienced in the absence of physical pathology, and are attributed to physical illness.

- Symptoms may be vague and unverifiable, an exaggeration of real symptoms (eg pain), excessive worry about real symptoms, or factitious self-inflicted/manufactured symptoms.
- Symptoms may be learned from others either by association or conscious mimicry.
- There may be discrepancy between reported symptoms and behaviour; inconsistent and inaccurate history.
- Patients often undergo multiple tests.
- Consider if vague/complicated medical history, multiple fluctuating symptoms and non-response to treatment.

Epidemiology

- **Onset** is usually pre-30 (from childhood to 35) and emotional symptoms are hotly denied.
- **Prevalence** 1%, 1–6% in primary care, 0.2–2% women, < 0.2% men.
- Makes up 3% of admissions to non-psychiatric wards, median 22-year old admissions.

- Co-morbidity with anxiety and depression, personality style in cluster B (DSM-IV), paranoid personality disorder, passive–aggressive or dependent.

Course and prognosis

Lifelong chronic illness with occasional remission.

Hypochondriasis

- A personality trait versus a psychological illness, primary versus secondary.
- Morbid preoccupation with health, including intrusive thoughts and images, focused attention and seeking of medical attention, with which they become dissatisfied.
- Associated with fear of ageing/death.
- Delusional form is a delusional disorder (monosymptomatic delusional hypochondriasis).
- Occurs in up to 10% of medical patients, prevalence 2–7% in general population.
- No increase in relatives or twins but more somatic complaints, hostility, poor social adjustment and anti-doctor sentiments.
- Young, non-white, female, poor education, low income.
- Co-morbid anxiety, depression and somatisation.
- Chronic, fluctuating course.

Somatoform pain disorder

- Persistent, severe and distressing pain that cannot be fully explained physically and occurs with sufficient emotional or psychosocial problems to explain it.
- Co-morbid anxiety and depression.
- Somatoform disorders occur in up to 50%.
- McGill Pain Questionnaire is used to evaluate.
- Outcome fair but not well evaluated; poorer in those seeking compensation.

Dysmorphophobia

- Also known as **body dysmorphic disorder.**
- Insight poor and delusional form described.
- Occurs in men preoccupied with body build, genitals, and hair loss; in women preoccupied with breasts, hips, and skin.
- **Prevalence**: annual 0.8%, at dermatology clinics 12%; cosmetic surgery occurs in 7–15%.
- Co-morbid with major depression in 60%, lifetime risk 80%; bulimia in women.
- Chronic relapsing remitting course.

Management

See Chapter 20.

EATING DISORDERS

Classification

ICD-10 recognises simply **anorexia nervosa** and **bulimia nervosa** with 'atypical' forms that do not satisfy the criteria fully or represent a milder picture.

DSM-IV recognises:

- **DSM-IV anorexia nervosa**:
  - **restricting type**: weight loss through dieting, fasting or excessive exercise
  - **binge-eating/purging type**: regular binge-eating with self-induced vomiting, laxatives, diuretics or enemas, differs from bulimia on body mass index (BMI).
- **DSM-IV bulimia nervosa**:
  - **purging type**: self-induced vomiting, laxatives, diuretics or enemata
  - **non-purging type**: fasting or exercise.

Clinical picture

Anorexia nervosa	Bulimia nervosa
Body weight at least 15% below expected BMI $\leq$ 17.5 kg/m^2	Weight usually normal but may be slightly under- or over-weight
Self-induced weight loss by avoiding fattening foods	Recurrent episodes of binge-eating, usually large amounts of high-calorie/carbohydrate foods
	Sense of lack of control during binging
Purging by self-induced vomiting, laxatives, enemata, appetite suppressants, excessive exercise and/or diuretics	
Damage to teeth, enlarged salivary and parotid glands, calluses on hands (Russell's sign) as a result of inducing vomiting	
Body image disturbance	
Amenorrhoea or impotence, loss of interest in sex	Menstruation normal or slightly irregular. Hyponatraemia, hypokalaemia, hypochloraemia, metabolic alkalosis due to vomiting
Abnormalities of growth hormone, cortisol, TSH and insulin	
Abdominal pain, cold-sensitive, lethargy, constipation	
Lanugo growth, bradycardia, peripheral oedema, anaemia, osteoporosis	
Delayed puberty if it occurs prepubertally	
Often preoccupied with food and cooking it for others	Often preoccupied with food and cooking

Table 12.11 Characteristics of eating disorders

Epidemiology

	Anorexia nervosa	Bulimia nervosa
Incidence	6–8/100,000 population 0.45–0.64/100,000 hospital inpatients	No reliable data
Prevalence	0.5–1% young women 6.5–7% ballet students 7% models 1% English private schools 0.2% English state schools	Lifetime 1% 1% women aged 16–35 years
Age of onset	8–15 years in children's study Peak 18 years, mean 15 years	
Ratio of women:men	10 : 1	10 : 1
Social class	I and II	I, II, IIINM
Personality disorder	72% meet criteria for 1+ OCD Borderline (40%) Histrionic (40%)	Borderline common

Table 12.12 Epidemiology of eating disorders

Aetiology

Common factors

- Genetics may account for 55–80% of variance.
- Adverse life events.
- Sexual experience
  - childhood sexual abuse in up to 30%
  - normal sexual experience plus conflict.
- Modern 'cult of thinness' in Western cultures (Russell)
  - increased incidence since 1950s
  - dread of fatness.
- Culture-bound syndrome
  - rare in developing world
  - increased incidence in immigrants
  - increased incidence in cultures undergoing rapid change.
- 30% mildly obese before onset and have early menarche.
- Regression to prepubertal asexualized state.
- High personal/parental expectations (neurotic perfectionist), low self-esteem.
  Perfectionism is less frequent in bulimia and vulnerability to obesity may override control.
- Regression to oral fixation.

Specific factors

- **Anorexia**
  - concordance in monozygotic to dizygotic twins = 56% : 7%
  - 4.1% first-degree relatives
  - hypothalamo–pituitary abnormality caused by limbic imbalance (some neuroimaging evidence)
  - parental personality disorder in up to 52%
  - sick role is adopted to avoid family conflicts.
- **Bulimia**
  - preceded by anorexia nervosa in 50%
  - 5-HT dysfunction: depleting brain 5-HT causes recurrence of symptoms in recovered bulimics
  - familial substance misuse and depression.

Differential diagnosis

- Physical illness (malabsorption syndromes, endocrine disorders, malignant disease, gastrointestinal disorders)
- Depression, alcoholism (may be co-morbid)
- OCD
- Personality disorder (borderline, obsessive-compulsive, histrionic).

Course and prognosis

Anorexia follows a long-term course with slow recovery.

- 30% recover in three years and a further 30% in 3–6 years
- at 33 years, the death rate was 18%, annual rate was 0.5–0.75% (54% anorexia, 27% suicide)
- poor outcome associated with older age of onset, chronicity, neurotic childhood traits, personality disorder.

Fifty per cent of bulimics recover with treatment

- 10% still meet criteria at 10 years, 15% have atypical eating disorder
- trend towards recovery, no known predictors of prognosis.

Obesity

- BMI = weight (kg)/height (m)^2: > 25 = obese
- **Prevalence**: 14% men, 16% women
- May represent abnormalities in the leptin system that provides satiety feedback
- Genetics accounts for 70%
- Associated with lower social class and sedentary lifestyle
- Also organic brain disease, medication
- Psychiatrist's role is minimal in management

	Anorexia nervosa	Bulimia nervosa
Drug treatments	Poorly evaluated but many have been tried Treat depression Low-dose neuroleptics for anxiety symptoms	All major groups effective in reducing binging/vomiting No long-term studies Fluoxetine at high dose (60 mg)
Family therapy	Conjoint 1. family meal 2. parents monitor weight improvement 3. patient responsible for continued gains Family counselling	May be useful but not a mainstay
Psychodynamic	Bruch: need to separate patient's autonomy from family ('sparrow in a golden cage') Crisp: supported escape from psychobiological regression to pre-pubertal growth stage	Not evaluated
Cognitive	Effective – challenge dysfunctional cognitions (Fairbairn) No established model	Most effective treatment 15% less drop-out than antidepressants 15–20 sessions over 5 months Reduces dysfunctional behaviours, increases self-esteem and social functioning Interpersonal also effective Exposure/response prevention ineffective
Inpatient	May need to restore weight	For 5% with severe depression no indication for bulimia alone
	Nursing role is supervisory and psychotherapeutic Dietary control to maintain positive energy balance of 1500–2250 kcal., giving weight gain of 200–300 g. daily Standardised weighing in same clothes with an empty bladder MHA can be used but associated with higher mortality risk (more severe, more suicide) Nasogastric feeding can be given compulsorily under a section	
Day hospital	Can be beneficial as part of a psychosocial programme	
Notes	Patient often avoids treatment	Patient usually co-operative

Table 12.13 Management of eating disorders

- Management comprises: (i) behaviour modification, (ii) pharmacotherapy, (iii) surgery
- Course is chronic, average weight increase 1 kg/year.

PERSONALITY AND ITS DISORDERS

Concepts

- Historical definition: 'Deeply ingrained and enduring behaviour patterns, manifesting themselves as inflexible responses to a broad range of personal and social situations' (ICD-10).
- Controversial area, recent work on treating personality disorders together with the concept of enduring personality change as a result of chronic illness/adversity, is challenging this definition.
- Stigmatising: 'Patients psychiatrists loved to dislike' (Lewis & Appleby).
- Treatability criterion for detention under Mental Health Act (legal concept of 'psychopathic disorder').
- Normal/abnormal rate vs disorder. Criterion of causing distress to self/others.

Classification

- Historically classified according to aetiological theory
- Dimensional
  - Jung: dispositions (traits)
  - Ketschmer: ectomorph, endomorph, mesomorph

ICD-10	DSM-IV
F60.0 Paranoid	301.0 Paranoid
F60.1 Schizoid	301.20 Schizoid
(F21 Schizotypal disorder)	301.22 Schizotypal
F60.2 Dissocial	301.7 Antisocial

F60.3 Emotionally unstable
  .30 impulsive
  .31 borderline
	301.83 Borderline

F60.4 Histrionic	301.5 Histrionic
F60.5 Anankastic	301.4 Obsessive-compulsive
F60.6 Anxious (avoidant)	301.82 Avoidant
F60.7 Dependent	301.6 Dependent
F60.8 Other specific	301.81 Narcissistic

Table 12.14 Classification of personality disorders

- ○ Eysenck: extroversion–introversion, neuroticism, psychoticism
- ○ Cloninger: temperament (novelty-seeking, harm avoidance, reward dependence, persistence) and character (self-direction, co-operation, self-transcendence)
- ○ Pilkonis & Frank: 'five-factor model' of openness, conscientiousness, extraversion, agreeableness, neuroticism (OCEAN).
- Categorical
  - ○ ICD and DSM
  - ○ Axis II disorders but move to axis I as biological correlates found (eg cyclothymic PD, schizotypal PD/disorder).

Epidemiology

- 10% population, 20% GP attenders, 30% psychiatric outpatients, 40% psychiatric inpatients
- 7% of all hospital admissions, 8.4% first psychiatric admissions
- Co-morbidity
- 57% affective disorders
- 41% anxiety disorders
- 56% substance abusers
- 50% any axis I.

Individual disorders

Cluster A

- Relationship (familial) to schizophrenia spectrum.
- Differentiate from psychosis, depression.
- Stress decompensation into psychosis, increased risk of schizophrenia.
- **Paranoid:**
  - ○ 0.6%
  - ○ pervasive suspicion and mistrust of others, grudges, jealousy. May be litigious.
  - ○ 'fanatics' (Schneider)
  - ○ co-morbid anxious, narcissistic, schizoid, schizotypal panic disorder.
- **Schizoid:**
  - ○ 0.4%
  - ○ 'shut-in' (Block), autism (Bleuler)
  - ○ cold, reserved, distant, interest in computers/mathematics/philosophy, unconcerned with everday activities and others
  - ○ distinguish from anankastic and anxious panic disorder.
- **Schizotypal:**
  - ○ 0.6%
  - ○ an axis I diagnosis in ICD
  - ○ pre-schizophrenic (Kretschmer)
  - ○ like schizoid but eccentric, odd behaviour, magical thinking and pseudohallucinations
  - ○ high co-morbidity with depression; Asperger's, autism.

Cluster B

- **Dissocial (Antisocial)**
  - 3%, M : F = 2–7 : 1
  - manie sans délire (Pinel), The Mask of Sanity (Cleckley)
  - selfish disregard for others and promotion of own welfare, lack of conscience, violation of societal norms; high-risk behaviour (substance misuse, self-harm, HIV, criminality)
  - genetic contribution, XYY karyotype
  - may involve MAOs, 'low serotonin model', subtle EEG changes
  - hyperactivity & delinquency in childhood (Robins: Deviant Children Grow Up)
  - exclude learning disability, hypomania.
- **Emotionally unstable** (Borderline)
  - 5% (10% outpatients, 20% inpatients)
  - women predominate
  - aetiology psychobiological, childhood abuse >75%
  - efforts to avoid abandonment, unstable relationships, unstable self-image, impulsive risk-taking, self-harming, affective instability, inappropriate anger and temper, emptiness, paranoid ideation/dissociation
  - suicide 8–10%
  - co-morbid affective, anxiety, somatisation, PTSD, substance abuse.
- **Histrionic**
  - 2–3%
  - genetic aspect to hysterical traits, different manifestation of antisocial genotype
  - oral/genetic developmental fixation
  - childhood deprivation/trauma
  - co-morbid dissociation/somatization/conversion disorders; exclude hypomania
  - narcissistic
  - 0.4%
  - ego-inflation (Reich), failure to internalise health self-esteem, 'God complex' (Jones).

Cluster C

- **Anankastic** (Obsessive-compulsive)
  - 1%, 10% psychiatric patients
  - biological factors, social learning
  - fixation at anal phase (Freud)
  - ordered, rigid, schedules/procedures/punctuality, humourless, unspontaneous, angry if lose control
  - differentiate from OCD, schizoid panic disorder.
- **Anxious** (Avoidant)
  - 0.7%
  - possible familial, parental rejection, social avoidance
  - extreme shyness, ineptness, self-doubting, insecure
  - exclude social phobia, schizoid panic disorder.
- **Dependent**
  - 0.7%
  - fixation at oral stage (Freud)

- ○ childhood deprivation
- ○ passive, avoiding responsibility/decision-making, subservient to others' needs.

Management

Managing personality-disordered patients is challenging. It is important to restrict contact to as few members of staff and locations as possible, avoid lone-working, keep careful notes, set clear and firm boundaries and be as consistent as possible in all interactions. The following may help:

- **Pharmacotherapy**
  - ○ antidepressants may help in anxiety and borderline, but unproven
  - ○ mood stabilisers (lithium, carbamazepine) have been claimed to help but are unstudied
  - ○ neuroleptics can help in some disorders (antisocial, borderline, narcissistic, histrionic schizotypal)
  - ○ other groups tried, no evidence.
- **Cognitive therapy**
  - ○ try to link biological and social factors
  - ○ claims made for Dialectical Behaviour Therapy (Linehan) in borderline personality disorder
  - ○ also Beck and Freeman's model.
- **Psychodynamic**
  - ○ little research, no robust evidence
  - ○ brief psychotherapies more likely to be helpful risk of dependence.
- **Therapeutic communities**
  - ○ run on democratic lines ('milieu therapy')
  - ○ open to abuse (eg Ashworth Inquiry)
  - ○ no reliable evidence although a number of studies claim effectiveness.

DANGEROUS SEVERE PERSONALITY DISORDER (DSPD)

The category of Dangerous Severe Personality Disorder is a political one, invented under proposed changes to the English Mental Health Act. Apart from human rights arguments, it is difficult to understand how such an individual would be treated, were they to be admitted to 'specialist units', one of which is being set up at Whitemore Prison. If the intention is simply incarceration, many groups have called for this to be made explicit so as to remove it from the realms of psychiatry.

Chapter 13

Psychiatric Treatment, Assessment and Prevention

Nick Kosky

CONTENTS

Psychiatric Treatment, Assessment and Prevention

PSYCHIATRIC ASSESSMENT

Psychiatric assessment can be instigated from a variety of sources, and the assessing psychiatrist will need to tailor the assessment accordingly. Common sources of, and reasons for, referral are given in Table 13.1.

Source	Reason(s)
Primary care	Determination of whether or not psychiatric disorder is present; diagnostic assessment; management or medication advice; ongoing care; risk assessment; gatekeeping to other care, eg plastic surgery; Mental Health Act assessment.
Other mental health professionals	Determination of whether or not psychiatric disorder is present; diagnostic assessment; management or medication advice; risk assessment; ongoing care; Mental Health Act assessment.
Other secondary care sources	Abnormal illness behaviour: determination of whether or not psychiatric disorder is present; diagnostic assessment; management or medication advice; risk assessment; ongoing care; gatekeeping to other care, eg plastic surgery; assessment of capacity to give consent; Mental Health Act assessment.
Courts/Prison	Determination of whether or not psychiatric disorder is present; fitness to plead/stand trial; assessment of *mens rea*; recommendations for disposal; risk assessment, including to dependent children; Mental Health Act assessment.
Social services	Determination of whether or not psychiatric disorder is present; risk assessment, including to dependent children; Mental Health Act assessment; management advice; ongoing care.

Table 13.1 Reasons for referral

The requirements of the referrer must be borne in mind, and responded to appropriately, through:

- engagement with the patient
- eliciting information sufficient to derive an initial formulation
- developing a management plan based on the initial formulation.

263

The interview

The success of the initial interview is highly dependent upon engagement with the patient.

Setting and physical environment

The setting should be quiet, comfortable and undisturbed if possible – warn the patient if you are on call or otherwise likely to be disturbed.

Remember your safety is a primary concern

- Make sure that both you and the patient can leave the room without obstruction.
- Make sure that you have telephone access or an alarm system and that you are familiar with the operation of both.
- If you are at the patient's house, try to ensure that the television is off and that children are being cared for by someone else. Make sure someone knows where you are and what time you are due to finish if possible. Take a mobile phone. If the patient is dangerous, do not go alone and have a plan for if things go wrong. Consider police back-up.

In general, see adults alone initially. For children over 16, parents do not have an automatic right to sit in. For learning disabled patients or patients with dementia, make sure the informant is available. This may also help with difficult situations – see the following.

Conduct of the interview

Introduce yourself and check that the patient has the same understanding as you as to the purpose of the interview. Explain the format and time constraints. You will probably need to repeat your name at least once, especially in the emergency setting.

General principles

Begin with open questions, narrowing down your questioning to elicit specific information. Take time to summarise and reflect. Avoid confrontation in the early part of the interview.

Sources of information

Be prepared to look at information about the patient **before** the interview if there is likely to be a risk to you. The role of information other than interview of the patient is now covered.

Difficult situations

Always be prepared to reassess if the time is not right

- **The unco-operative patient:** Talk over the circumstances of the referral. Point out the potential advantages of assessment. Highlight confidentiality as far as possible.
- **The unresponsive patient**: Consider mutism or stupor. Do not see the patient alone – stuporous patients can rapidly become overactive. Allow the patient adequate time

to reply. Try communication in writing. Observe and record the patient's behaviour, eg eye movements. A physical examination is essential.

- **The overactive patient**: Select the most important questions. Observe and record the patient's behaviour. There should be early recourse to an informant.
- **The confused patient**: Perform a cognition test early in the interview. Try to orientate the patient. Keep the interview short and relevant. There should be early recourse to an informant. A physical examination is essential.
- **The disinhibited patient**: Consider having a chaperone. Keep the interview short and relevant. If the patient is dangerous, read on.
- **The garrulous patient**: Propose to the patient that you will interrupt from time to time to help them focus.
- **The anxious patient**: Allow time for them to ventilate or habituate. Sometimes the presence of someone who the patient trusts can help allay anxieties.
- **The threatening patient**: Gather information, especially the views of nursing or accident and emergency staff **before** the interview. Keep the interview polite and formal. Allow adequate time for the interview. Consider having a chaperone – sometimes the presence of someone the patient trusts can help. **Do not put yourself in danger**. The assessment may have to wait until circumstances are right or until the patient has calmed down or sobered up.

History

A psychiatric history aims to understand and record the development of the patient's symptoms, putting them into a personal context.

- **Demographic details**. It is essential to record age, sex, racial/cultural background, marital status, employment status. Ask sensible questions about the home, community, job. These details are not only useful for 'getting a feel' for the patient, but also for building trust.
- **Presenting complaints**. Record your findings in chronological order. Summarise and reflect – make sure that you have got all the presenting complaints, especially the symptoms. Be aware of the difference between symptoms, impairment, disability and handicap. Patients and doctors inevitably have different perspectives on this!
- **History of presenting complaints**. Questions should investigate the following details before you start to formulate your diagnostic hypotheses. Use closed questioning judiciously to elicit other relevant symptoms that might support or refute your hypotheses:
  - Onset – was it sudden or insidious?
  - Relation to life events or illness.
  - Effect on patient (eg avoidant behaviour?)
  - Patient's efforts to cope (eg alcohol use?)
  - What makes things better?
  - What makes things worse?
  - Effect of any treatment?
- **Previous psychiatric history**. Enquire about previous diagnoses, treatment, and outcomes, hospitalisations. Ask about any previous use of the Mental Health Act.

Has there been any response to psychotherapy? Has there been any previous self-harm? What was it? Why? What were the consequences?

- **Previous medical history**. Enquire about previous diagnoses, treatment and outcomes.
- **Current treatments**. What are the physical/psychological treatments that the patient is currently taking? Ask about dose, duration, and effectiveness. Investigate the patient's ability to sustain relationships with professionals.
- **Systemic review**. Remember your duty to recognise organicity. A systemic review is also useful for spotting drug side-effects or contraindications. The following should be investigated:
  - Central nervous system: Headaches, fits, faints, funny turns, weakness, numbness, altered sensation
  - Cardiovascular system: Chest pain, palpitations, claudication
  - Respiratory system: Shortness of breath, cough
  - Endocrine system: Polyuria, polydipsia
  - Gastrointestinal system: Bowel habit, presence of blood in the faeces
  - Genitourinal system: Galactorrhoea, menstrual changes, prostatism. (Sexual function is usually covered elsewhere in the assessment.)
  - Musculoskeletal system: Mobility, pain
  - Skin: Rashes.
- **Family history**. The following questions should be asked.
  - **Parents**: Are they together or separated? What was the reason for the separation? Are they still alive? What is their age? What was the reason for death? Ask questions about the parents' jobs, personality and relationship with patient.
  - **Siblings**: Ask about their age, relationship with the patient, personality and jobs.
  - **Overall family culture**: Is the family secretive? Loving? Critical? Violent? What is its social position?
  - **Family history of medical and psychiatric disorder**: Enquire about suicide, substance use, or gambling in other family members.
- **Personal history**. An investigation of the patient's personal history should cover:
  - **Birth**: Was this a full-term, normal delivery?
  - **Developmental milestones**: Were the ages for reading/writing, walking/talking, and bladder/bowel control within the normal ranges?
  - **Childhood**: Were there prolonged separations; if so what were the reactions of both patient and parents? Were others involved in the patient's upbringing? What was the patient's capacity for attention and socialised play? Were there any serious illnesses or any 'neurotic' symptoms during childhood?
  - **Schooling**: What were the patient's academic, sporting, or other achievements? What were the relationships with peers and teachers like? Which exams were passed? Was there truancy, suspension, or expulsion?
  - **Occupation**: Make a list of jobs, with reasons for changes. Enquire about the relationship with employers and colleagues. Ask about work satisfaction, sick record and any appraisals and achievements.
- **Psychosexual history**. Ask about the patient's sexual orientation. Record the ages of onset of sexual interest and activity? What are the patient's present sexual practices? Is contraception used, if so, what form? What is the quality of the present relationship and past relationships? Is there any sexual abuse?

- **Substance use**. Does the patient use alcohol, tobacco, street drugs, or caffeine? Record their use chronologically. Look for adverse physical, mental, or social consequences, craving, tolerance, withdrawal, primacy given to use, stereotyped pattern of use, or reinstatement of use after abstinence.
- **Forensic history**. Record any arrests, cautions, convictions, or sentences (including motoring offences). Make a note of the role of alcohol in these offences and the motivation behind them, especially if they are serious or repeated. Are there any charges pending?
- **Premorbid personality**. The following should be investigated and recorded:
  - traits – impulsivity, avoidance/anxiety, aggression, orderliness, attention-seeking
  - mood
  - hobbies/leisure activities
  - membership of clubs/organisations
  - religious beliefs
  - non-sexual relationships – quality, number, ease of starting/maintaining.
- **Social circumstances**. Enquire about the following:
  - housing – type, size, adequacy, ownership?
  - finances – income, benefits, debts?
  - community involvement
  - household composition – are there children? What is their age, sex, progress/functioning, relationship?
  - home activities – way of spending typical day?
  - carers – family, friends, professionals, voluntary sector?

Mental state examination

The Mental State Examination is designed to access and describe the patient's behavioural, cognitive and emotional repertoire and world. It uses technical language to describe the patient's experience. The language used is described more fully in Chapter 6 (Psychopathology).

- **Appearance and behaviour**. Describe this fairly fully so as to 'paint a picture' for the listener. Give details of the patient's apparent age, sex, ethnicity, clothing, tattoos, piercings, scars, posture, and affect, ie perplexed, preoccupied, miserable, anxious, elated. Is the patient co-operative, tense, restless, or agitated? Are there any obvious mannerisms, tics, or stereotypes?
- **Speech**. What are the amount, volume, syntax, and rate of speech. Describe **form** not **content** of speech in this section. Include errors of production: Dysarthria, discursiveness, rhyming, punning, clanging. Consider whether there is formal thought disorder: Loosening of association, knight's move, word salad or verbigeration, thought block, perseveration, paraphrasing, neologisms.
- **Mood**. This should be assessed both objectively and subjectively.
  - **Objectively**. Does the patient appear elated, flat, incongruous, depressed, anxious? Is the mood labile during the interview?
  - **Subjectively**. How does the patient describe their mood and can this be explored further? For example, if the patient is elated do they sleep, are they irritable, spending, disinhibited (sexually); what are their thoughts like subjectively

267

compared to normal (richness, speed, etc). Look for depressive symptoms in these patients as well. If depressed, ask about their energy, hedonic capacity (ability to experience pleasure), sleep, appetite and weight, concentration, confidence, ideas of guilt or worthlessness, agitation or retardation, morbid ruminations.

- o **Suicide. Always** consider suicidal risk, looking for: Ideation and power or preoccupying nature of suicidal ideas, extent of planning, actual current intent, access to chosen method, barriers to completion, and any 'final' acts, eg writing a will or note. If the patient appears suicidal, check for ideas of harm to others, especially children. Read on for suicide risk assessment.
- **Thought content**. Ask about preoccupations, concerns, worries, phobias, obsessional ruminations, compulsions, and rituals. If there are abnormal beliefs investigate their content, onset (sudden or insidious), whether they are delusional or overvalued. You should know the definition of delusion, overvalued idea (see Chapter 6). Clarify whether the abnormality is in relation to the:
  - o world (ideas of reference, persecution)
  - o body (bodily change, disease, death)
  - o self (passivity, influence).
- **Perceptions**. Ask about any abnormal experiences: Their content, vividness, level of drowsiness when experienced, spatial location of experience (eg inside/outside the head), personal explanations, individual's response to the experience. Know the definitions of hallucination, illusion, and misinterpretation. Clarify whether the experience was in relation to the:
  - o world (hallucinations or illusions in all sensory modalities, including touch and deep visceral, déjà vu, derealisation)
  - o body (alterations in sensation, eg pain or deadness)
  - o self (depersonalisation, thought alienation or retardation).
- **Other common symptoms/syndromes** include:
  - o **anticipatory anxieties**: Avoidance
  - o **generalised/specific anxiety**: Muscle aches, palpitations, dry mouth, sweats, tremor
  - o **social anxiety**: Blushing, fear of embarrassment, observation, criticism
  - o **panic**: Fear of dying or collapse, non-cued, somatic symptoms
  - o **adjustment disorder or post-traumatic stress disorder**: Nightmares, flashbacks, hyperarousal/vigilance
  - o **excessive concern with weight/shape/certain part of body**: Eating pattern, body weight, laxative abuse, exercise, etc.
- **Cognition**. How closely this is examined depends on the presenting complaints and the age of the patient. As a minimum the following should be assessed.
  - o Orientation – time, place, person.
  - o Attention and concentration – days of the week, months of the year backwards, serial 7s, digit span forwards and backwards.
  - o Memory – **make sure you understand the definitions of different types of memory**, ie **immediate registration** – how many repetitions of a Babcock sentence, name and address, three common items, etc; **short-term memory** – recall of the above tests after a delay; and **long-term memory** – autobiographical data, current affairs/sports/entertainment, etc.
  - o Intelligence – make a general comment.

- **Insight**. What is the patient's view of their difficulties, their causes, proposed treatments? Phrases like 'full insight' or 'no insight' are particularly unhelpful and generally suggest that you have an inadequate knowledge of the concept.
- **Rapport**. Briefly comment on your reaction to the patient. Say why.

Other sources of information

Informant interview

The informant interview is the most important special investigation in psychiatry. The informant is usually a relative or friend. Other sources of information include primary care – scrutiny of general practitioners' notes is often revealing – schools, police, employers, probation and social services. Follow the above scheme in an abbreviated and appropriately tailored manner. Seek permission from the patient first. See the informant alone if possible. Remember the legal constraints surrounding confidentiality, and do not disclose information without permission.

Psychological assessment

Psychologists have expertise in the application and interpretation of psychometric instruments (see below).

Psychologists can often help to develop a psychodynamic, cognitive or schema-focused formulation.

Physical examination

A full physical examination should be undertaken for all day patients or inpatients. Examination can be tailored for other patients, eg thyroid signs/symptoms for patients with anxiety or depression, full neuropsychiatric examination for patients with cognitive problems. In an examination setting, always consider what you would or should examine.

Dysphasia

This is a partial failure of language function that is cortical in origin. It should be distinguished from dysarthria – which is a difficulty in production of speech by speech organs. Language disorders suggest a left-hemisphere lesion in right-handed people.

Type of dysphasia	Likely location of lesion
Expressive	Anterior
Receptive	Posterior
Auditory	Temporal
Visual	Posterior

Table 13.2 Cerebral origin of dysphasia

269

Dysphasia can be investigated by the following:

- **Receptive dysphasia**: Does the patient respond to commands, can the patient read and can the patient explain a passage of text?
- **Expressive dysphasia**: Can the patient name common objects and their parts, talk spontaneously about hobby/family and copy a passage?

Apraxia

Apraxia is the inability to perform volitional acts with intact motor and sensory systems. It is usually suggestive of a parietal lobe lesion. The following investigations will characterise apraxia.

- **Constructional apraxia**: Make figures with matchsticks, draw clock face.
- **Dressing apraxia**
- **Gait apraxia**: Heel-to-toe walking
- **Ideomotor apraxia**: Three-stage command ('take the paper with your right hand, fold it in half, place it on the table').

Agnosia

Agnosia is the inability to understand the meaning of sensory stimuli in the presence of an intact sensorium.

Type of agnosia	Description	Likely location of lesion
Astereognosia	Failure to identify three-dimensional form, eg coins, keys	Contralateral parietal lobe lesion
Atopagnosia	Failure to identify position on skin	Contralateral parietal lobe lesion
Finger agnosia	Failure to identify which finger has been touched	Dominant parietal lesion
Agraphognosia	Failure to identify letter traced on skin	Contralateral parietal lobe lesion
Anosognosia	Failure to identify functional deficits caused by disease	Usually unawareness of left-sided weakness/sensory inattention secondary to right parietal lesion

Table 13.3 Cerebral origin of agnosia

Physical investigations

These should be tailored to the diagnostic requirements of the patient. No set of investigations is routinely essential.

RISK ASSESSMENT

Risk can be defined as 'the chance of something undesirable happening'. The purpose of risk assessment is to allow risk management, which aims to reduce future harm by appropriate intervention.

Factor	Harm to others	Harm to self	Neglect/ exploitation
Demographic factors	Male Young Divorced or separated Unemployed	Male (suicide) Female (non-lethal DSH) Young or old Not married Unemployed Traditionally, social class I, V – suicide, V – DSH	Young or old Living alone
Historical factors	Antisocial or impulsive personality traits Previous violence Non-compliance Substance abuse	Substance abuse Previous DSH Impulsive personality Some forms of physical illness	Substance abuse Previous episode Low IQ Disturbance of sensorium Poor mobility
Situational factors	Poor social support or stability Recent life crisis Access to weapon Confrontation/ provocation	Evidence of planning Access to method Recent life crisis Poor social support or stability	Poor social support or stability
Mental state factors	Irritability/hostility/ anger Suspiciousness Agitation Suicidal ideas in severe depression Active intent to harm Disinhibition Delusions – jealousy, persecution, influence Command hallucinations	Depression Hopelessness Helplessness Agitation Suicidal ideas Command hallucinations Delusions about need to die etc	Depression Clouding of consciousness Disorientation Psychotic symptoms Memory disturbance Disinhibition

Table 13.4 Factors suggesting risk (this list is NOT exhaustive)

There are three types of risk:

- Risk to self: Usually regarded as deliberate physical violence, but can include starvation, etc.
- Risk to others: Violence, verbal aggression, predation, sexual offending, etc.
- Risk of neglect or exploitation.

Assessing and describing risk

You should describe precisely:

- **What** the risk is.
- **Who** is at risk.
- **How imminent** is the risk.

Risk management

It is **never** possible to eliminate risk but it **may** be possible to reduce it.

Effective risk management depends upon:

- addressing all the identified risk factors
- adopting a multidisciplinary approach
- ensuring that responsibility for aspects of the risk management plan is clearly allocated
- communicating the plan effectively – to patient, relatives, police, primary care, probation, housing, etc
- reviewing and adjusting the plan in a timely fashion.

Clinical versus actuarial risk

Clinical risk is based on interview. It often tends to emphasise mental state at the expense of historical factors. **Actuarial instruments** generate risk prediction measures or scores based on the application of epidemiological and statistical information. They are likely to be used increasingly in clinical practice but are currently the province of probation and forensic services.

When things go wrong

- Be open, do not alter records, do fill in adverse incident forms, do report to line manager.
- Be prepared to meet relatives.
- Be prepared to learn – take part in or implement an audit process to encourage reflection and debriefing.

All homicides and suicides by patients in contact with psychiatric services are referred to the *National Confidential Enquiry into Homicides and Suicides* based at the University of Manchester. This government-sponsored body is charged with developing safer psychiatric services. Their recommendations are published annually as *Safer Services* and all doctors involved in mental health services should be familiar with these.

Currently (in 2004), all homicides are investigated at a public inquiry, a process which has been subject to considerable criticism. This process first came to prominence after the murder of Johnathan Zito by Christopher Clunis. Themes common to most inquiry reports are:

- failure to take previous history into account
- poor record keeping
- poor risk assessment and management
- poor communication between different agencies
- lack of assertiveness in follow-up.

DEVELOPING A FORMULATION

A psychiatric formulation is a description of the case that includes those features that are necessary to distinguish it from other cases and that allow the construction of a management plan. It should include:

- demographic data
- name, age, occupation, marital status
- reason for referral
- descriptive formulation
- nature of onset (eg acute/insidious)
- total duration
- course (eg cyclic/deteriorating/static)
- main phenomena – including important positive findings from history and mental state.

Differential diagnosis

- List in order of probability those diagnoses that should be considered.
- Give evidence for and against each.
- Remember co-morbidity and that physical illnesses may also contribute to the clinical picture.

Aetiology

Try to answer the question: 'Why has this patient developed this particular disorder at this point in time?'.

The matrix shown in Table 13.5 may be helpful:

	Predisposing	Precipitating	Maintaining
Psychological			
Social			
Physical			

Table 13.5 Aetiological matrix

Investigations

List all the investigations that are needed to support your preferred diagnosis and rule out the others.

The most important investigation is an informant interview but other investigations include:

- **physical**: eg bloods, imaging, specialist examination
- **social**: eg police, school records, occupational or speech therapy assessment
- **psychological**.

Treatment (see relevant chapter)

The choice of treatment is driven by:
- diagnosis
- relevant aetiological issues
- consideration of risk.

Prognosis

When developing a formulation you should take into consideration both this episode and the future. Make some comment about overall functioning and provide evidence to support your opinion!

Management plan

The management plan should be written and a copy should be given to all involved parties (especially the patient). It will incorporate:

- setting overall objectives
- reducing symptom burden
- improving social functioning
- carer education
- relapse prevention
- treatment setting
- specific treatments proposed
- risk management.

You should determine with whom to share the plan, remembering that the plan is for the benefit of the patient, not you, so it is vital to discuss it with the patient.

The *Care Programme Approach* is the most widely used vehicle for planning and review in complex clinical situations.

- Allocate responsibilities clearly.
- Make sure you address common concerns.

Diagnosis

- What is it, or what might it be?
- Are any other information or investigations needed?
- What are implications?
- What is aetiology?

Medication

- Why this drug?
- What dosing schedule and duration of treatment?
- What are the possible side-effects?
- Is there an addictive potential?
- Are there possible interactions with other medications (including alternative and 'health foods')?
- Where can future supplies be obtained (general practitioner, day hospital, outpatient clinic, ward)?

Psychological treatment

- What is the purpose of treatment?
- Who will be giving the therapy?
- What will be the duration of treatment?
- What will be expected of the patient?

Relapse

- What are early warning signs of relapse?
- What should be done in an emergency?

STANDARDISED METHODS OF ASSESSMENT

This list is not exhaustive but you should ensure that you are familiar with these instruments at least before taking the exam.

Diagnostic interviews

- **Present State Examination (PSE).** A trained interviewer elicits abnormal phenomena and rates their severity. The CATEGO computer program generates a diagnosis.
- **Schedules for Clinical Assessment in Neuropsychiatry (SCAN).** This incorporates the tenth revision of the PSE. It allows diagnoses following the International Classification of Diseases tenth edition (ICD-10), and the Diagnostic and Statistical Manual of Mental Disorders third and fourth revisions (DSM-IIIR and DSM-IV).
- **Structured Clinical Interview for Diagnosis (SCID).** This is available for clinical use or as an epidemiological tool. It allows DSM-IIIR diagnoses. SCID-II allows diagnosis of personality disorder.

- **Composite International Diagnostic Interview (CIDI)**. This is for clinicians and non-clinicians. It generates DSM-IIIR and ICD-10 diagnoses.

Ratings to measure risk

- **HCR-20**. This is clinician rated. It is a 20-item scale taking into account historical and clinical factors to allow the generation of an overall score, predicting the likelihood of interpersonal violence over the next year.
- **Beck Suicide Inventory**. This questionnaire is based on historical and clinical factors predicting the likelihood of deliberate self-harm.

Rating scales to measure specific symptoms

- **Anxiety**
  - Hamilton Anxiety Scale (HAM-A) (clinician-rated)
  - Beck Anxiety Inventory (clinician-rated)
  - Hospital Anxiety and Depression Scale (HADS) (patient-rated)
- **Social anxiety**
  - Liebowitz (patient-rated)
  - Social Phobia Inventory (SPIN) (patient-rated)
- **Post-traumatic stress disorder**
  - Impact of Events Scale (patient-rated)
- **Depression**
  - Hamilton Depression Scale (HAM-D) (clinician-rated)
  - Hospital Anxiety and Depression Scale (HADS) (patient-rated)
  - Beck Depression Inventory (BDI) (patient-rated)
- **Obsessive-Compulsive disorder**
  - Leyton Obsession Inventory (clinician-rated)
  - Yale Brown Obsessional Compulsive Symptoms Schedule (YBOCS) (clinician-rated)
- **Schizophrenia**
  - Positive And Negative Symptoms of Schizophrenia (PANSS) (clinician-rated)
  - Schedule for the Assessment of Negative Symptoms (SANS) (clinician-rated).

Other scales

- Social Adaptation Self-evaluation Scale (SASS)
  - patient-rated
  - social functioning
- Global Assessment of Function (GAF)
  - clinician rated
  - forms Axis V of DSM classification.

Psychiatric subspecialties also have their own scales, some of which, especially in Old Age Psychiatry, aid clinical assessment and have a use in determining the beginning and end points of certain treatments, eg MiniMental State Examination (of Folstein) and 'cognitive enhancing' drugs for Alzheimer's disease.

PRINCIPLES OF PSYCHIATRIC TREATMENT

Primum non nocere (Hippocrates: 'First do no harm')

The treatment contract and therapeutic alliance

All contact with patients involves a set of implicit or explicit expectations on the part of both doctor and patient. Sometimes the nature of psychiatric illness and the lack of a common frame of reference make it difficult to find common ground. It is essential to find some areas of agreement to enable the construction of a **therapeutic alliance** (eg the doctor and patient agree that staying out of hospital is a good idea even though they may not agree on the diagnosis of schizophrenia).

It is important to be aware of the boundaries of the treatment contract and how this can be imperilled by distorted expectations, 'acting out' and other manifestations of transference; counter-transference also plays a part.

Aids to the treatment contract and therapeutic alliance include:

- honesty tempered with tact
- reliability
- reflection on transference/countertransference
- explicit boundaries of treatment, eg what therapeutic interviews will cover, etc.

Hindrances include:

- inflated claims for treatments
- collusion, dependence, enmeshment
- any exploitation, especially sexualised behaviour.

Treatment settings

Treatment can be as an **outpatient** (this covers treatment at your office and in the patient's home), a **day patient**, or as an **inpatient**.

Types of treatment

Psychological

Variables to consider include:

- length – number, duration and frequency of sessions
- focus on past vs here and now
- individual vs couple, vs family vs group
- focus on support vs change
- work between sessions
- evidence base
- model of therapy being employed

- therapist qualities (some therapies are now presented on computer or through guided self-help)
- patient requirements – YAVIS (young, attractive, verbal, intelligent, successful) and 'psychologically minded'
- work, previous therapy history may help you to assess the maturity of the defence styles.

Social

Do not forget that manipulation of the environment can be a very important part of management.

Physical (see Chapter 8 and specific specialty chapters)

- Drug.
- Non-drug: Electroconvulsive therapy, psychosurgery, vagal nerve stimulation, transcranial magnetic stimulation.

Treatment in special circumstances (see Chapters 10 and 21)

The following should be taken into account:

- Mental Health Act 1983
- Under Common Law
- Confidentiality, capacity and consent.

COMPLIANCE ('ADHERENCE')

There are a number of reasons why people comply with treatment.

- They fully understand the nature of their problem and appreciate how the treatment will help them.
- They partially understand and they trust their doctor.
- They are frightened or compelled.

The reliability of each can be speculated upon.

Non-compliance

The incidence of non-compliance is estimated at 20% of inpatients and 50% of outpatients. It is more common in primary care than in secondary care and partial compliance is more common than complete non-compliance.

- **Absolute non-compliance** is a deliberate decision that is not necessarily driven by psychosis or lack of insight. The patient's insight may be affected by cognitive deficit or it may be the first episode of illness.

- **Partial non-compliance** can be caused by forgetfulness and disorganisation (possibly secondary to cognitive deficit).

Reasons for poor compliance in schizophrenia (can be applied to other disorders)

Reasons for poor compliance according to professionals include:

- side-effects of drugs, especially extrapyramidal symptoms
- weight gain, sexual dysfunction less recognised by staff as reasons
- denial/lack of insight, especially during first episode.

According to patients side-effects are cited as the most common reason, especially sexual and weight changes (up to 90% women report menstrual disturbance with neuroleptics).

Other factors include:

- the complexity of the regime
- depot vs oral, once a day dosing vs three times a day or more
- degree of supervision
- lack of follow-up (eg lost to outpatient follow-up)
- views of friends
- perceived stigma (especially with extrapyramidal symptoms, drooling, etc)
- relationship with professionals
- substance misuse
- mental state: anxiety, grandiosity, depression, dementia.

Consequences of poor compliance

Non-compliance is associated with disease relapse.

Relapse is associated with increased cost to:

- the patient (social environment, chronic symptoms, stigma, more aggressive treatment)
- the NHS (25% of the cost to the NHS of schizophrenia is related to non-compliance). Drugs cost **only** 4% of the total direct health-care costs associated with schizophrenia
- others: Homicide, suicide.

In the first episode of schizophrenia there might be:

- sensitivity to extrapyramidal symptoms
- fear and apprehension
- days to therapeutic response and future relapse
- recognition of need for ongoing treatment.

Factors improving compliance

Factors improving compliance can be classified into three categories: The drug itself, the patient, family and carers, and the doctor.

In the case of **drugs**, variables to consider include the route of administration (depot, oral, dispersible, sustained release, liquid), the dosing regimen and the side-effect burden.

The patient, family and carers affect compliance through belief systems ('compliance therapy'). They can be helped by reputable self-help agencies, and by education on the diagnosis and mechanisms of the disorder, risks of relapse, side-effects and management strategies.

The doctor must find common ground to agree on with the patient (**therapeutic alliance**), ie there must be consistency of approach between all professionals, patience, a willingness to try out new treatments when appropriate, and move to the position of patient adherence rather than compliance.

PREVENTION

Prevention of illness in psychiatry comprises a spectrum of public health and patient/illness-specific interventions aimed to reduce incidence or minimise adverse consequences of a disorder.

Primary prevention

Population-based strategies aim to modify the risk factors for a given disorder. They can be aimed at the general population or at high-risk individuals, eg:

- education about substance misuse
- early intervention in psychosis
- *Antistigma Campaign* by the Royal College of Psychiatrists
- SANE campaign in the 1980s (to inform the general population about the existence and nature of schizophrenia).

Identifying the **at-risk** populations for primary prevention can be a problem.

- The relatively low incidence of disorders such as schizophrenia means that large populations would have to be included in primary-prevention strategies for a small reduction in incidence.
- Markers for psychiatric illnesses are often weakly predictive as screening measures, eg:
  - In Down syndrome a raised α-fetoprotein level during pregnancy gives an odds ratio of > 200 of positive caseness, which is very useful.
  - In schizophrenia the best indicator is positive history in a first-degree relative and this gives an odds ratio of only 8. Other indicators (birth complications, birth size for dates, cognitive impairment, social functioning, co-morbid psychiatric

disorder, schizotypal personality disorder, cigarette and cannabis smoking) all give odds ratios of around 3 to 5.
- There are considerable adverse consequences to a false positive, and 'screening' markers so far identified are not sufficiently specific.
- Considerable stigma exists, which not only contributes to the adverse consequences of false-positive identification, but also reduces help-seeking behaviour.
- Evidence that early intervention achieves substantial results over the long-term is uncertain. Cognitive dysfunction, predictive of social outcome, is established up to eight years before the first psychotic symptoms manifest.

Secondary prevention

Secondary prevention involves strategies aimed at an individual who is already expressing prodromal or actual signs/symptoms, eg:

- early intervention in schizophrenia
- optimising treatment strategies.

The possible problems met with in secondary prevention include:

- Some elements of optimal treatment (eg clozapine, CBT) are expensive and of restricted availability in the UK.
- Adherence to treatment can be a major problem.
- Treatment effect sizes in schizophrenia have not improved greatly with newer 'effective' treatments (eg atypical antipsychotics).

Tertiary prevention

Tertiary prevention describes those strategies that are aimed to keep well an individual who has already been treated, minimising handicap if recovery is not complete and reducing the potential for adverse consequences to others, eg:

- rehabilitation services for patients with schizophrenia (see Chapter 24)
- assessment of carer needs
- dry/clean environments for addicts.

Figure 13.1 expresses these strategies graphically for patients with schizophrenia.

However, there are problems in tertiary prevention for schizophrenia:

- rehabilitation services are under-resourced
- the cost-effectiveness of various models and some interventions (eg cognitive rehabilitation) is not established.

Similar problems exist with other serious, especially psychotic, mental illnesses. Substance misuse prevention strategies tend to be better developed, and regarded as more effective. Suicide rate (female only) has been demonstrated to be reduced in a Danish study as a result of general practitioner education although this was not replicated by the Hampshire depression project (Thompson *et al.*, 2000).

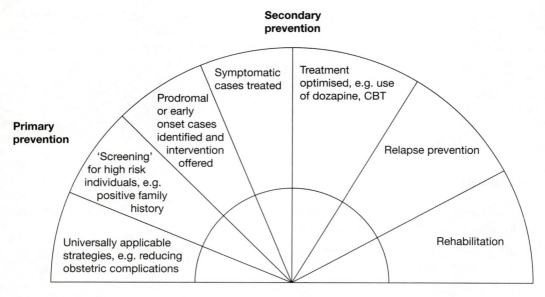

Figure 13.1 The spectrum of prevention in schizophrenia

Public health

Generally, public health measures in mental health are characterised by:

- lack of information on how to develop and implement interventions in particular contexts
- lack of information on the short-term outcomes and longer and deeper impacts of interventions
- lack of information on the cost-effectiveness, cost–benefit and cost–utility of the interventions
- response to problems after they have developed, rather than anticipating them and giving primacy to prevention.

The **Prevention Paradox** (Geoffrey Rose 1981) states that 'A preventive measure that brings large benefits to the community offers few benefits to each participating individual.'

Measures can involve litigation (eg alcohol prohibition in 1920s America) or education (eg sex education).

An example of the prevention paradox is **Motorbike Accidents and Head Injuries**.

- **Individual perspective** is that the likelihood of a motorcycle accident is low.
- **Population perspective** is that the likelihood of serious brain injury among those involved in a motorbike accident is high. Head injuries account for 67% of motorcycle-related hospital admissions, 33% of Accident and Emergency Department visits and 62% of deaths.

Mandatory helmet laws clearly benefit society but have only a small benefit to the individual. Similar arguments can be advanced for immunisation, seatbelt legislation and for drugs and alcohol.

The **Prohibition Paradox** would suggest that litigation is unlikely to reduce these activities to desired levels but makes consenting adults into criminals. Who benefits from this?

Chapter 14

Gender Issues and Psychosexual Disorders

Chris Fear

CONTENTS

Gender Issues and Psychosexual Disorders

GENDER AND DEVELOPMENT

Definition

Gender is the lifelong masculine/feminine status of an individual.

Sex is the phenotype of gender.

Biological determinants

The biological determinants of gender are the genotype – XY male and XX female.

In rare **intersex** states, socially-assigned sex overrides the biological gender. The fundamental mammalian gender is female in the absence of hormones.

Psychosocial determinants

Gender role is reinforced by parents and society.

The **core gender identity** is established by 18 months of age.

- 2–3-year-olds prefer their mother, but boys shift preference to the father at 4 years of age
- same-sex peer preference occurs from 3½ years
- sex stereotypes and greater aggression are present in boys from the age of 2
- fathers give gender-stereotyped toys from 12 months
- the perceived sex of the child influences parenting.

WOMEN'S MENTAL HEALTH

Historically, a male medical establishment has seen feminine gender and madness as equivalent in diagnostic labels such as 'hysteria' (same root as hysterectomy – ie pertaining to the womb). 'Deeply ingrained sexism characterises much psychiatric practice' (Allen, 1986).

Current emphasis is upon empowering women through:

- development of specialised services, especially liaison between psychiatry and obstetrics
- information about resources, access for pushchairs, childcare

- improving the gender balance of staff in senior positions and paying attention to patient safety
- privacy and freedom from harassment on wards (this reverses the short-lived fashion for mixed sex wards and has caused major problems for short-sighted modern hospital design)
- access to female staff
- women's groups and services for women are a priority for the *National Service Framework for Mental Health* (1999)
- public policy issues around tax/welfare and family issues
- recognition that women are more vulnerable to common mental health problems as a result of greater exposure to acute/chronic social stressors, smaller social networks, lower social status and income.

More common in women	More common in men	No gender difference
Anorexia nervosa (9 : 1)	Alcohol abuse	Bipolar affective disorder
Bereavement reactions and psychiatric consequences	Anankastic personality disorder (5 : 1)	Histrionic personality disorder
Borderline personality disorder	Antisocial personality disorder	Obsessive–Compulsive disorder
Bulimia nervosa	Paraphilias	
Deliberate self-harm	Tourette's syndrome	
Depersonalisation disorder (2 : 1)		
Depression (2 : 1)		
Dysthymia (2 : 1)		
GAD		
Panic disorder and agoraphobia (2 : 1)		
Post-traumatic stress disorder following road traffic accident		
Schizoaffective disorder		
Social phobia		
Specific phobia (2 : 1)		
Schizophrenia (2 : 1 for onset over 40 years, 4 : 1 for over 60 years)	Schizophrenia (onset < 30 years)	Schizophrenia (overall)

Table 14.1 Epidemiological gender differences

Childhood and adolescence

Boys are twice as likely to be seen by child psychiatric services, despite the higher incidence of childhood sexual abuse in girls. In community and primary-care clinics, the balance begins to equalise. In education, provision for special needs tends to be biased towards 'problem behaviour', favouring boys. Adolescent girls are more likely to present with deliberate self-harm or eating disorders.

Perinatal and menstrual mental health problems

See Chapter 26.

Camberwell Study

The Camberwell study by Brown and Harris (1978) found that four factors, in women, lead to 'the provocation and generalisation of hopelessness':

- loss of mother before age 11
- 'lack of an intimate, confiding marital relationship'
- no paid employment outside the home
- three or more children under 14 years.

Depression of mothers in inner cities has a prevalence of 30–40%.

Effect of maternal (or paternal) mental illness on children

In general parental mental illness has the following effects on children:

- incorporation of the child into the psychopathology (eg delusion or obsession)
- withdrawal and non-availability to the child
- family environment/discord
- economic and social deprivation
- resilience of the child is determined by coping style, intellectual ability and sociability
- child's behaviour will have an effect on the course and outcome of the parental mental illness.

More specifically, in **depression** there may be:

- insecure attachment
- emotional problems related to severity or duration of illness
- higher rates of phobia (three-fold), panic disorder and alcohol dependence (five-fold)
- boys externalise (conduct disorders), girls internalise (neurosis)
- poorer cognitive performance for children of postnatal depressives.

Eating disorders in the parent can cause:

- failure to thrive and less close contact during feeding as a baby
- vulnerability to the body image perception of the mother in adolescence.

Schizophrenia in the parent can cause:

- increased obstetric complications
- non-specific cognitive/attentional problems in childhood

- less sociable behaviour with peers/teachers
- deviant family communication.
- It may be related to a higher genetic risk of schizophrenia spectrum disorders in the child.

Anxiety and **personality disorders**, **substance misuse** and **physical illness** also affect children.

SEXUAL ORIENTATION AND IDENTITY

Cultural context

Homosexual orientation was a sexual deviation in the second edition of the Diagnostic Statistical Manual of Mental Disorders (DSM-II; published in 1968) but now it is only pathological if ego-dystonic. Gay activist groups have made discussion of many aspects of homosexuality politically incorrect and it is now viewed as a minority sexual orientation.

In non-Western cultures 64% see male homosexuality as normal and socially acceptable, while 36% disapprove. There are no data for female homosexuality.

Intercourse is the most common cross-cultural sexual behaviour.

Prevalence

In 1948 Kinsey stated that 10% of men and 5% of women were exclusively homosexual, 37% of men reported a homosexual experience, 4% had had only homosexual orgasms (Kinsey, 1948).

Of British men, 6.1% report lifetime experience of homosexuality; the US Census Bureau gives a prevalence of 2–3%.

Aetiology

There is a smaller interstitial nucleus of the anterior hypothalamus-3 (INAH-3) and a larger suprachiasmatic nucleus in homosexual men (although what the relevance of these differences might be is unclear).

There are critical periods during fetal development when future sexual behaviour can be influenced by the presence of **fetal gonadal androgenic substances**.

- congenital virilising adrenal hyperplasia
- less evidence in boys exposed to female hormones
- increased prevalence in brothers of male and sisters of female homosexuals.

SEXUAL DYSFUNCTION

Normal sexual cycle

The stages of the normal sexual cycle have discrete pathophysiological mechanisms:

- **Desire**: testosterone-driven in men; mechanism is unclear in women
- **Arousal**: penile erection in men, vaginal lubrication/labial tumescence in women
- **Orgasm**: ejaculation/vaginal contractions, release of muscular tension, pleasure
- **Satisfaction**.

Disorders of sexual desire

Disorders occur in 33% of women and 16% of men. **Sexual aversion** is an extreme form.

- Disorder can be associated with negative emotions, higher lifetime prevalence of depression (childhood sexual abuse in women).
- There is no objective measure of normality, diagnosis based on incompatibility.
- For diagnosis: Review pharmacological history, testosterone and prolactin levels (men), relationship, sexual relationship/identity/abuse.
- Treatment can be psychotherapy (eclectic) or testosterone can be given to men with low levels.

Erectile dysfunction

Erectile dysfunction occurs in 10% of men; 17% have some anxiety about their performance.

- It can be lifelong or acquired.
- A history/examination should be taken to exclude physical causes.
- Physical causes (drugs, vascular, neuropathies) should be treated.
- Treatment for dysfunction with non-physical cause can be:
  - first-line: Psychotherapy, drugs (sildenafil), vacuum devices
  - second-line: Self-injection (papaverine, phentolamine, prostaglandin E_1)
  - third-line: Prosthesis.

Arousal in women

Seventeen per cent of women have arousal disorders. This can be for various reasons.

- It can be confused with desire/orgasm disorders.
- A lack of foreplay or cultural/social/religious ideas may be the cause.
- Medical conditions (ie menopause!) should be excluded and/or treated.
- Topical lubricants can be used. There is no evidence for psychological treatment.

Orgasmic disorder in men

Premature/rapid ejaculation	Delayed ejaculation
Occurs in 29%	
Anxiety, hostility to women, conflict with partner, masturbatory practices, early sexual experiences	Insufficient stimulation vs lack of desire
Increased penile sensitivity? (Unproven.) Damage to sympathetic system from pelvic trauma, urethritis, drugs (trifluoperazine)	Neurological disorders, drugs (selective serotonin reuptake inhibitors)
Lifelong or acquired	Lifelong or situation-specific
Assess performance against expectations, voluntary control, coital positions, life events (if recent), attitudes relationship, sexual dysfunction in partner	Assess physically, history of when ejaculation can occur, societal/religious
Drugs (serotonergic antidepressants, antipsychotics, α-blockers). Psychotherapy, couples work	Treatment is psychological depending on model followed: increase stimulation vs acknowledge and work with lack of desire

Table 14.2 Orgasmic disorders in men

Orgasmic disorders in women

In women 24% have some level of orgasmic disorder: 10–15% are anorgasmic (primary), no orgasm through intercourse.

- 21% of women find sex 'not pleasurable'.
- Control, fear of pregnancy/rejection/vaginal damage can be causes.
- The doctor should assess requirements to achieve orgasm, societal/religious values, and relationship, neurological, and medication (antidepressants) factors.
- Medical problems should be treated; psychological approaches can involve directed masturbation, **sensate focus.**
- 70–90% have an initial improvement but this falls to 15% at 2 years.

Sexual pain disorders

Fourteen per cent of women suffer pain with intercourse.

Dyspareunia	Vaginismus
Male/female persistent genital pain during intercourse	Involuntary spasm of lower part of vagina, preventing intercourse
Women: Anatomical (atrophy, rigid hymen) Iatrogenic (episiotomy) Pathological (endometriosis, infection) Men (rare): Infection Peyronie's disease Prostatitis Drugs (selective serotonin reuptake inhibitors can cause painful ejaculation)	May affect insertion of tampons or vaginal examination Does not necessarily prevent sexual arousal Trauma, infection, dyspareunia etc. Anticipatory fear of pain.
No evidence for psychological causation but may be psychological sequelae.	Childhood trauma, adult conflict, penetration anxiety, resistance to male sexual prerogative, fear of pregnancy, social or religious mores, warding off castration urges/father's incestual threat.
Gynaecological/urological referral Psychosexual/social investigation if no demonstrable physical pathology. Treat disease. Sex therapy.	Gynaecological referral Psychosexual/social investigation if no demonstrable physical pathology. Psychotherapy. No intercourse, graded vaginal dilators, systematic desensitisation, Kegel exercises.

Table 14.3 Sexual pain disorders

GENDER IDENTITY DISORDERS

Gender identity disorders are heterogeneous disorders featuring a strong and persistent preference for the status and role of the opposite sex. They may manifest verbally, or non-verbally (cross-sex behaviour).

Gender dysphoria is a discontent (affective) with one's own gender.

Transsexualism is an extreme form. The patient acts as a member of the opposite gender, and/or undergoes hormonal/surgical procedures.

Classification

Classification is problematic. These disorders have been placed with paraphilias but they may be present in childhood. Currently they appear in a separate category in DSM-IV and under disorders of adult personality and behaviour in the International Classification of Diseases (ICD-10). These exclude physical intersex conditions (eg hermaphroditism).

Epidemiology

Gender identity disorder is more common in children referred with behaviour problems.

* 50–65% of homosexual men and 50% of homosexual women recall childhood cross-dressing.
* The ratio of male to female referrals is 5 : 1 (possibly reflecting parental concerns with boys).
* Cross-dressing is apparent by the age of 3.
* Adult transsexualism occurs in 1 per 50,000 of the population at a ratio of 2 : 1 in men to women.
* Homosexuals present in their mid-20s, heterosexuals in their mid-30s.

Aetiology

For biological aetiology see page 304.

Psychosocial aetiology can be divided as follows:

* **Psychodynamic**
  * boys with excessive mother–son symbiosis
  * girls with distant mothers (depression), unsupportive fathers (girl becomes substitute husband)
  * traumatic psychological losses may be related to onset
* **Social learning**
  * reinforcement of sex-typed behaviours
  * imitative/vicarious learning
* **Cognitive**
  * child labels itself as male or female and is rewarded by associated behaviours
* **Psychoanalytic**
  * unresolved separation anxiety/reparative fantasy of symbiotic fusion with mother
  * penis envy as a result of unresolved transsexualism in the mother causes her to treat male infant as an extension of herself; unresolved oedipal complex; 'blissful symbiosis'.

Clinical features

In **children** there may be an intense desire or preference for:

* being of the opposite sex

- cross-dressing (boys) or wearing stereotypical masculine clothing (girls)
- cross-gender roles in play
- stereotypical games of the opposite sex
- disgust with sex organs/secondary sexual characteristics
- desire to be treated as, or conviction that he/she has the typical feelings of the opposite sex
- request for hormones/operations to change sex.

In adults there is:

- a persistent sense of being born into the wrong sex
- rejection of social role, cross-dressing, trying to emulate opposite sex
- search for 'heterosexual'-type relationships with members of the same sex
- aversion to secondary sexual characteristics
- narcissistic and borderline personalities.

Differential diagnosis

In **children** it may be:

- normal behaviour
- monosymptomatic cross-dressing (which may lead to adult transvestitism)
- anatomical intersex (which should be excluded).

In adults there may be:

- psychosis
- internalised homosexual homophobia in adolescence.

Treatment

In children treatment is rarely needed, nor is it beneficial.

- Family therapy and individual education can be given.
- It may resolve into adolescent homosexual feelings.
- Ethical/legal issues surround adult treatments.

In adults treatment can involve:

- individual psychotherapy
- gender reassignment for intractable cases:
  - oestrogens or testosterone
  - live in the cross-gender role for 1–2 years
  - vaginoplasty for males, hysterectomy and bilateral salpingo-oophorectomy for females (phalloplasty rarely successful).

Prognosis

It follows a chronic cyclical course. Non-homosexual patients are more likely to pursue gender reassignment surgery to its conclusion.

INTERSEX DISORDERS

- **Congenital virilising adrenal hyperplasia** (adrenogenital syndrome): An enzyme defect in cortisol production; increased boy-type play and homosexuality in affected females.
- **Turner's syndrome**: XO karyotype, female genitalia, small infertile ovaries, short stature; gender identity disorder is rare.
- **Klinefelter's syndrome**: XXY, eunuchoid males, gynaecomastia, low testosterone, small testes, infertile.
- **5-α-reductase deficiency**: XY born with female genitalia; virilisation and phallus growth at puberty.
- **Androgen insensitivity syndrome**: XY, insensitive to testosterone; develops as female but infertile and no menses.

PARAPHILIAS

Paraphilias are intense sexual fantasies and urges leading to their acting out for sexual gratification. A 'disorder' of personality occurring in men.

- 50% have onset before age 18
- average three to five paraphilias over a lifetime
- peak age is 15–25 years
- rare after age 50 years.

Aetiology

- **Biological**: Androgen sensitive; sex ratio (more males to females); possible temporal lobe abnormalities.
- **Social**: Familial tendencies in form and substance; up to 50% of paedophiles were abused as children; weak, dominated fathers
- **Psychological**: Infant sexuality unchallenged by parental representations in the superego; protection against castration and separation anxiety; covers flaws in sense of bodily integrity and reality; outlet for aggression and sexual drives.

Clinical features

Exhibitionism

Exhibitionism involves exposing genitals to an unsuspecting stranger:

- 75% of sufferers are under 40
- they often have premature ejaculation, erectile problems
- Rooth (1971) classified them into:
  - type 1 – 80%; inhibited, emotionally immature, struggle against impulse, flaccid penis, guilt, good prognosis

- type 2 – 20%; sociopathic, erect penis, often masturbate, little guilt, sadistic pleasure, poorer prognosis
- Victims are usually unknown, pubertal girls
- 80% are deterred by being caught for the first time
- Good prognosis: Type 1, stable work, normal personality, heterosexual, supportive wife
- Poor prognosis: Type 2, victim child under 10, previous offending (any kind), physical contact with victim, onset during psychosis or organic brain disease.

Fetishism

Fetishism involves sexual activity towards object or an object used in sexual activity; 58% involve clothing, 23% rubber, 15% footwear, and 10% leather. Fetishism is rarely harmful.

Hypoxyphilia

This is also known as 'sexual asphyxia'. It can be solitary or with a partner and may involve sado-masochism. There is a significant mortality rate (in adolescents).

Necrophilia

Necrophilia describes an erotic interest in the dead or dying. It is rare but may occur with homicide.

Paedophilia

Paedophilia is preferential sexual activity with pre-pubertal children:

- victim is usually under 13, perpetrator must be >3 years older
- 10–20% of children are molested
- homosexual (boys, 12–15 years old), heterosexual (girls, 6–11 years old) or indiscriminate (6–11 years old)
- 50% are relatives or friends of the victim
- 70% of children participate actively
- if incestuous, it may not be true paedophilia (the child is often older): The father is endogamic (all sexual and social energies confined to the family), paedophilic, or promiscuous
- aggression and sadism are inherent
- paedophiles may be immature adolescents, middle-aged with marital problems, or elderly and socially isolated
- murder is rare (only four per year in UK).

Sadism/masochism

Sadism is the infliction of suffering or humiliation upon others for sexual gratification.

Masochism is being made to suffer passively for the same purpose.

Fantasies are common in both sexes, violence and acting out are diagnostic. There are sado-masochistic elements in most paraphilias.

Transvestism

Transvestism involves dressing in women's clothing for sexual gratification. Between 50% and 75% have cross-dressed by age 10. It may be symbolic in a homosexual relationship or possibly be part of exhibitionism.

Voyeurism

Voyeurism describes the act of observing unsuspecting women undressing, grooming, or having sexual intercourse. It often occurs with masturbation. Up to 20% of women are targeted by voyeurs/exhibitionists. The problem is associated with poor sexual performance.

Other paraphilias

- **Coprophilia/urophilia/klismophilia**: Abnormal interest in faeces/urine/enemas, respectively
- **Frotteurism**: Fondling/rubbing against an unfamiliar woman in a public place, with surreptitious masturbation
- **Partialism**: Sexual focus on a part of the body
- **Telephone scatalogia**: Obscene phone calls, usually with masturbation.

Differential diagnosis

- Gender identity disorder.
- Sexual dysfunction.
- Anxiety.
- Personality (eg borderline).
- Psychosis.
- Normal.

Treatment and prognosis

- Cognitive behavioural therapy.
- Covert sensitisation.
- Imaginal desensitisation.
- Thought stopping.
- Masturbatory/aversive conditioning.
- Sexual addiction programmes.
- Psychoanalytic and psychodynamic psychotherapies.
- Drugs (neuroleptics, fluoxetine, imipramine, lithium).
- Anti-androgens (hypertension, diabetes, etc are possible adverse effects).
- Interest decreases with age but spontaneous recovery is unlikely.
- Prognosis is guarded or poor.

FURTHER READING

Allen, H. 1986. 'Psychiatry and the construction of the feminine.' In P. Milner & N. Rose (eds), *The power of psychiatry*. Cambridge: Polity Press.

Brown, G. W. & Harris, T. 1978. *Social origins of depression: a study of psychiatric disorder in women*. London: Tavistock.

Kinsey, A., Pomeroy, W. & Martin, C. 1948. *Sexual behaviour in the human male*. Philadelphia, PA: W B Saunders.

Rooth, F. G. 1971. 'Indecent exposure and exhibitionism.' *British Journal of Hospital Medicine*. April: 521.

Chapter 15

Psychiatric Services and Management

Sarah Price

CONTENTS

Psychiatric Services and Management

CURRENT SERVICE PROVISION

The history of mental health service provision is covered in Chapter 27. Current services are directed towards the management of acute episodes (crises) together with a strategic approach to the management of chronic illnesses in community settings.

Inpatient services

Inpatient service provision differs according to the population served.

- **Acute wards**. Patients with acute episodes of mental illness are admitted, assessed and treated over relatively short time periods, ranging from days to several weeks or a few months. Admission may be informal or under mental health legislation.
- **Rehabilitation wards**. Patients with chronic and relapsing illnesses, complicated by treatment resistance, poor compliance or limitations to independence spend longer periods, sometimes several years, on these wards. Focus is on rehabilitation rather than acute treatment.
- **Therapeutic communities**. A community environment where all residents contribute to decisions about daily life, support one another, and set boundaries for behaviour. Emphasis is on interpersonal interactions rather than medication. Therapeutic communities provide:
  - permissiveness
  - reality-confrontation
  - democracy
  - communalism; and
  - can be effective for people with borderline personality disorder.
- **Halfway houses**. Community housing which is staffed but outside the hospital setting. They provide places of refuge for patients in crisis who require short-term support but do not need to be admitted to hospital.

Emergency psychiatric services

In an emergency, mental health services can be accessed through referral by a general practitioner, self-referral, or other agencies (social services, housing association, NHS Direct etc).

- **Hospital assessment**
  - allows assessment by duty doctor/nurse.

- **Crisis team/home treatment**
  - teams are developed in the community
  - self/general practitioner/other agency referral
  - covers patients who would otherwise need admission
  - is rapid
  - is intensive
  - has family and carer involvement
  - is assertive with regard to maintaining contact
  - is time-limited.

Primary care

Mental health services are mostly provided by Mental Health or Partnership Trusts. A few Primary Care Trusts provide services themselves. Other sources of services include:

- non-statutory agencies, eg MIND, Rethink, some providing day-centre facilities
- voluntary sector
- user/carer groups
- housing associations specialising in services for people with mental health problems
- mental health in-reach services in prisons and sometimes police cells.

Improving communication and partnership between agencies in primary care is essential for efficient, seamless patient care. Some models now exist that use integrated 'primary-care liaison teams' to provide specialist mental health care in a primary-care setting for problems that cannot be dealt with by primary care alone. Teams are coming together and boundaries are being broken down. There are also implications for the relationship between health and social care.

Social care

Historical boundaries between health and social care have led to problems with inefficiency and 'holes' through which patient care may fall. The Health Act (1999) enabled Health and Local Authorities to bring resources together in pooled budgets, allowing easier allocation of resources to those in need. The NHS Plan provides for Care Trusts to evolve from Mental Health Trusts and/or Primary Care Trusts with powers to commission and provide both health and social care.

Community-based services

Community mental health teams are often based in the communities they serve and are geographically distant from inpatient units. They are multidisciplinary teams of professionals providing care to patients and support to primary-care teams. Functions include:

- liaison with primary-care teams
- assessment
- accessing and advising on local resources

- social work assessments
- care co-ordinator responsibility
- outpatient services
- provision of medication
- psychological therapies
- family and carer support and advice.

Patient care is reviewed and monitored through the Care Programme Approach, regular team meetings, and supervision.

Day hospitals

Day hospitals are often located with the community mental health teams. They provide an environment for multidisciplinary assessment and therapeutic work, phased reintegration of discharged inpatients and an alternative to admission.

Other services

- Assertive outreach/assertive community treatment teams have:
  - 'difficult to engage' patients
  - small caseload
  - complex cases
  - high frequency of contact.
- Early intervention teams have:
  - contact as early in illness as possible
  - assertive medical treatment
  - insight, compliance, relapse prevention therapy
  - moderate frequency contact.
- Outreach to hostels (eg Salvation Army, homeless).

Provision of mental health services must accommodate socio-demographic factors, such as age, gender, race, socio-economic class, employment status, household structure, homelessness, etc. Toolkits have been developed and disseminated by the Department of Health with the Sainsbury Centre and Institute of Psychiatry as well as the Office of National Statistics (ONS) Psychiatric Morbidity Surveys.

Ethnic minorities (see Chapter 30)

Patients from ethnic minority communities have specific needs for services that are culturally sensitive and non-discriminatory. The following factors must be considered:

- language barriers (requiring interpreters)
- cultural sensitivity
- racial discrimination
- social isolation.

HEALTH SERVICE MANAGEMENT

The management structure of the NHS has undergone several changes over recent years, one of the most significant being the key aim of the NHS Plan (2000) to provide for more locally driven service developments, steering away from the traditional top-down, centrally led approach.

Development of NHS management

- **Early days**: Matron, medical superintendent, medical secretary
- **1974–1984**: Accountability within a team of equals: Consensus management
- **1983**: Griffiths challenged this model – 'Who is in charge?'
- **1984**: Recruitment of managers from outside the NHS, often ex-military
- **1990s**: Formation of NHS Trusts, chief executives introduced to:
  - provide direction
  - make decisions
  - lead the organisation
  - ensure 'doing the right things and also doing things right'.

NHS Plan

This is a 'radical action plan' to modernise the NHS over a 10-year period. A 'Modernisation Board' headed by the Secretary of State for Health with the 'Modernisation Agency' working with NHS regional executive offices and trusts to devolve power away from the Department of Health into 28 Strategic Health Authorities (replacing Local Health Authorities). These will operate as local headquarters for the NHS.

Its key aims are:

- increased capacity
- power shifted to frontline Primary Care Trusts
- independent inspection
- open working
- financial resources driven by patient choice (eg by 2005 all patients choose which hospital treats them)
- common standards of care, process and methods of inspection.

Strategic Health Authorities are accountable to the Department of Health, which provides overall direction of standards, resources, investment decisions and patient choice. The Secretary of State for Health is supported by junior ministers, a Permanent Secretary, Chief Executive, Board of Directors, Chief Medical and Dental Officers and National Clinical Directors for different areas of health.

Primary Care Trusts

The 303 Primary Care Trusts covering England hold 75% of the NHS budget, giving them the power to purchase services for patients from different providers. Key responsibilities involve planning and securing services, improving the health of the community, and local integration of health and social care.

Local delivery plans

Each Primary Care Trust must produce a local delivery plan outlining the health service improvements that are planned to bring services in line with the NHS Plan. Each NHS trust is also required to produce its own plan which will fit with the Primary Care Trust delivery plan.

Other contributors to local planning are:

- strategic health authorities
- workforce development confederations.

The local delivery plans must identify milestones (annual or quarterly) over a three-year period and each three-year plan must be supported by a financial plan and a strategy plan.

Amendments may be made to plans as necessary at any time during the implementation process.

MAINTAINING STANDARDS

A number of concepts and organisations have been introduced to set and maintain consistent standards of excellence in service development and clinical practice.

National Institute for Clinical Excellence (NICE)

NICE was launched in 1999 to advise on the clinical and cost effectiveness of new and existing treatments, promote clinical audit (see Chapter 28) and develop evidence-based clinical guidelines (eg atypical neuroleptics, electroconvulsive therapy, schizophrenia).

National service frameworks

These frameworks are evidence-based guides for local service development that outline the care and treatment patients can expect to receive from the NHS. The frameworks each relate to a major area of care or a disease group (eg mental health, cancer, diabetes, older people).

Quality and performance assessment

Procedures and agencies to audit and ensure adherence to the guidelines and frameworks. Further information can be found in the websites listed at the end of this chapter.

- The Commission for Health Improvement awards trusts star ratings (0–3) according to their performance and compliance with National Service Framework and NICE guidelines and practice of clinical governance. The aim is to reduce clinical variation across the country and eliminate malpractice.

- Modernisation Agency
- Patient surveys
- National Clinical Assessment Authority
- Performance Assessment Framework.

Clinical governance

This concept was introduced in 1999. It is the process of using the evidence base and peer review to improve clinical practice. Responsibility rests with chief executives. The main areas of focus include:

- continuing professional development
- procedures for reporting concerns about professional conduct
- clear risk management policies
- programme of quality improvement activity
- participation in the National Clinical Audit
- ensuring implementation of national service framework and NICE guidelines
- clear lines of responsibility and accountability with regard to clinical care
- internal/external scrutiny.

Finance

Just over 5% of public spending is on the NHS and social-care services. Over £72 billion was budgeted for NHS spending in 2003/4. The main sources of these monies are tax and national insurance.

The main expenditure sources are:

- Primary Care Trusts (75%), which purchase and provide local health services. The amount allocated to each Primary Care Trust is weighted according to socio-demographic factors (social deprivation, age, morbidity and mortality rates).
- Department of Health
- centrally purchased services.

NHS trust income is negotiated from Primary Care Trusts in the form of service agreements designed to deliver against targets and priorities in the local delivery plan. Trusts are also funded centrally for health professional training. If a trust fails to break even at the end of the financial year, they must agree a recovery plan with their Strategic Health Authority, to run over a five-year period. The NHS Bank holds funds to provide NHS trusts with an overdraft facility. Loans are also available for reforming working practice or setting up new methods of service delivery.

It is anticipated that national tariffs will be introduced for health-care procedures to move the emphasis from negotiating the price of health care to providing adequate and appropriate services to meet the needs of patients, introducing patient choice as advocated by the NHS Plan.

To aid financial health-care planning, patients are divided into health-care resource groups that are clinically similar and will therefore require similar levels of health-care resources.

USEFUL WEBSITES

www.audit-commission.gov.uk
www.chi.nhs.uk
www.doh.gov.uk/clinicalgovernance
www.doh.gov.uk/nhsplan
www.doh.gov.uk/nsf
www.modernnhs.nhs.uk
www.nao.gov.uk
www.nhsconfed.org
www.nice.org.uk

Chapter 16

Psychiatry in Relation to Neurology and Medicine

Hugh Rickards

CONTENTS

Psychiatry in Relation to Neurology and Medicine

DELIRIUM (TOXIC CONFUSION STATE)

Delirium is an acute or subacute condition usually resulting from a medical or surgical event. Prevalence is 20% in general medical patients and 80% in medical Intensive Care Units.

Clinical symptoms and illness course

- Onset is acute or subacute.
- It is usually polysymptomatic at onset.
- There is fluctuating consciousness.
- It is worse in the evenings.
- The patient shows distractibility.
- There is disturbance of the sleep–wake cycle.
- There is psychosis (mainly visual hallucinations and mood-incongruent delusions).

Delirium of gradual onset can be caused by:

- Lewy body disease
- indolent tumours
- chronic poisoning (including occupational poisoning)
- sub-dural haematoma.

The **differential diagnosis** is from **dementia** (gradually progressive clinical course with clear consciousness) and **depression** (prominent affective symptoms, less acute onset, diurnal mood variation).

Risk factors

Some risk factors imply a direct causation (such as organ failure) while others imply complex causation (such as post-surgery or old age):

- polypharmacy
- older age
- pre-existing brain disease
- substance abuse
- organ failure (eg hepatic failure).

Specific risk factors for delirium in the elderly include:

- low albumin
- polypharmacy

- use of psychoactive drugs
- dementia
- visual impairment
- social isolation.

Classification

In the **International Classification of Diseases** (ICD-10) delirium is classified under F05 (organic disorders), with separate sections for withdrawal and intoxication delirium.

In the fourth revision of the **Diagnostic and Statistical Manual for Mental Disorders** (DSM-IV) there is a specific category (239.0 'Delirium due to general medical cause'), with separate sections for intoxication and withdrawal from specific substances. There are also the categories:

- delirium of multiple aetiologies
- delirium NOS (not otherwise specified; either cause not found or 'unusual or unlisted cause').

Clinical assessment

Clinical assessment should include:

- clinical observation
- serial testing of orientation (using Galveston Orientation and Amnesia Test)
- Delirium Rating Scale (use the currently most valid and reliable version)
- electroencephalogram (EEG) shows diffuse slowing (low-voltage fast-activity in delirium tremens and benzodiazepine intoxication)
- complex partial status can present with delirium (fronto-temporal spike and wave or generalised seizure activity)
- attempt to find and treat causative factors.

Good discriminating tasks include orientation to passage of time (what time is it now? how long have we been talking?), planning tasks (clock drawing, Luria three-step task) and 'Trail making' test. In delirium, performance of these tests can be seen to fluctuate.

Aetiology

The following mnemonic is useful:

Infections (systemic or central nervous system (CNS))

Withdrawal (including nicotine, drugs of abuse and prescribed drugs)
Acute metabolic changes (in Na, K, Ca, Mg)
Trauma
CNS pathology (tumours, neurodegenerative)
Hypoxaemia (pulmonary disease)

Deficiency (vitamin B_1, B_6, B_{12}, folate, B_2, and hypervitaminoses A and D)
Endocrinopathy (pancreas, thyroid, adrenal, pituitary, parathyroid)
Acute vascular (myocardial, heatstroke)
Toxins (including iatrogenic and substance abuse)
Heavy metals (Pb, Hg, Mn, Th, As and others).

A second mnemonic is indicated in Table 16.1.

Diagnosis	Clinical symptoms apart from delirium	Diagnostic tests	Treatment
Wernicke's	Ataxia, Opthalmoplegia		Parenteral thiamine
Hypoglycaemia	Pale, sweaty	Blood glucose	Glucose
Hypertension	Papilloedema	Diastolic blood pressure ≥140	
Hypoxaemia	Depends on cause	Blood gases	
Hypoperfusion	Depends on cause	Blood pressure	
Intracranial bleed	Headache, focal Neurology	CT/MRI of head	
Meningitis/ Encephalitis	Fever, headache, focal neurological signs	Lumbar puncture CT/MRI head	Antibacterial/ antiviral
Poisons	Dysarthria, ataxia, nystagmus	Test for specific substance	Depends on cause

CT/MRI, computed tomography/magnetic resonance imaging.

Table 16.1 A Mnemonic useful in Emergency departments to exclude major causes of delirium needing immediate treatment

Even after thorough investigations there are a small number of people for whom the cause is still unknown. Delirium in these people may be:

- feigned ('factitious')
- self-induced (self-administration of insulin)
- a result of another person (poisoning)
- a truly idiopathic neurological syndrome (cf. mitochondrial encephalopathy with lactic acidosis (MELAS), a recently discovered cause of encephalopathy).

Treatment

- Identify risk factors and treat them.
- Identify aetiology and treat.

- Nurse consistently in a side room with natural light.
- Adequately hydrate the patient.
- Give haloperidol (oral or parenteral) for agitated and psychotic symptoms.

NEUROPSYCHIATRY OF BRAIN INJURY

The most commonly affected brain areas following traumatic brain injury are the medial and anterior temporal lobes and the basal part of the frontal lobes. These are the parts of the cortex most implicated in the development of mental disorder. People are at risk of mental disorder following brain injury for three main reasons:

- damage to parts of brain controlling perception and mood control
- experience of major life events and loss events
- impaired cognitive ability to process life events.

A pre-existing mental disorder may be a risk factor for brain injury.

Types of injury

- **Traumatic brain injury**. One in 10,000 people suffer severe and persistent disability following head trauma. Closed, deceleration brain injury can lead to damage of the orbito-frontal and anterior temporal lobes. Penetrating head injury increases the risk of post-traumatic epilepsy.
- **Sub-arachnoid haemorrhage** incidence is 6 per 100,000 people per year. It often affects medial frontal lobes.
- **Herpes simplex encephalitis** incidence is 1 per 100,000 per year. It most commonly affects the medial temporal lobe.

Anoxic or hypoglycaemic injury

- **Diffuse injury** affecting areas of brain with highest oxidative metabolism (basal ganglia and hippocampus). It may be the result of self-harm attempts.

Depression following brain injury

Prevalence of depression after brain injury is between 25 and 50% but diagnosing post-brain-injury can be difficult:

- vegetative functions may be impaired without depression (disturbance in sleep and appetite, irritability)
- emotional expression may be impaired (right hemisphere, basal ganglia and thalamic lesions)
- dysphasia
- unhappiness is common following brain injury.

Look for a pre-injury history of depression and deterioration in function following some degree of recovery. Diurnal variation in mood, pervasive low mood with depressive cognitions and indications of depressive pseudo-dementia on cognitive testing are useful discriminators.

Treatment of depression following brain injury:

- There are no good treatment trials. Antidepressants with anti-cholinergic actions have problematic side-effects (increased confusion, constipation, blurred vision). However, tricyclic antidepressants have been used effectively in headache and sleep disturbance after traumatic brain injury.
- Selective serotonin reuptake inhibitors (SSRI) should be the first choice antidepressants. Citalopram has less effect on the cytochrome p450 system so has a role in the treatment of depression in people on anticonvulsants.
- Other treatments:
  - cognitive behaviour therapy
  - electroconvulsive therapy (ECT; avoid in first 6 months after injury)
  - family and carer support.

Psychotic symptoms following brain injury

The patient may have had a pre-existing psychosis.

Psychotic symptoms may be part of epilepsy (ictal, post-ictal) or part of delirium (including post-traumatic delirium).

Appraisal of the world can be affected following brain injury, which can mimic psychosis:

- amnesia leading to confabulation
- damage to perceptual systems (hearing, vision, taste, smell)
- impaired self-awareness and understanding (anosagnosia)
- receptive aprosodia (misunderstanding of another's emotional intent through speech inflexion)
- agnosias
- complex partial seizures.

Treatment of psychotic symptoms following brain injury:

- exclude toxic, metabolic and infective aetiologies
- careful assessment of cognition
- relationship to seizures
- in post-traumatic delirium, minimise or avoid medications
- avoid 'typical' anti-psychotics (impairment of cognition, rigidity, abulia)
- 'atypical' anti-psychotics cause less rigidity and less cognitive impairment.

Irritability after brain injury

Irritability is an 'excessive response to a relatively minor stimulus'. It is a normal response, common to many psychiatric disorders and very common after brain injury.

The **causes** of irritability are:

- general physical conditions (constipation, infections)
- primary psychiatric disorders (depression, anxiety, psychosis)

- specific cognitive impairments (aprosodias, amnesia, misidentification)
- drug treatments (including treatments for irritability)
- epilepsy
- premorbid state.

Treatments of primary irritability include:

- anticonvulsants and propranolol are the mainstay of treatment
- drugs that include gabapentin, carbamazepine, valproate, SSRIs, methylphenidate and amantidine.

There are six good random controlled trials on the treatment of agitation/aggression after brain injury: Four trials on high-dose β-blockers (up to 3g/day), one trial on methylphenidate and one trial on amantidine.

Case series have been reported for amitryptilline, sertraline and carbamazepine.

There is no clear evidence to support any treatment.

Abulia

Abulia is the 'abnormal lack of ability to act or to make decisions' or 'lack of volition in the absence of depressed mood'.

It is caused by damage to the orbito-frontal cortex or mid-brain diencephalic structures.

Abulia **treatment** involves the use of dopamine agonists like bromocriptine with the following caveats:

- Do not overlook depression
- Use caution if there is a previous history of psychosis
- Hypotension is a possible side-effect
- It can increase inappropriate behaviours
- There can be a potential problem in patients with physical disability who begin to initiate movement.

Post-traumatic stress disorder

(See Chapter 20.)

Post-concussional syndrome

This is a controversial diagnosis in which headache, impaired concentration, irritability, fatigue and tinnitus follow brief concussion.

Look for a temporal relationship between the onset of symptoms and the initiation or dosage change of a specific medication

- corticosteroids (can cause depression, mania, psychosis)
- muscle relaxants (including baclofen, dantrolene and tizanidine)
- anticonvulsants
- topiramate (irritability, psychosis)
- vigabatrin (psychosis)
- other anticonvulsants can dull cognition

Table 16.2 Drugs used in brain injury rehabilitation which can cause mental symptoms

Managing mental disorder after brain injury

- Was there a pre-existing mental disorder?
- What is the current mental disorder?
  - symptomatic?
  - idiopathic?
- Avoid polypharmacy.
- Perform one intervention at a time.
- Explore broader social/carer support issues.

NEUROPSYCHIATRY OF MOTOR DISORDERS

Co-morbidity of motor and mental disorder

Disorders of movement and mental state co-exist for different reasons.

- Drugs used to treat a motor disorder can lead to mental disorder (eg drug-induced psychosis in Parkinson's disease)
- Drugs used to treat mental disorder can lead to motor disorder (eg tardive dyskinesia)
- CNS pathology can lead to motor and mental disorder (Huntington's disease, Wilson's disease)
- Psychological disorder can present with 'psychogenic movement disorder' (eg dissociative motor disorder)
- Motor and mental disorders can be coincidentally co-morbid (eg co-morbidity of schizophrenia and Parkinson's disease).

Parkinson's disease

Mental disorders currently account for the greatest morbidity in Parkinson's disease.

Affective disorders account for 40% in variance of quality of life in Parkinson's (vs 17% for motor disorder). Psychosis is the single greatest cause of family breakdown and nursing home placement.

Depression

- Vegetative symptoms are common in Parkinson's disease with no depression so do not distinguish well between Parkinson's disease and depression.
- Non-verbal communication often appears 'depressed' in Parkinson's disease.
- Affect and thought content are better discriminators (eg Beck's cognitive triad).
- Mood can fluctuate with motor state (non-motor fluctuations).

Differential diagnosis is between Parkinson's disease and:

- non-motor fluctuations
- delirium
- adjustment reaction (to diagnosis)
- drug-induced psychosis
- Lewy body disease.

There are no randomised controlled trials of treatment:

- SSRIs are first-line treatment (but can produce nausea with anti-Parkinson's therapy)
- tricyclic antidepressants are not commonly used
- ECT is a useful treatment and can lead to transient improvement in motor symptoms.

Psychosis

The psychosis of Parkinson's disease:

- is often preceded by vivid dreams/nightmares
- is often visual hallucinations/illusions
- can include persecutory delusions or Othello syndrome.

Differential diagnosis is from delirium, Lewy body disease and depression with mood-congruent psychosis.

Psychosis in Parkinson's disease should be managed by:

- reducing anti-Parkinson's disease medication as much as possible
- treating metabolic/infective problems
- assessing whether the symptoms are disabling.

If antipsychotics are needed, quetiapine first-line, then clozapine (two randomised controlled trials support this). Avoid sulpiride and risperidone. Rivastigmine is useful for Lewy body disease (one randomised controlled trial).

Huntington's disease

Huntington's disease is an inherited neuropsychiatric disorder.

- Inheritance is autosomal dominant (short arm of chromosome 4).
- It is progressive.
- Prevalence is one per 10,000.
- The young onset (Westphal) variant is more akinetic/rigid.

There is a triad of symptoms:

- dementia
- movement disorder
- psychiatric disturbance (mood and personality change, psychosis).

Cognitive impairment involves:

- impaired planning
- impaired multitasking
- disinhibition.

The **movement disorder** is usually chorea or dystonia but can include tics and myoclonus. Management of movement uses dopamine blocking/depleting drugs (sulpiride, risperidone, tetrabenazine). Depression is a common side-effect of these medications.

The **mood disorder** is common and is treated similarly to standard depression. Psychosis is schizophrenia-like and tends to be less responsive. Huntington's disease can be misdiagnosed as schizophrenia (movement disorder is attributed to tardive dyskinesia and cognitive impairment to 'negative symptoms').

Individual **genetic testing** is available with a standard testing protocol (including psychiatric screen and genetic counselling). Pre-natal testing is also available but is not widely utilised.

Management involves the following:

- holistic management by MDT
- CPA-based care
- attention to feeding, swallowing and weight loss
- some patients make advanced directives or refusals.

Tourette syndrome

Tourette syndrome is an inherited neurobehavioural disorder.

Diagnostic criteria are:

- multiple motor tics
- one or more vocal tics
- onset before 18 years
- not caused by other detectable neurological pathology.

About 0.1–1% of school-aged children fulfil these criteria. It has been recorded in all major cultural groups worldwide.

Tics:

- are stereotyped
- are experienced with a premonitory urge
- are suppressible at the expense of inner tension
- rebound after suppression.

The **clinical course** of the syndrome is:

- typical age of onset between 6 and 9 years
- initial symptoms are simple tics
- tends to become more complex
- symptoms typically wax and wane
- peak severity occurs between 12 and 14 years
- tendency to improve into adulthood.

Co-morbidity and associated symptoms include:

- echolalia in 30% of clinic sample
- coprolalia/praxia in 30% of clinic sample
- self-injurious behaviours in 30% of clinic sample
- attention deficit and hyperactivity disorder is very common in children with Tourette syndrome in a Tourette clinic.

Obsessive compulsive behaviours and obsessive-compulsive disorder is very common in Tourette syndrome patients:

- tics and compulsions share similar phenomenology
- patients with Tourette syndrome have more exploratory, symmetrical and counting compulsions and more sexual and aggressive ruminations than in pure obsessive-compulsive disorder.

Treatment of Tourette syndrome involves:

- illness education and working with education providers
- counselling and family therapy to help adjustment to diagnosis
- risperidone/sulpiride for tics
- SSRIs for obsessive-compulsive disorder
- stimulant medication for attention deficit disorder (the most current evidence is that tics are not worsened by stimulant medications)
- consider using no medication as an option (self-limiting illness).

Wilson's disease

Wilson's disease is an autosomal recessive illness (on chromosome 13).

Elevation of serum free copper occurs with deposition in liver and brain, in particular there is atrophy of the basal ganglia.

Clinical features of Wilson's disease are as follows:

- onset in childhood or early adulthood
- presents as motor disorder, psychosis, personality change, or dementia
- motor disorder mostly dystonic but can be choreic, tremulous, or akinetic-rigid.

The **diagnosis** is by:

- Kayser–Fleischer rings on slit-lamp examination
- impaired hepatic function
- caeruloplasmin low but free copper is elevated in serum
- elevated 24-hour free copper in urine
- T2-weighted MRI shows high signal in putamen.

Treatment involves:

- dietary changes
- zinc or potassium iodide may bind copper in the gut
- penicillamine can chelate copper (sometimes leading to a worsening of symptoms)
- tetrathiomolybdate has been used.

NEUROPSYCHIATRY OF EPILEPSY

Epilepsy and mental illness can interact in different ways. Psychiatric symptoms can be ictal or peri-ictal, mental disorders may look like epilepsy, anticonvulsants can change mental state and treatments for mental disorders can affect epilepsy.

Faints (myoclonus may occur)
Responding to hallucinations
Flashbacks
Dissociative states
Psychogenic fugue (the longer and more complex an episode, the less likely it is to be epilepsy)
Hyperventilation attacks
Staring tics

Table 16.3 Disorders that can look like epilepsy

Anxiety and epilepsy can be related in the following ways:

- Anxiety can lead to hyperventilation, thus lowering seizure threshold.
- People can overbreathe on purpose to induce a seizure.
- Hyperventilation attacks (carpopedal spasm and hypersalivation) occur.
- Fear can be part of the ictus itself.

Differential diagnosis is by good history and EEG (preferably with video) during an attack.

Epileptic seizure	NEAD
Short-lived (<5minutes)	Longer
Stereotyped and restricted to one or two presentations	Less stereotypical; multiple seizure types
Back-arching, thrashing and pelvic thrusting can occur in frontal seizures but less commonly seen	Back-arched, thrashing, non-synchronous jerking, carpet-burns on face and crying out all common
Incontinence	Incontinence
Post-ictal confusion	Post attack distress more common
Serum prolactin raised 20 minutes post attack (not 100% sensitive or specific)	Post-attack serum prolactin rarely raised
Anoxia and up-going plantar reflex during seizure	'Eye sign': Eyes are held forcefully shut during seizures. If the patient is placed on their side and the eyes opened, they may appear to be looking down, if turned on the other side, the eyes still look down
	Childhood emotional trauma is a risk factor

Table 16.4 Differences between epilepsy and non-epileptic attack disorder (NEAD)

Frontal seizures

These can be misdiagnosed as NEAD. Features of frontal seizures include:

- abrupt onset and offset
- short duration
- often occurring many times nocturnally
- bicycling, thrashing, or pelvic thrusting
- head turning, posturing
- often no rise in post-ictal prolactin
- medial frontal foci may not show on inter-ictal or ictal EEG.

Diagnosis often requires overnight videotelemetry.

Epilepsy and psychosis

Psychotic symptoms occur at different times in relation to the ictus (seizure).

Ictal psychotic symptoms include olfactory or gustatory hallucinations, elementary visual hallucinations and complex hallucinations involving hallucination in different modalities (temporal lobe focus).

Other visual phenomena which occur as part of the ictus include teleopsia, dymegalopsia and palinopsia. Complex psychic phenomena including *déjà vu* and *jamais vu* (or *entendu*); depression and fear may also occur as part of the ictus.

These phenomena tend to be stereotyped with short duration (ranging from seconds to a few minutes).

Post-ictal confusional states can occur after complex partial or generalised seizures. They can involve complex, automatic behaviours with amnesia for events afterwards.

Post-ictal psychosis typically occurs following a lucid period of around 24 hours after a seizure or cluster of seizures. There are no demonstrable EEG abnormalities. The psychosis tends to be affective in nature and can last for days or weeks. Treatment is aimed at aborting clusters of seizures.

Interictal psychosis describes a psychosis occurring between ictal events and having no clear relationship to the ictus. Symptoms are more like 'nuclear schizophrenia' but with better preservation of insight and affect. Treatment is with atypical antipsychotics (avoid clozapine if possible as it lowers seizure threshold to a greater degree).

Forced (paradoxical) normalisation was first described by Landoldt in the 1950s. The patient usually has complex partial seizures. Following treatment with anticonvulsants (usually etho-suximide or vigabatrin), the EEG normalises and the patient becomes acutely psychotic. Treatment may involve changing the anticonvulsant or using antipsychotic treatment.

Epilepsy and depression

Depression is common in epilepsy. Occasionally depressed mood can occur as part of the ictus (stereotyped, short lived). Antidepressants can alter the seizure threshold and interact with anticonvulsants.

Citalopram is least likely to interact with anticonvulsant medication and its effect on seizure threshold is relatively modest.

NEUROPSYCHIATRY OF MULTIPLE SCLEROSIS

Multiple sclerosis is the most common neurologically disabling condition of adulthood. Symptoms occur as a result of inflammatory plaque formation in the CNS in relation to damage to myelin.

Symptoms are episodic (lasting days or weeks) and include:

- optic neuritis
- vertigo
- diplopia
- parasthesia and anaesthesia
- paralysis
- sphincter disturbance.

The **clinical course** can be:

- benign
- relapsing remitting
- primary progressive
- secondary progressive.

Diagnosis is by:

- clinical history and examination
- MRI: Periventricular and other CNS white matter lesions are visible on T2 scan
- cerebrospinal fluid contains oligoclonal bands, but serum does not
- visual evoked potentials show conduction delay.

Depression in multiple sclerosis

Lifetime prevalence of depression in multiple sclerosis patients is 30–50%. Depression is associated with advanced disease. Diagnosis can be difficult as patients with multiple sclerosis often have somatic symptoms (weight loss, sleep and appetite distubance, anergia, fatigue). Better discriminating factors include pervasive low mood, anhedonia, diurnal variation in mood or function, depressive cognitions.

Suicide in multiple sclerosis:

- 3% in a six-year follow-up study
- 15% of deaths in people with multiple sclerosis
- 25% of outpatients have had suicidal ideation within the last week.

Risk factors for depression in multiple sclerosis are:

- male
- young onset of disease
- significant depression
- social isolation
- substance abuse.

There are no randomised clinical trials of **treatment**. Tricyclic antidepressants may worsen the autonomic symptoms and anticholinergic side-effects may worsen existing problems (eg constipation). SSRIs can worsen nausea or sexual dysfunction.

ECT produces an adverse neurological outcome in 20% of people (particularly if there are contrast-enhancing lesions on MRI).

Mania in multiple sclerosis

Mania is relatively rare but may be:

- a pre-existing bipolar disorder
- iatrogenic (steroids, baclofen, dantrolene, tizanidine)
- related to drugs of abuse.

Paroxysmal changes in mental state

- **Pathological laughing and crying**
  - sudden onset and offset
  - in response to non-affect laden stimulus
  - associated with chronic multiple sclerosis and cognitive impairment
- **Emotional lability**
  - excessive emotional response to minor stimulus
  - brief in duration.

Psychosis in multiple sclerosis

Psychosis is relatively uncommon. Schizophreniform symptoms are common in men, related to bilateral temporal horn lesions.

Differential diagnosis needs to exclude:

- dementia related to multiple sclerosis
- delirium
- drug-induced psychosis
- depression with mood-congruent psychosis.

Treatment is with atypical antipsychotics. The prognosis for psychotic symptoms is relatively good.

Cognition in multiple sclerosis

Cognitive impairment is present in around 40% of people with multiple sclerosis in the community. Typically there are reduced processing speed and impaired executive functions, which are positively correlated with total lesion load on MRI and quality of life. The Folstein Mini Mental State Examination is not sensitive to cognitive change in multiple sclerosis. Suggested tests include the **Addenbrookes Cognitive Examination (ACE)** and the **Frontal Assessment Battery (FAB)**.

NEUROPSYCHIATRY OF SLEEP DISORDERS

Normal sleep

Sleep is divided into rapid eye movement (REM) and non-REM sleep. Non-REM sleep is further subdivided into Stages 1–4.

The following are generalisations about sleep in the normal young adult.

- The normal human adult enters sleep through Stage 1 NREM sleep.
- REM sleep does not occur until 80 minutes or longer.
- REM and NREM sleep alternate through the night with an approximately 90-minute cycle.

- Slow-wave sleep (stages 3 and 4) predominates in the first third of the night.
- REM sleep predominates in the last third of the night.
- Wakefulness during sleep usually accounts for less than 5% of the night.
- Stage 1 sleep constitutes around 2–5% of sleep.
- Stage 2 sleep constitutes around 45–55% of sleep.
- Stage 3 sleep constitutes around 3–8% of sleep.
- Stage 4 sleep constitutes around 10–15% of sleep.
- REM sleep constitutes around 20–25% of sleep, occurring in four to six discrete episodes.

Stage 1 sleep is light sleep from which a person can be roused easily. **Stage 2 sleep** shows sleep spindles and K-complexes on EEG (lasts 10–25 minutes) and a person is less easily rousable. **Stage 3 sleep** involves high-voltage slow- (delta) wave activity; and **Stage 4 sleep** comprises more than 50% high-voltage slow-wave activity.

Sleep disorders

Sleep disorders include:

- narcolepsy
- parasomnias (REM sleep behaviour disorder, somnambulism, confusional arousals, nightmares, sleep paralysis, periodic limb movements of sleep)
- sleep apnoea
- sleep phase disturbance.

Narcolepsy

Prevalence of narcolepsy is between three and six people per 100,000.

Symptoms of narcolepsy include (because of the intrusion of REM sleep into wakefulness):

- sleep attacks (100%)
- cataplexy (70%)
- hypnogogic hallucinations (20–40%)
- sleep paralysis (25–50%).

Diagnosis is through **polysomnography** and **multiple sleep latency testing** (short sleep latency, sleep onset REM).

Treatment is with stimulant medication (modafinil, dexamphetamine) and clomipramine for cataplexy.

REM sleep behaviour disorder

This is REM sleep without atonia, leading to the acting out of dreaming behaviour. It may be a first symptom of akinetic–rigid syndromes such as Parkinson's disease or it can be related to alcohol or drug use.

Treatment is with clonazepam.

Somnambulism

Somnambulism occurs when there is abrupt arousal out of slow-wave sleep. A strong family history is common. It may be related to emotional stress.

Treatment is through risk management, benzodiazepines, imipramine and stress reduction.

Night terrors (pavor nocturnus)

Sudden arousal from slow-wave sleep in first third of the night can cause night terrors. There may be a loud scream, no memory of a dream and intense autonomic arousal. It can be related to sleep walking.

Treatment is with psychotherapy, benzodiazepines and tricyclic antidepressants.

Nightmares

These are fearful, vivid dreams associated with REM sleep. They are more common in children. They can be caused by certain medications (eg propranolol). Reassurance is the best treatment.

THE ELECTROENCEPHALOGRAM (EEG)

The EEG is predominantly used to detect the presence of seizure activity but can also detect changes in alertness and stages of sleep. The recording is a measure of voltage between electrodes usually placed on the scalp.

The waveforms generated are usually described in terms of amplitude and frequency as in Table 16.5:

Name	Frequency (Hz)
Delta	0.5–4
Theta	4–8
Alpha	8–14
Beta	14–32
Gamma	32–48+

Table 16.5 Frequency of different waveforms

Alpha rhythm is the predominant frequency of the normal, awake brain and is recorded maximally in the posterior regions of the brain. It tends to appear on eye closure and disappear on eye opening.

Evoked potentials

These are summations or averages of mostly post-synaptic potentials following some kind of stimulus (auditory, visual, or proprioceptive). They can be useful in the diagnosis of a number of neurological disorders including multiple sclerosis.

Actions of drugs on EEG

Different groups of drugs affect the EEG recording in different ways depending on the situation (therapeutic dose, acute intoxication, or withdrawal).

Barbiturates at normal doses often increase fast activity but overdosing leads to a predominance of slower frequency waves.

Antipsychotics can lead to an increase in both fast and slow frequencies with a reduction in beta activity. The EEG in people with epilepsy can deteriorate, particularly with clozapine, which can lead to EEG deterioration in over 50% of patients with epilepsy.

Tricyclic antidepressants can also lead to increases in fast and slow activity on EEG and a reduction in seizure threshold.

The effect on EEG of **SSRIs** is less clear and does not show any specific patterns.

Benzodiazepines at therapeutic doses enhance beta activity and raise the seizure threshold. Intoxication with benzodiazepines can lead to predominant fast activity.

Chapter 17

Critical Appraisal Skills

Katie Kelly

CONTENTS

Critical Appraisal Skills

Critical appraisal of a scientific paper is an important skill in informing clinic practice and has a prominent place in the Part II examination. It can only really be learned through practice and should be a key part of postgraduate training. Some aspects of study design have been covered in Chapters 4 and 11. This chapter will offer a framework of questions to consider and an overview of statistical concepts.

APPRAISING STUDY REPORTS

Research reports follow a similar format wherever they are published. The following questions provide a framework for determining how seriously to take the findings of a given study.

Study design

- Does the title describe the study accurately (what and who is it about)?
- Is there a clear rationale?
- Is the literature reviewed fully?
- Is the sample population relevant and large enough (are any power calculations stated)?
- Was ethics approval received and were ethical concerns addressed?

Data presentation

- Were the methods of measurement and data collection reliable and valid?
- Are the statistics appropriate and clearly explained?
- Are the results described adequately?
- Was statistical significance discussed (for quantitative research)?
- If there is a valid statistical association is it due to chance, bias, or confounding?

Conclusions

- Are the main findings explained and the results analysed sufficiently?
- Is the interpretation of hypothetical findings sound?
- Are the conclusions logical and well described?
- How do the findings compare with other research?
- Are the results clinically useful/discussed in terms of cost–benefit analysis?
- Have the authors discussed directions for future research?

BASIC STATISTICAL CONCEPTS

Descriptive: Describe characteristics of a given sample (mean, median).

Inferential: Quantify certainty when making inferences about a general population from a given sample of that population. Only works if each individual of the target population has the same chance to be sampled.

Types of data

Data can be **categorical:**

- binary (ie dead or alive)
- ordinal (ie social class I–V)
- nominal (ie married, single, or divorced)

or it can be **quantitative**:

- discrete (ie number of siblings)
- continuous (ie weight).

Descriptive statistics

These can be measures of location or measures of spread.

Measures of location are:

- **mean**: Average = $(\Sigma\chi)/n$
- **median**: Middle value in the range
- **mode**: Most frequently occurring value.

Measures of spread are:

- **range**: Difference between highest and lowest value
- **centiles**: Two values which encompass most rather than all of the data values (eg inter-quartile range, from 25th to 75th centiles)
- **standard deviation** (σ): Standardised measure of data dispersion (spread around the mean)
  - in a normal distribution this would be: 67% of values lie between ± 1SD; 95% of values lie between ± 2SD; and 99% of values lie between ± 3SD
- **variance** (s)$=\sigma^2$
- **$n - 1$**=degrees of freedom of the variance
- **standard error** = (standard deviation/$\sqrt{n}$)
- difference between the sample and population means
- when distribution curve is symmetrical the mean approximates to the median

The normal distribution

Normal distribution (many continuous) variables are analysed using parametric statistics. A typical normal distribution is shown in Figure 17.1.

Transformations: Data that do not form a normal distribution can be transformed to approach normal:

- Skewed data (left- or right-hand tail of distribution is longer than expected) can be plotted as $\log_e$.
- When the ratio of the standard deviation to the mean is similar among several groups of observations, use $\log_{10}$.
- When variable is a count, square root can be used.
- For extremely skewed distributions try a reciprocal (1/data).

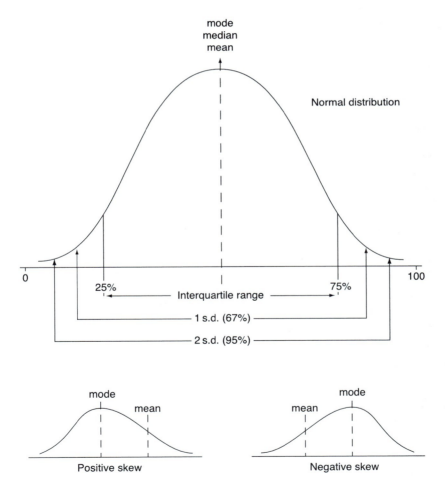

Figure 17.1 Normal distribution and skewness

335

Central Limit Theorem: Even when the original variable is not part of a normal distribution, the sample mean approaches normal distribution as sample size increases.

Inferential statistics

Certainty can be quantified in making inferences from a sample.

- **Hypothesis Testing** involves the testing of a hypothesis about a population to see whether experimental data support or refute it. Suppose researchers believe there is no difference between populations A and B.:
  - The **Null hypothesis** (H_0) says that there is no difference (H_0 : A=B)
  - The **alternative hypothesis** (H_A) is that there is a difference (H_A : A=B).
- **Errors** can be type I or type II.
  - **Type I error**: False rejection of null hypothesis where no true difference exists ('backing a loser')
  - **Type II error**: False acceptance of null hypothesis where a true difference exists ('missing a winner').

Researcher's decision	Yes	No
Reject H_0	Type 1 error (α)	Correct decision (power)
Accept H_0	Correct decision	Type 2 error (β)

Table 17.1 Is H_0 really true?

- **Power**: The probability of demonstrating significant difference between groups where one exists ($1 - \beta$).
  - Type I error = significance level of the test = α
  - By calculating beforehand how many observations are needed, a statistician sets the significance level of a test at 5% and the power at 80%.
- **Bonferonni Correction**. When multiple statistical tests are used on the same data, some significant results will be due to chance (1 in 20 if α is set to 5%). Bonferonni corrected for this: Bonferonni correction = α/ (number of times statistical tests are used on same data).
- **Statistical significance** is arbitrarily assigned to events which would occur by chance less than once in 20 times (ie < 5% or P (probability) < 0.05). So H_0 would be rejected if $P < 0.05$.
  - P measures the strength of evidence against H_0, the lower the P value the greater the evidence.
- **Confidence intervals** (CI). A range of values within which the true value lies to a specific degree of confidence (eg 95%).
  - CI should be quoted with P values
  - smaller samples have wider CIs (less certainty)
  - 95% CI = mean + (1.96 × Standard Error of the Mean)
  - ie 95% CI = $\mu + [1.96 \times (\sigma/\sqrt{n})]$.

Parametric and non-parametric statistical techniques

- Parametric tests assume normal distribution and comparable standard deviations.
- Non-parametric tests do not require normal distribution ('distribution free').
- Parametric testing is more powerful and makes the calculation of CIs easier.

APPLYING STATISTICAL TESTS

Continuous data, one variable measured

Number of samples	Parametric	Non-parametric
One sample eg average weekly blood pressure in ten students (one average from each student)	One sample *t*-test	Wilcoxon signed rank sum test
Two samples Paired (average weekly blood pressure before and after exams)	Paired *t*-test	Wilcoxon matched pairs signed rank sum test
Unpaired (average weekly blood pressure in students who exercise regularly vs those who do not)	Two-sample *t*-test	Mann–Whitney *U*-test
Three or more samples (average weekly blood pressure in French, German and History students)	One-way ANOVA	Kruskal–Wallace test

Table 17.2

For **Analysis of Variance** (ANOVA) the variability between different group means is compared with the variability of observations around the mean within the group. Ratio is the F statistic.

ANOVAs differ depending on number of factors/independent variables (*n*-way ANOVA: *n* = number of factors).

Categorical data (including binary data or proportions)

Number of samples	Test	
2	Paired samples	McNemar Test
	Unpaired samples (two independent groups)	χ^2 test
3 or more	Unpaired samples (three or more independent groups)	χ^2 test

χ^2 test is non-parametric

Table 17.3

Binary data can also be represented in contingency or frequency tables:

Sex	Admitted	Not admitted
Male	25	75
Female	40	60

Table 17.4 Cross-tabulation of sex vs admission

Correlation

- Correlation measures degree of association between two sets of variables and provides a measure of strength of association.
- Correlation coefficients range from −1 to +1
  - +1: perfect positive association (one variable increases with the other in a linear fashion)
  - −1: perfect negative association (one variable increases as the other decreases in a linear fashion)
  - 0: no correlation at all.
- **Parametric data**: Use Pearson's (product moment) *r*.
- **Non-parametric data**: Spearman's ρ or Kendall's τ.

Regression

Regression determines the nature of the relationship between two or more variables and allows predictions to be made from this.

- **Simple linear regression.** If a linear relationship can be seen between two variables, when plotted on a graph, one is designated the dependent variable (*y*) and calculated from the other, the independent variable (*x*), by the equation: $y = a + bx + e$, where (a = constant, b = regression coefficient, e = residual or error).

- **Multiple regression** determines relationship between a dependent variable and two or more independent variables.
  - **linear**: Continuous variables
  - **logistic**: Continuous variables and binary outcome (weight, blood glucose, presence/absence of diabetes).
- Other types of regression.
  - **n-way ANOVA**: For categorical variables
  - **Analysis of co-variance** (ANCOVA): categorical and continuous variables
  - **Multi-variate ANOVA** (MANOVA): number of dependent variables
  - **Multi-variate ANCOVA** (MANCOVA): multiple independent and dependent variables.

Factor analysis

Factor analysis identifies groups of variables (factors) that are highly inter-correlated. It can be used to reduce large, complex data sets to a smaller number of explanatory variables.

Survival analysis

A regression analysis for survival data used in longitudinal cohort studies to determine time interval until there is an outcome (eg death, relapse).

- It can be plotted as a survival curve.
- It can compare two populations differing in treatment received or exposure to risk factors.
- For more than one variable, use Cox's proportional hazards regression analysis.
- Kaplan–Meier method is also used in survival analysis.

SOURCES OF ERROR IN STUDY DESIGN

Bias

A systematic, as opposed to random error that distorts the data obtained from a clinical trial.

- **Information bias**: Information is tainted by the subject's own beliefs and values.
- **Observer bias**: Objectivity of researchers varies greatly.
- **Interviewer bias**: Unblinded researchers may (consciously or unconsciously) alter their approach to certain subjects.
- **Ascertainment bias**: Results systematically distorted by knowledge of which intervention each participant is receiving.
- **Selection bias**: Recruitment of an unrepresentative study population.
- **Recall bias**: Systematic error due to differences in accuracy or completeness of recall of past events (especially in retrospective studies).

Confounding

The effects of two relevant exposures have not been separated (eg age and social class in epidemiological studies).

Confounding variable: One associated with **both** exposure and outcome, giving a spurious association.

In a study, coal miners who worked at the coal face were found to have twice the incidence of lung cancer that was present in surface workers. This apparently higher risk might be explained by the fact that coal-face workers smoke more than surface workers. Smoking would therefore be a confounding variable.

Dropouts/Attrition

Subjects leaving a study early can skew subsequent results and their interpretation. This can be approached by:

- targeted refreshment sampling approach: New data is collected from the original sampling population
- statistical methods (eg last observation carried forward)
- analysing the dropouts for differences from completers and deducing reasons (ie is there a common adverse effect?)

Assessment of treatment effects

Reviewing published literature alone may result in bias where a sample of a particular trial's results (which might be clinically important but statistically modest) is unpublished precisely because they are not exceptional. In rigorous meta-analyses, this selective exclusion of certain randomised trial results is overcome through a systematic review of all (or an unbiased subset of) randomised trials ever undertaken, published and unpublished.

RANDOMISED CONTROLLED TRIALS (RCT)

Subjects are randomly allocated to experimental and control groups to investigate treatment effects. The effect can be small; a 10–20% risk reduction is often clinically important. Smaller expected differences are more susceptible to bias or confounding. It is essential to calculate sample size based on power to eliminate these factors.

Simple randomised controlled trials

Advantages of simple randomised controlled trials are that:

- assignment to treatment can be concealed
- confounders are equally distributed

- blinding is more likely
- randomisation facilitates statistical analysis
- when well-designed, they have high internal validity.

Disadvantages of simple randomised controlled trials are that:

- they are expensive
- large samples are required
- rigorous exclusion and selection criteria improve validity but complicate recruitment
- subjects consenting may differ from average (volunteer bias). Psychiatric patients with co-morbidities or concurrent substance abuse are often excluded.
- they are limited by ethical constraints
- a poorly designed randomised controlled trial wastes resources, exposes patients to risk of treatment without advancing medical knowledge and can mislead clinicians
- findings may not be relevant to everyday practice
- researchers may benefit from special expertise or facilities
- subjects may not comply.

Crossover randomised controlled trials

Subjects are initially assigned to intervention or control group but crossover to the other group at a given point.

Advantages of crossover randomised controlled trials are that:

- subjects are own controls
- sample size is reduced
- all subjects receive some treatment
- 'within-subject' comparisons are possible.

Disadvantages of crossover randomised controlled trials are that:

- all subjects receive placebo or alternative treatment at some point
- washout period is lengthy or unknown
- cannot be used for a treatment which has permanent effects.

Relevance of randomised controlled trials to everyday practice

Pragmatic randomised controlled trials have been designed to answer clinically relevant questions in relevant settings and on representative groups of patients. The treatment, patients and services involved should be representative of what is available in everyday practice. Scientific quality can be compromised and blinding and dropouts can be problematic.

Consort statement

All randomised controlled trial publications should follow the Consort Statement, specifying the following:

- **Title/abstract**: Number of subjects allocated to interventions ('random allocation', 'randomised', or 'randomly assigned').
- **Introduction**: background, scientific background, rationale.
- **Method**
  - subjects: Inclusion/exclusion criteria
  - settings/location for study
  - details of interventions and how/when administered
  - objectives and hypotheses
  - outcomes: With clearly-defined primary and secondary outcome measures and methods of enhancing measurements (multiple observations, training of assessors)
  - sample size: How calculated, explanation of interim analyses and stopping rules
  - randomisation: Method (sequence generation) and restrictions (eg blocking, stratification)
  - allocation concealment: eg numbered containers, central telephone and whether sequence hidden until interventions assigned
  - implementation: Who produced allocation sequence, enrolled subjects, assigned subjects to groups
  - blinding: Single, double, evaluation
  - statistical methods.
- **Results**
  - flow of subjects through each stage (with diagram). Numbers of participants randomly assigned, receiving intended treatment, completing, analysed for primary outcome in each group
  - protocol deviations with reasons
  - periods of recruitment and follow-up
  - baseline demographic data and clinical characteristics
  - numbers analysed and whether by 'intention-to-treat'. Results stated as absolute numbers where feasible (10/20, not 50%)
  - primary/secondary outcomes with a summary of results for each group, estimated effect size and its precision (95% CI).
  - ancillary analyses: including subgroup analyses, adjusted analyses, pre-specified and those exploratory
  - all important adverse events in each group.
- **Discussion**
  - interpretation of results, taking into account hypotheses, bias, imprecision and dangers of multiple analyses and outcomes
  - external validity (do the findings generalise?)
  - general interpretation of the results in the context of current evidence
  - suggestions for further investigation.

OTHER QUANTITATIVE STUDIES

Cohort (longitudinal, follow-up) study

Sample is selected **before** the onset of disease and followed over time to establish who develops the disease and the associated factors. Subjects are divided at the outset into two groups: Those who received the exposure of interest and those who did not. This allows conclusions to be drawn about the association between an exposure and a disease.

- It is an observational study.
- Prospective or retrospective.
- It can evaluate rare exposures, temporal relationships and multiple outcomes.
- It requires large samples so best suited to studying relatively common diseases.
- It is useful where researchers would be likely to lose contact with large numbers of subjects.

Advantages of cohort studies include:

- they are ethically safe
- subjects are matched (exposed/unexposed cohorts should be as similar as possible)
- establishes timing and directionality of events (causation and exposure)
- they are easier and cheaper than randomised controlled trials
- can examine many outcomes for a single exposure (allows natural history of a disease to be studied)
- can calculate incidence rates
- historical cohort studies can offer a short-cut to studying diseases with a long interval between exposure and disease.

Disadvantages of cohort studies include:

- controls are difficult to identify
- exposure may be linked to a hidden confounder
- blinding is difficult
- can still be expensive
- no randomisation
- for rare diseases, large sample size or long follow-up is necessary (delay before results are available)
- losses to follow-up can affect validity.

Case–control study

Compares people with a condition ('cases') to others from the same population who do not have that condition ('controls'). Outcomes are compared that establish associations and causal relationships.

- Suitable for studying rare diseases.
- Evaluates distant and multiple exposures.

Advantages of case–control studies include:

- they are quick and cheap
- fewer subjects are needed.

Disadvantages of case–control studies include:

- it is not possible to calculate incidence rates
- rare exposures are difficult to investigate
- rely on recall or records to determine exposure status
- susceptible to selection or recruitment bias (unrepresentative study population)
- cases and controls must come from the same population
- susceptible to recall bias (ie patients forgetting or looking at things with hindsight and trying to find an explanation for an illness).

QUALITATIVE RESEARCH

Concerned with personal feelings, experiences and opinions, this is subjective rather than numerical. Data are usually gathered using semi-structured interviews or simple observation. Of particular value in psychiatry/psychology (eg when examining reasons for non-compliance or stigma).

Advantages of qualitative research are that it can:

- illuminate complex issues
- complement quantitative research by helping in questionnaire development.

Disadvantages are that:

- it is difficult to plan data collection and analysis
- researcher's interests can influence data collection.

Frequencies are used to summarise **qualitative data**. A **frequency** is the number of observations in each category, usually tabulated or presented as a bar or pie chart.

Proportions are the fraction of observations in each category of a binary variable. Binary variables are usually presented by showing the percentage in just one of the categories.

OTHER STUDY DESIGNS

Single case studies or case series

These identify priorities or hypotheses for more comprehensive study. They may be the best available information on very rare diseases.

Disadvantages are that:

- they are prone to bias and chance associations
- no comparison group (cannot test hypotheses) is available.

Cross-sectional surveys

See Chapter 11.

Randomised controlled trial	strong
Cohort	moderate
Case control	moderate
Cross-sectional	weak
Ecological	weak

Table 17.5 Relative ability of studies to 'prove' causation

Economic analyses

Inform the best use of resources by comparing effects ('outputs') of competing interventions with their costs ('inputs'). There are four main types:

1 Cost minimisation

- o only the inputs (costs) are considered
- o outputs are assumed equal
- o eg using the cheaper of two equally effective treatments.

2 Cost–benefit

- o inputs and outputs are measured in monetary terms
- o eg costs of drugs, nursing staff etc versus time off work with and without treatment.

3 Cost-effectiveness

- o costs are related to a clinical output measure (life years gained)
- o cannot distinguish between interventions providing more benefit at greater cost or less benefit at lower cost.

4 Cost utility

- o an output combines quantitative and qualitative information about amount and relative quality of life gained
- o eg Quality Adjusted Life Year (QALY).

STATISTICAL CONCEPTS IN EVIDENCE-BASED MEDICINE

Screening and diagnostic studies

For example, a study investigating the usefulness of a test.

	Disorder present	Disorder absent	Totals
Diagnostic test positive	A True positive	B False positive	A + B
Diagnostic test negative	C False negative	D True negative	C+D
Totals	A + C	B + D	A + B + C + D

Table 17.6

- **Sensitivity**: Proportion of true cases correctly identified [A/(A + C)]
- **Specificity**: Proportion of true negatives correctly identified [D/(B + D)]
- **Positive predictive value**: Proportion of test positives with the target disorder [A/(A + B)]
- **Pre-test probability**: Probability of a subject having the disorder before testing [(A + C)/(A + B + C + D)]. For a screening test, disease prevalence.
- **Pre-test odds**: The odds that a subject will have the disorder before the test, this is calculated as pre-test probability/(1 – pre-test probability).
- **Likelihood ratio for a positive result** (LR+): The odds that a positive test result will be present in a patient with the target disorder compared to a patient without the target disorder = sensitivity/ (1 – specificity)
  - LR+ ≥ 10: Positive test result indicates a big change from pre-test to post-test probability. Test is useful for ruling in the diagnosis (especially when pre-test probability is ≥ 30%).
- **Likelihood ratio for a negative result** (LR–): The odds that a negative test result will be present in a patient with the target disorder compared to a patient without the target disorder = (1–sensitivity)/specificity.
  - LR– ≤ 0.1: Positive test result indicates a big change from pre-test to post-test probability, making the test useful for ruling in the diagnosis (especially when pre-test probability < 30%)
  - **Post-test odds** = pre-test odds × likelihood ratio
  - **Post-test probability**: Probability that a subject will have the disorder after the test is calculated as post-test odds/(post test odds + 1).
- **Bayesian probability**: Investigator estimates the prior probability of an event occurring, includes this in a hypothesis and conducts a study to test that hypothesis. The probability is subsequently modified according to the findings.

Randomised controlled trials

| | Outcome event (eg improved) | | |
	Yes	No	Total
Control group	a	b	a + b
Experimental group	c	d	c + d
Totals	a + c	b + d	a + b + c + d

Table 17.7

- **Control Event Rate** (CER): Risk of outcome event in the control group (a/a + b)
- **Experimental Event Rate** (EER): Risk of outcome event in the experimental group (c/c + d)
- **Relative Risk Reduction** (RRR): Equals CER – EER/CER
- **Absolute Risk Reduction** (ARR): Equals CER – EER
- **Absolute Risk Increase** (ARI): Equals EER – CER
- EER and CER are not rates but proportions.
- **Number Needed to Treat** (NNT): The number of patients who must be exposed to an intervention before the clinical outcome of interest occurs (the number of patients needed to treat to prevent one adverse outcome). The lower the NNT the better the intervention.
  - Number needed to treat: = 1/ARR.
  - Number needed to harm(NNH) = 1/ARI.
  - CI should be stated.

Harm/aetiology

Ratio measures are used in interpreting possible causal associations and estimating strength of association between exposure and disease.

	Disorder present (cases)	Disorder absent (controls)	Totals
Exposed to risk	a	b	a + b
Unexposed to risk	c	d	c + d
Totals	a + c	b + d	a + b +c + d

Table 17.8

Cohort studies show that Relative Risk (RR) = (a/a + b)–c/c + d

If RR = 1, risks of exposed and non-exposed populations identical.

If RR > 1, exposed group at greater risk.

If RR < 1, exposed group at less risk.

- Should always show CI (usually 95%).
- CI encompasses 1, H_0 is accepted.
- CI does not include 1, H_0 is rejected (there is a difference in risk between exposed and unexposed populations).

Case–control studies show that the Relative odds = odds ratio (OR) = (a/b)/(c/d) = ad/bc.

Notes about relative risks and odds ratios.

- Relative risk is more useful in cohort studies.
- OR is useful in case–control studies where events are usually rare and RR is difficult to estimate.
- When risk (or odds) in the two groups is small for both (< 20%), then, OR = RR.
- OR as an approximation to RR is unreliable when events are common, especially when the event rate is high in only one group. The OR overestimates the strength of the association.

Intention to treat (ITT)

A technique used in trials to try to reduce bias from withdrawals, dropouts and protocol violations. All study participants are included in the analyses as part of the groups to which they were originally randomised, regardless of whether they completed the study or not.

- If there is missing follow-up data, data from the last available time point are used (last observation carried forward).
- For drop-outs, a poor outcome is assumed (worst case scenario).
- It reflects real clinical practice.
- Failure to perform ITT analysis may bias results.

Reliability

The level of agreement between repeated measurements.

- **Inter-rater (intra-rater)**: Degree to which different raters (or the same rater at different times) give consistent estimates of the same phenomenon.
- **Test–retest**: Consistency of a measure from one time to another.
- **Parallel (alternative) form**: Consistency of two tests constructed in the same way from the same content domain.
- **Split-half**: Consistency between two halves of the same test.
- **Internal consistency**: Consistency across items within a test.

Statistical measures of reliability include kappa (diagnostic agreement corrected for chance) and Cronbach's alpha (measures internal consistency).

Validity

Whether a test measures what it aims to measure. This depends on reliability. Predictive and incremental are the most important.

- **Face**: Whether a test looks as if it is valid (basic but unsatisfactory test).
- **Concurrent**: Correlated with an available test that is known to be valid.
- **Construct**: Internal consistency in construction (similar questions correlate well).
- **Predictive**: Test can predict future behaviour (must have evidence of correlation > +0.7).
- **Incremental**: Test improves on decisions made from existing information or simpler techniques.
- **Internal**: Integrity of experimental design.
- **External**: Appropriateness of applying results to non-study populations.

SYSTEMATIC REVIEWS AND META-ANALYSES

A systematic review tries to access and review, systematically, all relevant articles in the field being studied. A meta-analysis generates a quantitative summary of the evidence, enabling the results of similar studies to be summarised as a single overall effect with confidence intervals.

Publication bias

Trials included in a systematic review are a biased sample because negative or weak positive studies are less likely to be published or because non-English language journals are excluded. A Funnel Plot can be used to look for publication bias.

Heterogeneity

Systematic differences between the results of studies that cannot be attributed to chance. Substantial heterogeneity between studies in a meta-analysis can bias the summary effect, may reflect important methodological differences and may mean there are distinct sub-groups of patients.

- **Heterogeneity** can be measured by calculating the Q statistic or with a Galbraith Plot (identifies which studies contribute most to heterogeneity).
- **Random effects** modelling does not assume a single underlying population treatment effect and takes into account the heterogeneity among studies.
- **Fixed effects** modelling does assume a single underlying population treatment effect.
- Generally, the results from both models are reported and the smallest overall effect is regarded as most likely to be true (usually the random effects result).

Meta-analysis

A meta-analysis calculates the summary effect size (as an odds ratio) by taking a mean of all the individual study effect sizes weighted by the individual study size. A Forest Plot is a pictorial representation of a meta-analysis. Cochrane reviews are examples of rigorous, large-scale meta-analyses in which published and unpublished data are included.

Chapter 18

Child and Adolescent Psychiatry

Alka Ahuja and Jane Scourfield

CONTENTS

Child and Adolescent Psychiatry

OVERVIEW

Child and adolescent psychiatry has, historically, been a multidisciplinary speciality. This reflects the multifactorial causation of psychiatric disorders, the fact that a number of agencies are concerned with the welfare of children (parents, schools, social services, the health service, courts, police and voluntary agencies, eg NSPCC), and the frequent use of psychological treatments.

It is important to consider the developmental perspective:

- symptoms are quantitative deviations from normality, eg too much, too intense, etc
- children are continuously developing, eg 3-year-olds are different from 14-year-olds.

CLASSIFICATION

The International Classification of Diseases (ICD-10) and the fourth revision of the Diagnostic and Statistical Manual of Mental Disorders (DSM-IV) have similar approaches to child and adolescent psychiatry. There are separate sections for disorders typical of childhood and for developmental disorders.

ICD-10

The ICD-10 includes the major psychiatric disorders as **Behavioural and emotional disorders with onset usually occurring in childhood and adolescence** (Table 18.1).

ICD-10 employs a multiaxial framework for psychiatric disorders in childhood and adolescence.

- Axis I: Clinical psychiatric syndromes
- Axis II: Specific disorders of development
- Axis III: Intellectual level
- Axis IV: Associated medical conditions
- Axis V: Associated abnormal psychosocial conditions
- Axis VI: Global social functioning.

There is increasing consideration of vulnerability or risk factors, protective factors and their interactions in predisposing and perpetuating childhood psychiatric disorders.

Diagnoses are based on the fact that the emotions or behaviour lie outside the normal range for age and sex, and that ordinary personal functioning or development is impaired or that the child experiences significant suffering.

Children and adolescents can also be affected by adult psychiatric disorders such as obsessive-compulsive disorder, schizophrenia, depression, eating disorders, etc.

Behavioural and emotional disorders with onset usually occurring in childhood and adolescence	Disorders of psychological development
Hyperkinetic disorders Disturbance of activity and attention Hyperkinetic conduct disorder Other hyperkinetic disorders Hyperkinetic disorder, unspecified	**Specific developmental disorders of speech and language** Specific speech articulation disorder Expressive language disorder Receptive language disorder Acquired aphasia with epilepsy (Landau–Kleffner syndrome) Other developmental disorders of speech and language Developmental disorder of speech and language, unspecified
Conduct disorders Conduct disorder confined to the family context Unsocialised conduct disorder Socialised conduct disorder Oppositional defiant disorder Other conduct disorders Conduct disorder, unspecified	**Specific developmental disorders of scholastic skills** Specific reading disorder Specific spelling disorder Specific disorder of arithmetic skills Mixed disorder of scholastic skills Other developmental disorders of scholastic skills Developmental disorder of scholastic skills, unspecified
Mixed disorders of conduct and emotions Depressive conduct disorder Other mixed disorders of conduct and emotions Mixed disorder of conduct and emotions, unspecified	**Specific developmental disorder of motor function**
Emotional disorders with onset specific to childhood Separation anxiety disorder of childhood Phobic anxiety disorder of childhood Social anxiety disorder of childhood Sibling rivalry disorder Other childhood emotional disorders Childhood emotional disorder, unspecified	**Mixed specific developmental disorder**
Disorders of social functioning with onset specific to childhood and adolescence Elective mutism Reactive attachment disorder of childhood Disinhibited attachment disorder of childhood Other childhood disorders of social functioning Childhood disorder of social functioning, unspecified	**Pervasive developmental disorders** Childhood autism Atypical autism Rett's syndrome Other childhood disintegrative disorder Overactive disorder associated with mental retardation and stereotyped movements Asperger's syndrome Other pervasive developmental disorders Pervasive developmental disorder, unspecified

continued opposite

Behavioural and emotional disorders with onset usually occurring in childhood and adolescence	Disorders of psychological development
Tic disorders Transient tic disorders Chronic motor or vocal tic disorder Combined vocal and multiple motor tic disorder (de la Tourette's syndrome) Other tic disorders Tic disorder, unspecified	**Other disorders of psychological development**
Other behavioural and emotional disorders with onset usually occurring in childhood and adolescence Non-organic enuresis Non-organic encopresis Feeding disorder of infancy and childhood Pica of infancy and childhood Stereotyped movement disorders Stuttering (stammering) Cluttering Other specified behavioural and emotional disorders with onset usually occurring in childhood and adolescence Unspecified behavioural and emotional disorders with onset usually occurring in childhood and adolescence	**Unspecified disorder of psychological development**

Table 18.1 ICD-10 classification of disorders of childhood

DSM-IV

The DSM-IV describes the major psychiatric disorders of childhood and adolescence as **'Disorders usually arising in Infancy, Childhood, or Adolescence'**. This section of the classification is according to age at presentation. It is not absolute because children and adolescents can be affected by adult psychiatric disorders such as depression, eating disorders, etc. However, the DSM-IV gives additional guidelines for children in some of these disorders, eg depressive disorders, anxiety disorders, etc.

The DSM-IV and ICD-10 have some minor differences while diagnosing certain childhood disorders, eg attention deficit and hyperactivity disorder/hyperkinetic disorder.

It has a multiaxial framework similar to the ICD-10.

- Axis I: Clinical disorders
  - other conditions that may be a focus of clinical attention
- Axis II: Mental retardation
  - personality disorders
- Axis III: General medical conditions

355

- Axis IV: Psychosocial and environmental problems
- Axis V: Global assessment of functioning.

EPIDEMIOLOGY

Classic studies

Pre-school period

The study by Richman *et al.* (1982) of 3-year-olds in Waltham Forest showed the following details.

- Common abnormalities of behaviour were bedwetting (37%), daytime wetting (17%), poor appetite (17%), night waking (14%), difficulty settling at night (13%), soiling (13%), fears (13%) and overactivity (13%).
- 7% had moderate to severe behaviour problems.
- 15% had mild behavioural problems.
- Prevalence rates were found to be equal in boys and girls.
- Associated factors were:
  - speech and language delay
  - maternal depression
  - poor parental marriage.
- Psychosocial adversities predicted a poor outcome.

Middle childhood

Rutter *et al.* (1970) carried out the Isle of Wight Study on 10- and 11-year-olds.

- 6.8% had a psychiatric disorder.
- 4% had a conduct disorder; 2.5% had an emotional disorder.
- Boys outnumbered girls by 1.9 : 1.
- 2.5% had an IQ < 70 and 5.7% had a physical disorder.
- Child psychiatric disorders in Inner London outnumbered those in the Isle of Wight by 2 : 1.

Adolescence

Prevalence of psychiatric disorders in adolescence is 10–20% and disorders in boys outnumber girls by 1.5 : 1.

More recent studies

A recent study by the Office for National Statistics (Melzer *et al.*, 2000) investigated 10,438 children and adolescents aged 5–15 years.

- 10% had a mental disorder.
- Conduct disorder was found in 5%, emotional disorders in 4%, and hyperkinetic disorder in 1%.

- Less common disorders (autistic disorders, tics and eating disorders) occurred in 0.5%.
- Prevalence of mental disorders was greater among children and adolescents:
  - in one-parent families
  - reconstituted families
  - families with five or more children
  - with uneducated and unemployed parents
  - in social class V and where parents were social sector tenants.

AETIOLOGY

Predisposing factors (that increase vulnerability to disorders), **precipitating factors** (that trigger the onset of the disorders) and **perpetuating factors** (that maintain the symptoms) may be found in the individual, family or environment.

	Individual	Family	Environment
Predisposing factors			
Precipitating factors			
Perpetuating factors			
Protective factors			

Table 18.2 Factors involved in the aetiology

Individual factors

- **Genetics**: There is evidence for genetic factors in childhood autism, Tourette syndrome, adolescent depression, schizophrenia, nocturnal enuresis, hyperkinetic disorders and mental retardation.
- **Gender**: Usually boys outnumber girls 2 : 1.
  - **Conduct disorders**: More boys than girls
  - **Emotional disorders**: In childhood boys and girls are equally represented but girls outnumber boys in adolescence.
  - **Anorexia nervosa**: Girls outnumber boys.
- **Cognition**: There are more psychiatric disorders in children with low IQ. Children with specific learning difficulties (eg specific reading retardation) show increased conduct disorder.
- **Temperament**: 'Difficult' temperament is associated with behavioural difficulties and attachment problems.
- **Chronic illness and disability**: Associated with increased psychiatric disorders (especially in children with central nervous system disorders and perceptual difficulties).

Family factors

The quality of family relationships is more important than the organisational structure of the family.

- **Early attachment**: Inadequate early attachments result in behavioural and emotional problems, difficult peer relationships and increased psychosocial problems in females. Positive changes are possible if the right environmental supports are provided.
- **Brief separations**: There are more problems following separation from a family with chronic difficulties than from a healthy family. Better parenting from adoptive or foster parents can have a positive impact. Multiple hospital admissions are a risk factor for later conduct disorder.
- **Divorce**: Increased emotional and conduct disorders occur, more in boys than in girls. However, children in well-functioning single-parent families do better than those in conflictual two-parent families.
- **Life events**: Disrupted early attachments, divorce, parental mental illness and criminality are associated with childhood psychiatric disorders. Four or more stressful life events between the age of 3 and 4 years double the chances of enuresis.
- **Family structure**: There is little evidence that any family structure per se is associated with greater incidence of child psychiatric disorders. Increased conduct and emotional disorders are found in single-parent families (but these families are more likely to be socio-economically disadvantaged).
- **Family size (see Table 18.3)**: Children from large families (more than four children) are twice as likely to develop conduct disorders. Lower intelligence and lower levels of reading attainment are found in children from large families.
- **Ordinal position**: Eldest children and only children tend to do better at school and work. Youngest children have higher school refusal.
- **Parenting style**: A disorganised approach to discipline, and harsh parenting lead to conduct disorder and aggression in children.
- **Marital discord**: There is increased risk of conduct disorder and delinquency, especially in boys.
- **Parental mental illness**: Alcoholism, personality disorder, chronic depression and other chronic emotional difficulties in parents are high risks to children. Children of parents with non-psychotic illness, especially depression, may be at greater risk than those with psychotic parents. Depression during the post-partum period affects the infant's cognitive and emotional development.

Mental disorders occur more in

- families with five or more children (18%) compared with two children (8%)
- families with neither parent working (20%) compared with both parents working (8%)
- families with gross weekly household income of < £200 (16%) compared with ≥ £500 (6%)
- families of social class V (14%) compared with social class I (5%)

Table 18.3 Family demographics and mental disorders
(Source: Melzer et al., 2000)

- **Parental criminality**: This is associated with a two- to threefold increase in child psychiatric disorder.

Environmental factors

- **Neighbourhoods**: Rutter *et al.* (1975) compared rates in the Isle of Wight and an inner-London borough and found higher rates in the latter area. The high rates are associated with higher rates of family and social risk factors. Social cohesion among neighbours is associated with decreased violence.
- **Social class and disadvantage**: Weak association of social class with childhood disorders but definite association with social adversity. Mild generalised learning difficulties are strongly associated with children from working-class families. Financial adversities and unemployment are important risk factors.
- **Schools**: Children do worse in schools where there is a high proportion of other children with behavioural difficulties. Bullying affects 10% of primary school children and may lead to emotional difficulties.

CLINICAL SYNDROMES

Temper tantrums

Tantrums are normal in toddlers. They are only a problem if severe, persistent and the parents are unable to deal with them. They tend to increase if the child gets attention or benefits through its tantrums.

Behavioural methods are helpful in the management of temper tantrums.

Sleep disorders

Wakefulness

Wakefulness is the most common sleep difficulty; 10% of children wake up every night.

- Peak incidence is at 12–24 months.
- It is associated with child's temperament, family stressors and parental factors (maternal depression).
- Behavioural methods are useful in management.

Night terrors

Night terrors occur in 3% of children (in older pre-school children but may persist into middle/later childhood).

- They often occur every night.
- The child suddenly sits up during sleep, shouts, screams and is terrified.
- There is no memory of the event.
- There is a fault in slow-wave sleep.
- Behaviour techniques are used for night terrors (child woken up every night before onset of the symptoms).

Sleep walking

The child gets up and walks about the house but is unresponsive.

- Family history is common, possible genetic basis.
- Most resolve spontaneously.

Nightmares

The child gets up frightened but is **able to describe** the dream, and it occurs in rapid eye movement sleep.

- Peak age for occurrence is 5–6 years.
- Associated with physical disorder (eg fever) or an emotional disorder (eg post-traumatic stress disorder).
- A rarer cause is **nocturnal epilepsy**.
- Reassurance and cognitive behavioural approaches ('rehearsal-relief') are useful.

Eating disorders

Food refusal and faddiness

Twelve per cent of children and adolescents have moderate or severe feeding problems.

- They may refuse to eat a wide range of foods or want it to be prepared in a specific way.
- Consider the child–parent relationship and family circumstances.

Non-organic failure to thrive

This is defined as being consistently below the third centile in weight or a reduction in growth velocity.

- 2% of inner city White children are affected.
- role of environmental deprivation, abuse and maltreatment and impaired mother–child interactions
- developmental counselling, family support and behaviour management programme are useful.

Pica

Pica is the persistent eating of non-nutritious substances, eg soil, paint chippings, inedible plants, etc.

- It is higher in young deprived children, the mentally handicapped, and those with pervasive developmental disorder.
- Associated with iron deficiency.
- Usually improves if associated anaemia is treated.

Anorexia nervosa

A condition characterised by excessive dieting and weight loss accompanied by a morbid fear of weight gain. Associated with disturbed perception of body image and widespread endocrine disorder involving the hypothalamic-pituitary-gonadal axis manifesting and primary or secondary amenorrhoea or delayed onset of puberty.

- Occurs in 0.5% of 12–19 year olds.
- Peak age of onset is around 14 years.
- Girls outnumber boys.
- **Aetiology**: Cultural factors (models, athletes, ballet dancers), abnormal family processes (over-involvement, promotion of dependence, emotional suppression) and premorbid perfectionism and histrionic traits. Higher heritability compared to bulimia.
- **Clinical features**: Failure to acknowledge an eating problem, weight loss (weight 15% below that expected for age and height or body mass index ≤ 17.5), intense fear of gaining weight, disturbed body image, delayed onset of puberty, growth retardation and amenorrhoea.
- **Associated features**: Obsession with size of body parts, preoccupation with food, calories etc, secret vomiting, abuse of laxatives and diuretics and excessive exercise.
- **Physical features**: Pallor, emaciation (disguised by baggy clothing), lanugo hair, skin dry and cold, loss of or failure to develop secondary sexual characteristics, bradycardia, hypotension and hypothermia.
- **Investigations**:
  - decreased luteinising hormone and follicle-stimulating hormone
  - increased cortisol and basal growth hormone
  - thyroxine normal but decreased triiodothyronine
  - decreased potassium
  - increased liver enzymes
  - decreased phosphate and magnesium
  - calcium is normal or raised
  - increased urea.
- **Treatment**: Structured programme of targeted weight increase (about 0.2kg/day) on outpatient or inpatient basis, psycho-education, family therapy and individual psychotherapy (cognitive behavioural therapy, psychodynamic therapy).
- **Prognosis**: Poor if chronic presentation, pre-pubertal age, repeated vomiting and purging, 5% become bulimic and about 5% die either through suicide or medical complications.

Bulimic disorders

Recurrent episodes of overeating in which a huge amount of calories are consumed in a short time. These episodes are followed by compensatory behaviours including self-induced vomiting or purging, laxative or diuretic abuse, alternate periods of starvation and excessive exercising. Associated weight and shape concerns.

- Affects 1% of adolescent girls.
- Peak age of onset is 19 years.
- **Aetiology**: Occurs as part of anorexia nervosa or as part of a pattern of normal weight regulation in people with low self-esteem and insecure gender roles, may be secondary to depression.

- **Clinical features**: Irresistible urge to overeat followed by self-induced vomiting and purging, or alternate periods of starvation with a morbid fear of becoming fat. Guilt, anger, shame and depression may occur.
- **Physical features**: Normal body weight, calluses on fingers, damage to tooth enamel and parotid enlargement as a result of frequent vomiting.
- **Treatment**: Cognitive behavioural therapy, family therapy, antidepressants (selective serotonin reuptake inhibitors).
- **Prognosis**: Episodic course and depression seen in 15–36% cases.

Pervasive refusal syndrome

A potentially life-threatening condition in which there is profound refusal to eat, drink, walk, talk or attend to basic needs. The children are usually underweight, dehydrated and resistant to all forms of help.

- Very rare.
- Affects girls (8–14 years old).
- Stop eating, walking, talking or self-care.

Food avoidance emotional disorder

A primary emotional disorder in which food avoidance is a prominent feature.

- Marked food avoidance and weight loss.
- No distorted body image or preoccupation with weight.

Functional dysphagia

This describes a fear of vomiting and difficulty in swallowing.

- No associated body image disturbance.
- Identifiable trigger present usually but no organic cause.

Attention deficit disorder (Hyperkinetic disorder)

- Affects 1.7% of a male sample.
- It is more common in boys than girls.
- **Aetiology**: Genetic factors, developmental factors, perinatal risk factors, food additives and immunological factors, increases with social adversity.
- Continuing maternal criticism and hostility lead to persistence of the disorder.
- **Clinical features**: triad of overactivity, inattention and impulsivity.
- Pervasive across different situations (ICD-10 criteria more rigid) and occurs before age of 7 years.
- Activity levels tend to fall with age but impulsivity continues.
- Associated with low IQ, antisocial behaviour, specific learning disorders and motor clumsiness.
- **Treatment**: Information from school as well as parents is essential for diagnosis.
- Behavioural interventions, stimulants (MTA study and NICE guidelines suggest methylphenidate and dexamphetamine), other drugs (atomoxetine clonidine in co-

morbid Tourette's syndrome, if sleeplessness is a problem; and/risperidone if there is associated aggressive behaviour), dietary modifications and educational support.

- **Prognosis**: May predict later antisocial disorder and substance misuse. Prognosis is poor if there are associated conduct problems, depression and maternal criticism.

DAMP, a disorder comprising **D**eficits in **A**ttention, **M**otor control and **P**erception, is a distinct disorder seen in some children.

Specific developmental disorders

Specific motor retardation (clumsiness)

Impairment in development of motor co-ordination with normal intelligence.

- Associated perceptual difficulties and delayed motor skills.
- Difficulties in writing, drawing and handling things (ball games, crockery).
- Educational and emotional problems common.
- Lower performance IQ.

Specific delay in language development

- **Causes**: Delayed maturation, family history, social environment (abuse, large families, twins, and lower social class) but **rule out hearing defects.**
- Deviant and delayed language occurs in infantile autism.

Specific reading disorder

Discrepancy between attainment and reading age as predicted on the basis of age and IQ.

- More common in boys than girls, raised levels in working-class families.
- Affects 4–10% of 9–10 year olds.
- Associated with speech delay, family history, **conduct disorder** (33%), brain injury, poor visuospatial ability, large family, overcrowding, low birth weight, episodic hearing impairment, visual defects and impulsivity and school refusal.
- Appropriate remedial teaching and prevention of secondary handicaps are needed.

Specific disorder of arithmetical skills

Serious impairment in the development of arithmetic skills which is not explicable in terms of general intellectual retardation or inadequate schooling. Sufferers misread signs or set out work incorrectly.

Pervasive developmental disorders

This is a triad of qualitative impairments in **reciprocal social interactions**, patterns of **communication** (verbal and non-verbal) and **restricted stereotyped repetitive repertoire of non-adaptive interests and activities**.

- Onset in infancy or early childhood.
- Intellectual handicap and developmental delay common (usually lower verbal IQ).
- Predictors of good prognosis: Early speech acquisition and high intelligence.

Infantile autism

This is an organic neurodevelopmental disorder described by Kanner.

- Prevalence is 4 per 10,000 population.
- Boys outnumber girls.
- There is no clear period of normal development and delay or deviant development is seen in the first three years of life.
- It is associated with infections such as congenital rubella and cytomegalovirus, perinatal factors, epilepsy and genetic conditions such as fragile X, phenylketonuria, tuberous sclerosis and neurofibromatosis. No social class bias.
- **Speech and language**: 50% do not develop any speech. Speech delays and lack of social use of language (pragmatics) are seen.
  - **Speech**: often stilted, lacks emotional expression; neologisms, pronominal reversal and echolalia are present and child is unable to appreciate metaphors.
- **Social abnormalities**: Aloofness, poor understanding and lack of response to social and emotional cues (lack of spontaneous affection), avoidance of eye contact, lack of empathy and shared play.
- **Behavioural abnormalities**: Unusual preoccupations, interests in parts of objects, rigid daily routines, unusual attachments to odd objects and manneristic behaviours. Often circumscribed interests in sterile topics, eg train timetables, numbers, etc.
- Detailed neurodevelopmental assessment is important.
- **Treatment**: Behavioural and educational interventions and medication for any associated conditions, eg anti-epileptics.

Asperger's syndrome (schizoid disorder of childhood)

- Prevalence is 2.6–3 per 1000 children.
- Male preponderance.
- **Intelligence** is usually within normal range.
- **Absence of delay in early language development** and appropriate use of grammar and vocabulary present.
- Oddities in communication may occur, such as peculiar prosody and abnormal facial and emotional gestures.
- Circumscribed interests and imposition of routines are common.
- Usually detected later in life when child enters more socially demanding environments such as school.

Rett syndrome

- Deteriorating condition characterised by **progressive loss of acquired abilities**.
- Only seen in **girls**.
- Normal development occurs in the first 1–2 years of life.
- Associated social withdrawal, dementia, stereotyped hand-washing movements, **deceleration of head growth**, broad-based stance ataxia, profound mental handicap, limb contractures and kyphoscoliosis common.
- Prognosis is poor.

Childhood disintegrative disorder (Heller syndrome; disintegrative psychosis)

- Normal development up to two years of age followed by **loss of previously acquired skills**.
- Seen in both boys and girls.
- Profound regression occurs with loss of language, regression of play and loss of social skills and adaptive behaviour.
- Motor mannerisms emerge and loss of bowel and bladder control may occur.
- Organic in origin and deterioration is fatal.

Disorders of social functioning

Reactive attachment disorder

Persistent abnormal pattern of relationships with carers present since before 5 years of age.

- **Aetiology**: Prematurity, congenital malformations and temperamental characteristics in the infant, childhood experience of abuse in carers or presence of a physical or mental illness.
- **Clinical features**: Contradictory and ambivalent social responses with carers, inappropriate sociability and affection with less familiar adults, fearfulness and hypervigilance (frozen watchfulness) seen.
- **Differential diagnosis**: Mental retardation, autism.

Disinhibited attachment disorder

- **Aetiology**: Disrupted early experiences (inadequate parental care, multiple placements in care), brain damage.
- **Clinical features**: Unable to make specific attachments to primary carer, persistent abnormal social functioning and indiscriminately friendly behaviour towards any adult. May show attention-seeking behaviour, overactivity, emotional lability and poor toleration of frustration and aggression.
- Improvement or establishment of a settled consistent environment for the child is important.

Emotional disorders

Separation anxiety disorder

This is a preoccupying worry that something might happen to the principal attachment figure (usually the mother) or that something may separate the child from him/her.

- Repeated nightmares, social withdrawal and physical symptoms (stomach aches or headaches) occur.
- School refusal and co-morbid depression are common.

Phobic disorder of childhood

- Equal incidence in boys and girls (but animal phobias are more common in girls).
- 2% of children are affected.
- **In pre-school children**: Related to actual events (animals, dark) and resolve spontaneously.
- **In middle childhood**: Specific fears (eg of animals, darkness) lessen but specific fears of school and social situations appear.
- **In adolescents**: Social phobias, agoraphobia, panic disorders and generalised anxiety disorders occur.
- One-third have a **family history** of panic or phobic disorders.
- It may be a learnt response if present in the family or it may develop following a traumatic event.
- **Treatment**: Behavioural methods (desensitisation, modelling and relaxation).

Social anxiety/sensitivity disorder

Persistent and recurrent fear of, or avoidance of, strangers.

- Occurs before 6 years of age.
- Equivalent to social phobia.

Sibling rivalry disorder

Persistent jealousy or emotional disturbance causing psychosocial impairment; occurs within a month after birth of a sibling.

Depression

- In childhood boys outnumber girls but in adolescence this is reversed and girls outnumber boys.
- 0.5–2.5% among children and 2–8% among adolescents.
- Prevalence increases with increasing age (more common in adolescents).
- **Aetiology**: Genetic (especially for bipolar disorder) and environmental factors contribute, loss (past or recent) may be a triggering event but physical illness, normal bereavement reactions and ordinary sadness must be excluded.
- **Clinical features**: presentation varies with age, **depressed mood and vegetative symptoms are uncommon in childhood**. Anhedonia, feelings of anger, poor memory and boredom are prominent.

- Other symptoms seen are social withdrawal, anger, irritability, somatic complaints, sleep difficulties and academic deterioration. Suicidal ideas are common in adolescents.
- **Co-morbid conditions**: Eating disorders, separation anxiety, school refusal, social phobia, conduct disorders, physical disorders.
- **Treatment**: Ensure the young person's safety (risk of self-harm), cognitive behaviour therapy, family therapy and antidepressants in severe cases.
- Most respond well but some develop recurrent and chronic depression.

Suicide

- More boys than girls commit suicide but self-harm is more common among girls.
- It is the third most common cause of death in adolescents.
- Sustained hopelessness, planning and premeditation are ominous signs.
- 15–25% repeat self-harm within a year and 1–2% will eventually succeed with suicide.
- **Increased risk of repetition**: Older males, disturbed family relationships, alcohol abuse, and psychiatric problems.
- **Associated factors**: Early loss of parent, poor family relationships, physical and sexual abuse, media models, mental illness in parents, school (bullying) or work problems.

School refusal

Non-attendance at school may be the result of truancy (conduct disorder) or school refusal (emotional disorder).

- It is equally common in boys as girls.
- **Three main incidence peaks by age**: Age 5 (school entry – separation anxiety), age 11 (most common age of presentation at time of transfer to secondary school – personality problems common) and at age 14–16 (first manifestation of depression or specific phobias).
- **Clinical features**: Inability to go to school or to stay in school because of anxiety and in spite of parental or other pressure, somatic symptoms occur to avoid going to school.
- May be of acute onset or follow an event (eg illness, bereavement, etc).

School refusers	Truants
Other emotional symptoms plus family history of neurosis	Other antisocial symptoms plus family history of antisocial behaviour
Academic performance satisfactory	Academic performance poor
Small family size	Large family size

Table 18.4 Differences between school refusers and truants

- **Treatment**: Rule out problems at school (bullying, or fears about physical activities or learning difficulties). Aim is to get the child back to the current school as soon as possible (Kennedy approach); if it is a chronic problem then graded return using support from parents, teachers, etc can be useful. Supplementary interventions for specific problems may be needed.
- Prognosis is better in younger children and if diagnosis is early.

Obsessive-compulsive disorder

- Affects 1% of clinic populations (1 in 250 adolescents).
- Onset is insidious and occurs in middle childhood.
- **Aetiology**: A family history is common (5% of parents), neurobiological factors.
- **Clinical features**: Grooming and washing rituals (younger adolescents), ruminations, doubts and obsessional slowness (older adolescents).
- Obsessions may occur in depression, anorexia nervosa, autistic disorders and tic disorder.
- **Treatment**: Behaviour therapy (response prevention, modelling and real-life exposure), family therapy and antidepressants (especially selective serotonin re-uptake inhibitors and clomipramine).
- **Prognosis** is better if duration of illness is shorter and if illness is part of an affective illness rather than in pure obsessive-compulsive disorder.

Elective mutism

Child has ability to speak but does not do so in some situations and with some people.

- Very rare (0.8 per 1000 children).
- More common in girls than boys.
- **Aetiology**: Electroencephalogram (EEG) abnormalities, parental mental illness, and parent's first language different from the child, traumatic events. Rule out hearing and language difficulties.
- **Clinical features**: Often starts with the onset of school. Normal speech is usually present but 50% have minor speech problems. Shyness, emotional and conduct problems are common.
- Family work and behavioural methods are used for treatment but it is important to exclude any organic cause.
- Poor prognosis if it persists at age of 10 and if there is a family history of psychiatric problems.

Conversion disorder

Loss of physical functioning as a result of a psychological cause.

- Incidence is the same in boys and girls.
- Epidemic hysteria is common in boarding schools, nurses homes, etc.
- There may be previous or current experience of physical illness (epilepsy and other neurological disorders).
- Commonly there are disorders of gait, loss of limb function and pseudoseizures (associated with incest).
- Consider possible sexual abuse.

- Treatment aims to reduce the secondary advantages of the sick role and increase the advantage of 'wellness behaviour'.
- Follow-up studies indicate that 46% have an organic illness.

Recurrent abdominal pain

- Seen in 25% of 5–6 year olds.
- Equal incidence in boys and girls.
- **Aetiology**: Temperamental difficulties, poor communication in families, mental illness in family.
- It is associated with emotional disorders, especially **school refusal**.
- Characterised by severe diffuse recurrent pain which is poorly localised; it sometimes has a cyclical nature (periodic syndrome or abdominal migraine).
- Good short-term prognosis but may recur in adult life.

Post-traumatic stress disorder

- Clinical features depend on child's age and development and the nature of the trauma.
- It may occur following chronic stresses (sexual abuse).
- Anxiety, fearfulness, repetitive play, recurrent intrusive memories and dreams occur. Numbing is uncommon.

Conduct disorder

Severe and persistent antisocial behaviour, such as excessive fighting, stealing, destruction of property, cruelty (especially to animals), fire setting, or truancy.

- Can be pervasive or situation specific.
- Incidence is 8.3% in 4–11 year olds and 14% in 12–16 year olds.
- Half to one-third present from childhood.
- More common in boys than girls.
- Conduct disorder may be:
  - **Unsocialised**: Acts performed alone.
  - **Socialised**: Acts performed along with peer group.
  - **Mixed disorder of conduct and emotions**: Co-existence with emotional symptoms.
  - **Oppositional defiant disorder**: Milder form with provocative, angry and disobedient behaviour to adults.
- Associated with emotional problems, **hyperactivity** (hyperkinetic conduct disorder), specific reading retardation, low IQ, life events eg death of a family member ('sleeper effects'), family discord, large family size, disadvantaged backgrounds, antisocial behaviour, mental illness and alcoholism in parents.
- **Treatment**: Behavioural training packages for parents and group therapy, individual psychotherapy (cognitive therapy, anger management, interpersonal problem solving) and family therapy.
- Prognosis is poor but those with good peer relationships do better.

Fire setting

- A severe form of conduct disorder with younger peak age and high male preponderance.
- Two groups:
  - younger group (boys with lower IQ, set fires on their own at home)
  - older group (operate in gangs and show other antisocial behaviour).
- Family history of antisocial problems, alcoholism and low intelligence.
- Motives are of two types, ie set fire in anger or for revenge and curiosity about fires.

Stealing

Stealing is the most common antisocial act at all ages.

- **Comfort stealing** is common, associated with emotional problems.
- **Marauding offences** are part of socialised conduct disorder in adolescence.
- **Proving offences** are rebellious and represent bids for a stronger self-identity.

Truancy

Voluntary non-attendance at school before the age of 16 years.

Solitary truanting is associated with later personality and social difficulties.

Delinquency

Delinquency is not a psychiatric diagnosis.

- This is a social rather than a medical form of deviance.
- Sexual offences, eg prostitution, are common in girls whereas sexual inadequacies, eg exhibitionism, are more common in boys.

Developmental disorders

Enuresis

Enuresis is the repeated involuntary passing of urine after age of 5 years with no organic cause.

- It may be diurnal/nocturnal, primary/ secondary (following a dry period).
- 10% of 5-year-olds and 5% of 10-year-olds.
- More common in boys than girls.
- **Aetiology**: Genetic factors (70% first-degree relatives are enuretic), environmental factors (family discord, large family size, problems over toilet training, acute stresses like birth of sibling), immature bladder, small functional bladder and low mental age.
- Increased rates of psychiatric disorders if daytime wetting is also present.
- **Treatment**: Behavioural methods (star charts, bell and pad method) and medication (tricyclic drugs and desmopressin).

Encopresis

Encopresis describes disorders of bowel function and control over the age of 4 years in the absence of physical abnormality or disease.

- It is present in 1% of primary schoolchildren.
- It is more common in boys than girls.
- **Aetiology**: Coercive or premature toilet training, developmental delay, family conflicts, sexual abuse, or neglect.
- Presents as failure of bowel control, depositing faeces in abnormal places, or excessively fluid faeces (constipation with overflow incontinence).
- Behavioural techniques along with contingency plans are useful.

Tic disorders

Tics are rapid, involuntary, purposeless, repetitive movements involving the face, neck and arms.

- 20% of children have tics at some time in their childhood and they persist in 1% of children.
- **Aetiology**: Neurological basis, family history is common, other associated psychiatric problems, EEG abnormalities and associated developmental delays.

Tourette syndrome

- Tourette syndrome is more common in boys than girls.
- Present with **motor** (posturing, echopraxia, smelling or touching objects) and **vocal tics** (throat clearing, coughing, explosive exhalations); 30–40% develop obscene utterances. Associated with **attention deficit hypertension disorder** and **obsessive-compulsive disorder**. It has a fluctuating course.
- **Treatment**: Includes behavioural interventions (muscle relaxation, massed practice) and pharmacotherapy (low-dose antipsychotics like haloperidol, risperidone or sulpiride).

Psychoses

Schizophrenia

- Onset is insidious and developmental delay is common.
- It is more common in boys than girls.
- **Clinical features**: Schneiderian first-rank symptoms and formed delusions are uncommon. Exaggeration of normal anxieties may occur. Vagueness of thought, circumstantial and tangential thinking, blunted affect, social withdrawal and educational difficulties occur.
- Manic episodes may be diagnosed as schizophrenia in adolescents.
- Prognosis is poor, especially in the presence of neurological impairment.

Manic-depressive illness

About a fifth to a quarter of adult bipolar illness begins in adolescence.

Associated with more frequent episodes, higher risk of suicide and strong family history of bipolar illness.

Substance abuse

- The three most common drugs used by adolescents are tobacco, alcohol and cannabis.
- Often used in the context of conduct disorder and antisocial problems.
- Peer pressure, poor parent–child relationships and boredom are common causes.

Gender identity disorders (see Chapter 14)

- Between 3 and 4% of children have gender identity difficulties.
- **Treatment**: Consider the child's uncertainty about gender identity and limit the child's cross-sex behaviour. Individual psychotherapy is useful in older children.

CHILD ABUSE AND NEGLECT

Physical abuse

Children may present with physical injuries or psychological features (unhappiness, aggression, or poor academic achievement).

Causes include:

- difficult temperament in child
- parental mental illness
- parent's own childhood experience of violence
- negative attitude towards the child.

Abuse is underestimated in clinical practice.

Emotional abuse

Emotional abuse is characterised by overt verbal abuse, rejection, blame, threats of abandonment, mocking, or taunting. Children may show psychological symptoms, such as abnormal attachment behaviour, poor self-esteem, defiant behaviour, social withdrawal and underachievement.

Causes include:

- negative feelings towards what the child represents
- parental mental illness.

Sexual abuse

Sexual abuse is defined as the involvement of a child by an adult in sexual activity.

Causes include:

- blurred family boundaries
- child's needs being undervalued
- parent's own childhood experience of abuse
- poor sexual satisfaction in parental marriage.

It is more frequent in girls than boys. Most cases arise within the family where the abuser is usually a male relative or a co-habitee of the girl's mother.

Abuse may present as:

- a crisis (overdose)
- disclosure to a trusted person outside the family (eg teacher)
- disclosure to a professional following a medical or psychological problem (vaginal discharge, sexually transmitted disease, conversion disorder, depression, inappropriate sexualised behaviour).

Any disclosure of sexual abuse should be taken seriously.

The child's welfare and protection are of paramount importance. The obligation to protect the child overrides medical confidentiality and the doctor can initiate action from police/social services. It is a not a psychiatric disorder but is a **risk factor** for many psychiatric conditions.

Neglect

Neglect is a lack of physical care-taking and supervision and a failure to fulfil the developmental needs of the child. It may present with physical (non-organic failure to thrive) or psychological symptoms (disturbed attachment, emotional disorder).

Munchausen's syndrome by proxy is a specific type of neglect.

- Symptoms or signs of illness are fabricated/induced by the carer.
- Child may present with fits, bleeding, fever, or breathing problems.
- Perpetrator is usually the mother and there may be previous history of an undiagnosed or unusual condition in another child.
- Immediate protection of the child is important.

CONTENTS

Learning Disability Psychiatry

DEFINITIONS

Learning disability (LD)

Originally a statistically derived term describing people who were two standard deviations below the norm (Intelligence Quotient (IQ) < 70). Broadened to include **functional** and **communication** elements occurring before age 18 (**developmental period**).

In the 2001 White paper, **Valuing People (DoH)**, LD includes:

- a significantly reduced ability to understand new or complex information, to learn new skills (impaired intelligence), with
- a reduced ability to cope independently (impaired social functioning) which started before adulthood, with a lasting effect on development.

The presence of a low intelligence quotient, for example an IQ below 70, is not, of itself, sufficient to decide provision of additional health and social care support; assessment of social functioning and communication skills should also be taken into account. Many people with LD also have physical and/or sensory impairments. The definition covers adults with autism who also have LD, but not those with a higher level autistic spectrum disorder who may be of average or even above average intelligence (eg some people with Asperger's syndrome).

The terms **mental handicap**, **mental retardation, mental deficiency and mental subnormality** were considered derogatory and replaced in the UK by LD (1992). This has caused confusion since, in the Americas, LD describes people with specific LD (eg specific reading disability (dyslexia)). A term gaining international credence at the present time is **Intellectual Disability**.

Term	IQ range	% of the LD population
Mild LD	50–69	75
Moderate LD	35–49	20
Severe LD	20–34	3
Profound LD	< 20	2

Table 19.1 Categories of LD

World Health Organisation

Impairment: Any loss or abnormality of psychological, physiological or anatomical structure or function.

Disability: Any reduction or lack (resulting from impairment) of ability to perform an activity in the manner or within the range considered normal for a human being.

Handicap: A disadvantage for an individual, resulting from impairment or disability that limits the fulfilment of role that is normal for that individual (age, gender, culture dependent). Includes dimensions of: physical independence, occupations with/without economic self-sufficiency, social integration, orientation or other.

MENTAL HEALTH ACT 1983

See Chapter 10.

The history of LD service provision

This is best understood either as an acceptance of or reaction to the prevailing societal attitudes and legislation. Two significant themes are framed in the thinking of the time:

- people with disability are blessed or cursed (or abandoned) by their god (good versus evil dichotomy)
- the inclusion of people with disability in society is a mark of a society's civilisation versus people with disability being the evidence of incipient degeneracy (normalisation versus eugenics).

The following chronology replays these themes, based on developments in the UK and demonstrating the oscillations between exclusion/inclusion, supervision/support, organisationally between ownership and partnership. The template could be applied almost anywhere in the world:

- 1329 Edward II's law differentiates between 'natural fools' (LD) and 'lunatics' (mental illness). The estate of a fool can be taken by the Crown and only their care funded but a lunatic's estate can only be managed by the King on their behalf, with profit used to fund their care, in the expectation that they will recover.
- 1886 Idiots Act: Authorities must establish asylums for the care, education and training of people with mental disorder.
- 1890 Lunacy Act: Did not distinguish between idiots and lunatics.
- 1913 Mental Deficiency Act: Local authorities responsible for supervising those with a 'defect of reasoning present from birth'.
- 1927 Mental Deficiency Act reclassified asylums as hospitals.
- 1944 Education Act: Defined a group of children with LD as 'uneducable'.
- 1946 NHS Act: Local authorities lost responsibility for hospitals and colonies but retained responsibility for community services.
- 1959 Mental Health Act: Contributed to the development of informal treatment and community care for health needs while identifying the local authority as the appropriate provider of social care.

- 1970 Education Act: Local authority given responsibility for providing education to all children. Power of health authorities to provide training for the 'uneducable' removed.
- 1972 *Normalisation* introduced by Wolfensberger to describe the processes by which people with LD could become a valued part of society. Subsequently renamed *Social Role Valorisation* (1982). Identified:
  - isolation v integration
  - dehumanisation v dignity and respect
  - age inappropriateness v age appropriateness.
- 1979 *Jay Report,* a Committee of Enquiry into mental handicap nursing and care identified that people with LD should:
  - make their own decisions
  - take risks
  - live in family type groups
  - have medical care provided by generic services with an interest in LD, physical and mental ill health.
- 1980 *An Ordinary Life* (King's Fund) stated that 'Mentally handicapped people should live in the mainstream of life, living in ordinary houses, in ordinary streets with the same range of choices as any citizen mixing as equals in the community'.
- 1981 John O'Brien published his five accomplishments:
  1 Share ordinary places
  2 Make choices
  3 Develop abilities
  4 Be treated with respect
  5 Have relationships.

These ideals can be seen underpinning all subsequent thinking and service design.

- 1981 Education Act: Children with disabilities should be in mainstream education.
- 1983 Mental Health Act: Identifies mental impairment and severe mental impairment as forms of mental disorder but does not permit compulsory treatment unless they occur with 'abnormally aggressive behaviour' or 'seriously irresponsible conduct'.
- 1988 *Community Care Agenda for Action*: Social Services is the lead agency for assessment/funding of non-health care.
- 1989 Royal College of Psychiatrists' good practice guidance confirms Social Services as the lead agency for care with appropriate specialist medical and psychiatric services alongside.
- 1989 *Working for Patients* (White Paper): Established NHS Trusts, GP Fundholding and the Purchaser-Provider divide.
- 1990 Community Care Act: Local authority responsible for assessing need, designing care, and funding residential care.
- 1992 Health Service Guidelines: Purchasers must ensure access to service is not denied by disability, special provision is made where generic services cannot respond, and needs of long-stay patients included in such planning.
- 1992 *Services for People with LD and Challenging Behaviour or Mental Health Needs* (Mansell Report):
  - individual assessment and service plan
  - challenging behaviour services in addition to other services
  - local provision

- ○ small homes
- ○ day care
- ○ hospital only for short-term assessment and treatment
- ○ joint community teams, LD & health authority.
- 1993 Education Act: Integrate **unless** incompatible with wishes of parent.
- 1995 Disability Discrimination Act: Disability includes physical and mental impairments which have a substantial or long-term effect on ability to carry out normal day to day activities. Omitted education access.
- 1998 *Signposts for Success* (DoH, 1998): Good practice guidance for commissioning and providing health services for people with LD. Respect, rights, quality, use of personal health care records, equality of access.
- 1998 Human Rights Act: Article 2. No child shall be denied the right to education.
- 1999 *Facing The Facts* (DoH, 1999): Survey of service provision found intention good; planning, delivery, partnership and leadership poor.
- 1999 *Once a Day* (DoH, 1999): Good practice guidance for primary care teams.
- 2001 *Valuing People*. (2001): DoH White Paper:

Principles	Practice
Rights	LD Register
Choice	Health Education Factor
Independence	Health Action Plans
Inclusion	Housing
	Employment

Not a National Service Framework, but identified how LD should be included in development and supported in access of mainstream services by developments in specialist LD Services.

- 2004 Mental Capacity Bill. (June 2003 before Parliament.) Principles:
  - ○ assume capacity unless otherwise proven
  - ○ all practicable steps to be taken to improve capacity
  - ○ unwise decision does not equal incapacity
  - ○ must be in best interests
  - ○ least restrictive option.

Service design in the future should aim to be supportive and inclusive and in partnership.

AETIOLOGY AND DEVELOPMENT

The **developmental period** of brain development is considered to be the first 18 years. Connections within neural networks develop rapidly *in utero* and within the first three years the **developmental milestones** are reached. The more severe the LD, the more likely an **organic pathology** is to blame.

Social class

Mild LD is up to nine times more frequent in lower social class. Social factors, poor diet (breastfeeding may increase IQ by 10 points), poor education and emotional instability are thought to play a role in achieving appropriate developmental milestones.

Aetiologies

Various data exist regarding the causes of LD, but without population registers, the exact prevalence of the various causes remains poorly understood. In severe impairment, the following causes are listed:

- 33% Down's syndrome
- 19% other congenital abnormalities
- 18% perinatal injury
- 14% infection
- 4% biochemical disorders (inborn errors of metabolism)
- 15% aetiology unknown.

There is a high degree of additional disability: 30% visual impairment, 40% hearing impairment and 50% communication difficulties.

Primary disorders with direct effects

These disorders, the result of chromosomal abnormalities or inborn errors of metabolism directly affecting brain development are detailed in Table 19.2.

Chromosomal abnormality	Syndrome	Birth rate	Survival	Clinical features
Trisomy 13	Patau's	0.2/1000	18% survive first year	Severe LD, forebrain divides incompletely with midline defects (cleft lip/palate, ocular defects), microcephaly, limb flexion contractures, 'rocker bottom' feet, renal and cardiac malformations.
Trisomy 18	Edward's	0.3/1000 M : F = 3 : 1	10% survive first year	Profound LD, clenched fist with second and fifth fingers overlapping third and fourth, 'rocker bottom' feet, exomphalos, cardiac and renal defects.
Trisomy 21: nondisjunction (94%), translocation (3–5%) mosaics (1–3%)	Down's	1.4/1000 varies with maternal age from 1/1400 at 25 to 1/46 for ≥ 45	80% survive first year. Mean life expectancy 60	Mostly moderate LD (IQ 20–75 mean around 50) but some mosaics do not have LD. Craniofacial features present at birth: Brachycephalic skull, 3rd fontanel, short thick neck, upward sloping palpebral fissures, epicanthic folds, flat nasal bridge, apparently large tongue (relatively small mouth). Hands short and broad with simian crease (50% in both hands) and short incurved 5th phalanx. Cardiac lesions 40–60%. Associated duodenal atresia, leukaemia, hypothyroidism and, latterly, Alzheimer's dementia.

Table 19.2 *continued overleaf*

Table 19.2 *continued*

Chromosomal abnormality	Syndrome	Birth rate	Survival	Clinical features
4p deletion	Wolf-Hirschhorn	Rare, 2/3 female	2/3 survive first year	Profound LD and seizures (few adult survivors). Microcephaly, hypertelorism, coloboma (25%), cleft palate (30%), heart defects (50%) & common renal defects.
5p deletion	Cri du Chat	0.02/1000, 70% female but more males survive	50% survive first year	Severe LD, cat-like cry (hypoplastic larynx, improves with age). Microcephaly, micrognathia, down-slanting palpebral fissures.
15q12 deletion, maternally inherited	Angelman	0.033–0.066/1000		Severe LD, happy demeanour and smiling face (happy puppet syndrome). Frequently have abnormal gait/ataxia/tremor, seizures (EEG: Large amplitude slow spike wave), poor sleep, little verbal communication.
15q12 deletion, paternally inherited	Prader Willi	0.07/1000		Moderate to no LD, hypotonia, short stature, insatiable appetite (obsessional drive) with obesity, emotional lability.
16p deletion, autosomal dominant	Rubenstein-Taybi	0.008–0.01/1000		Moderate to no LD (IQ usually 35–50), broad thumbs, webbed fingers and toes, beaked nose, short upper lip, pouting lower lip, agenesis of corpus callosum, large foramen magnum, keloid formation, pulmonary stenosis, vertebral anomalies, chest wall anomalies, sleep apnoea, and megacolon.
17q deletion	Smith-Magenis	0.04/1000		Mild to moderate LD, broad square-shaped face, brachycephaly, prominent forehead, synophrys, upslanting palpebral fissures, deep-set eyes, broad nasal bridge, marked mid-facial hypoplasia, short full-tipped nose with reduced nasal height, micrognathia in infancy changing to relative prognathia with age, and distinctive mouth (fleshy everted upper lip with 'tented' appearance). Sleep disturbance, stereotypes, self-injury, is generally unrecognised until 18 months or older.

Chromosomal abnormality	Syndrome	Birth rate	Survival	Clinical features
Chr 21 X-linked mostly female	Aicardi			Severe LD, severe epilepsy (infantile spasms), retinopathy, agenesis of corpus callosum, microcephaly, hemivertebrae.
22q11.2	DiGeorge, Velocardiofacial, Shprintzen, Conotruncal Anomaly Face (CTAF), Caylor Cardiofacial, Autosomal Dominant Opitz G/BBB	0.16– 0.25/1000		Characterised by palatal defects, heart abnormalities, LD (25%), craniofacial abnormalities, and over 180 other clinical findings, which include schizophreniform psychosis, bipolar mood disorder, immune problems and hypocalcaemia (30%).
Xq27	Fragile X	1/1000 male births		Mild–moderate LD (borderline LD in females), floppy ears, macro-orchidism, hypertelorism, single palmar crease, joint laxity, autism.
45XO (60%) XX/XO mosaic (15%) Isochromosome Xq or Xp (10%) Xdel or Xring or Y abN (15%)	Turner's	1/3000 females		Mild (10%) – no LD (90%), short stature, webbed neck, low post hairline, wide spaced nipples, co-arctation of aorta (35%), renal tract abnormalities (60%), poor secondary sexual characteristics, poor social skills.
47XXY	Klinefelter's	1/500 men		Mild to no LD, slow secondary sexual characteristics, tall, gynecomastia, small atrophic testes, azoospermia.
3q26.3	Cornelia de Lange (Amsterdam dwarfism)			IQ 30–85, synophrys, long curly eyelashes, low front and back hairlines, turned-up nose, down-turned angles of the mouth and thin lips, small lower jaw/protruding upper jaw, microcephaly, eye and vision problems, excessive body hair, which may thin as the child grows (78%).
7q11.2 autosomal dominant	William's	0.13/1000		Mild LD, broad brow, bitemporal narrowness, periorbital fullness, short nose, full nasal tip, malar hypoplasia, long philtrum, full lips, wide mouth, malocclusion, small jaw, and prominent earlobes are observed, stellate/lacy iris pattern and strabismus, supravalvar aortic stenosis, hypothyroidism (10%).

Table 19.2 *continued overleaf*

Table 19.2 *continued*

Chromosomal abnormality	Syndrome	Birth rate	Survival	Clinical features
Autosomal dominant, incomplete penetrance (50%), sporadic mutation in the fibroblast growth factor gene	Apert's	0.00625/1000		Moderate LD. Under-developed middle third of the face with small nose, hypertelorism, strabismus, and proptosis. Acrocephaly, syndactyly.
Autosomal recessive, almost 50% chromosome 11q13 gene (mostly Whites), < 20% 16q21 and 15q22, 3p13 possibly implicated.	Laurence-Moon-Biedl	0.008/1000		Mild-moderate LD, obesity (post puberty), retinitis pigmentosa, hypogonadism, dwarfism, polydactyly and syndactyly.

Table 19.2 Primary disorders

Primary disorders with secondary neurological damage

Development is affected later as the secondary result of neurological damage from an inborn error (Table 19.3).

Defect	Disease	Birth rate	Clinical features
Protein metabolism	Phenylketonuria	0.05–0.2/1000	When untreated, progressive brain damage with 40–60 point reduction in IQ by 1 year, microcephaly, eczema, hypertonicity, epilepsy, dysphasia.
Carbohydrate metabolism	Galactosaemia	0.02/1000	Neonates present with vomiting, diarrhoea, failure to thrive and persistent jaundice. Cataracts and LD develop if left untreated and children may die of liver failure. Slight reduction in IQ if treated.
Lipid metabolism (gangliosidosis)	Tay-Sach's	0.04/1000 in Ashkenazi Jewish communities	Normal development to 4–6 months, then progressive deterioration: Feeding difficulties, abnormal startle response, worsening seizures, severe form die by 36 months. Late onset form: Presents age 2–10, possible misdiagnosis as multiple sclerosis. LD varies with severity.

Defect	Disease	Birth rate	Clinical features
Lipid metabolism (lipofuscinosis)	Batten's	0.025/1000	Normal development followed by worsening seizures, intellectual and visual impairment. Most die.
Mucopoly-saccharide metabolism Mucupoly-saccharoidosis I	Hurler syndrome	0.0125/1000	Presents 6–18 months with macrocephaly, course facies, hepatosplenomegaly, corneal clouding, claw hands and other contractures. Development plateaus at 2–4 years with progressive decline and death age 6–10.
Mucopoly-saccharide metabolism X-linked Mucupoly-saccharoidosis II	Hunter syndrome	0.0125/1000	Presentation 1–2 years, features as Hurler syndrome (but **no** corneal clouding), plus skin infiltration ('peau d'orange'), mild to moderate LD and longer survival.
Mucupoly-saccharoidosis IIIa, IIIc & IIId	Sanfillipo syndrome	0.01/1000	Early development normal with gradual coarsening of features, hyperactivity and aggression. Development plateaus at 6 and regresses to severe incapacity in the few who survive into adulthood.
Congenital hypothyroidism		0.1–2/1000	Age (months) at diagnosis IQ < 1 unaffected < 3 89 3–6 70 6+ 54 Umbilical hernia, placid, poor feeding, constipation, hypothermia, oedema, peripheral cyanosis, large tongue, hoarse cry, dry skin.
Assumed chromosomal disorder, many implicated: 16p13.3 site of gene product tuberin 11q22–23 and chr9 Family history (autosomal dominant) in 75%	Tuberous sclerosis	0.02/1000	Site and severity of tubers in the brain determines IQ; may show developmental delay from birth with epilepsy starting before 2 years. Autism common; adenoma sebaceum at puberty (sebaceous gland hypertrophy); other skin lesions (shagreen patches, café,-au-lait spots, icthyosis). Tubers may also arise in heart, kidney, lungs.
Chromosome 17q11.2 (peripheral) and 22q12 (central). Both autosomal	Neuro-fibromatosis	0.4/1000	< 10% have epilepsy, similar incidence of mild LD. Café,-au-lait spots are the hallmark with peripheral nerves also affected (plexiform neurofibroma). Sensory organs can be affected.

Table 19.3 Congenital disorders with secondary neurological damage

Secondary disorders

The effects of disease or injury on the fetus or baby.

Antenatal

- Neural tube defects (vitamin B_{12}), 1–8/1000 births, 10% mild LD.
- Rhesus incompatibility, impairment varies.
- Infection (rubella, cytomegalovirus, syphyllis, toxoplasmosis, listeria).
- Alcohol and drugs (fetal alcohol syndrome).
- Heavy metal poisoning.

Perinatal

- Hypoxia (hypoxic-ischaemic encephalopathy).
- Hypoglycaemia.
- Infection (encephalitis, meningitis).
- Trauma (birth).
- Cerebral thrombosis.
- Emotional/physical abuse.

Postnatal

- Nutrition.
- Trauma (accidental and non-accidental).
- Infection (encephalitis, meningitis).
- Encephalopathies (epilepsy).
- Metabolic.
- Emotional/physical abuse.

PREVENTION OF DISABILITY

Primary

Avoid development of condition

- Antenatal screening (Down's syndrome, PKU, galactosaemia, Rhesus screening, testing for infectious diseases).
- Rubella immunisation for all women of childbearing age.
- Accident prevention.
- Childhood immunisations (measles, mumps, rubella, pertussis, meningococcal meningitis).

Genetic counselling

- Tay Sachs disease eradicated amongst American Jewish families.

- Specific conditions noted with some general rules for recurrence:

  Disability of unknown cause   30% recurrence risk

  Balanced translocation   20% risk mother, 5% risk father

  Dominant   50% risk

  Recessive   25% risk

  X linked disorders   50% sons affected

     50% daughters carriers.

Environmental manipulation

- Folate supplementation in pregnancy.
- Improved nutrition.
- Improved antenatal infection control.
- Better obstetric care.
- Avoidance of maternal drug and alcohol misuse.
- Immunisations.

Secondary

Early detection and treatment

- Neonatal screening for hypothyroidism, Rhesus incompatibility, PKU and other metabolic conditions.
- Appropriate treatment of conditions like neonatal jaundice.
- Management of childhood infectious diseases.
- Better neonatal care (major increase in severe LD is prematurity).

Tertiary

Prevention of impairment developing into a disability and then into a handicap

- Education programmes for autistic children.
- Assessment of additional impairments (vision, hearing, communication).
- Physiotherapy for physical disability.
- Identifying and treating psychiatric conditions.
- Management of epilepsy.

Epilepsy

- A common co-morbidity affecting 15–30% of people with LD (increases with severity of LD).
- Complex and difficult to treat, marked differences from the general population:
  - generalised 62.5% (twice general population)
  - partial 32.5% (half general population).
- Sedating effects of anti-epileptic drugs are exacerbated in LD and side-effects difficult to interpret in people without verbal communication.

Differential diagnosis

- Hallucinations (non-verbal individuals responding to hallucinatory experiences).
- Panic attacks (fear is the most common psychic phenomenon in TLE).
- Behaviour disorders.
- Physical illness (gastro-esophageal reflux and pain may appear seizure-like).
- Epilepsy: Partial (simple, complex, secondary generalised).
  Generalised (absence, clonic, tonic, tonic-clonic, myoclonic and atonic).
- NEAD (non-epileptic attack disorder – more common).

Management

- Diagnosis: When, by whom, validity, are all attacks seizures?
- Physical injuries: Are these contributing to further disability (head injuries)?
- Psychological factors: Anxiety, stress, depression are all associated with epilepsy.
- Social factors: Care situation important in implementing management plans.
- Educational needs: Special educational opportunities for children with epilepsy.
- Status Epilepticus: Identify those who need rescue medication.

LD IN CLASSIFICATION

ICD-10

- F70 to F79. According to degree of LD.
- F70. Mild.
- F71. Moderate.
- F72. Severe.
- F73. Profound.
- F74–F77. Not used.
- F78. Other mental retardation where assessment of degree of impairment is unreliable because, for example, of co-existing blindness, deafness or physical impairments.
- F79. Unspecified mental retardation where there is insufficient information to assign to a specific degree of impairment.
- A brief description is given under each category of the predicted skills or functional level associated with the various degrees of LD but also notes the possibility of variable presentation with pockets of skills.
- Fourth character is used to note the presence or absence of impairment of behaviour.
- F7*.0. No or minimal impairment of behaviour.
- F7*.1. Significant impairment of behaviour requiring attention or treatment.
- F7*.8. Other impairments of behaviour.
- F7*.9. Without mention of impairment of behaviour.

- Separate use of appropriate coding where the aetiology of the LD is known is advocated as F70 PLUS and coded elsewhere typically not in the F section of ICD-10. Examples of common known aetiology are in Table 19.4.

Chapter heading	Aetiological examples
Endocrine, nutritional and metabolic diseases	E00. Congenital iodine deficiency syndrome E70.0 Classical phenylketonuria E71.0 Maple-syrup-urine disease
Disorders of the nervous system	G00 Bacterial meningitis G04 Encephalitis, myelitis G40 Epilepsy G91 Hydrocephalus G93.1 Anoxic brain damage NEC
Diseases of the circulatory system	I61 Intracerebral haemorrhage I63 Cerebral infarction
Congenital malformations, deformations and chromosomal abnormalities	Q02 Microcephaly Q85.1 Tuberose sclerosis Q86.0 Fetal alcohol syndrome Q90 Down's syndrome Q93 Other monosomies and deletions

Table 19.4 Classification of specific aetiologies

Psychiatric disorders in LD

Psychiatric diagnoses in LD can use standard classification systems such as ICD-10 or DSM-IV, but there are limitations in use for those who have impairments in communication and self-awareness. Many psychiatric diagnoses require self-reporting of symptoms to meet criteria. If someone has no speech, first rank symptoms of schizophrenia may be impossible to demonstrate. Developmental states may also carry some symptom presentation as a normal part of the process of maturation (eg the obsessional and repetitious behaviours associated with children aged below three years). If the brain development of an adult with LD has plateaued at this stage they may still present with obsessional behaviour which is not pathological but appropriate to their stage of development.

The DC-LD (Diagnostic Criteria for psychiatric disorders for use with adults with LD/mental retardation. Royal College of Psychiatrists, Occasional Paper OP48), developed by LD specialists, classifies mental illness taking into account the different presentations and difficulties in making the full range of diagnoses for people with LD. It is a multiaxial scale, incorporating information about degree of LD, aetiology and simplified psychiatric disorder groupings with greater detail for developmental disorders and behavioural problems.

Axis I: Severity of LD
Axis II: Cause of LD
Axis III: Psychiatric disorder
           DC-LD Level A: Developmental disorder
           DC-LD Level B: Psychiatric illness
           DC-LD Level C: Personality disorders
           DC-LC Level D: Problem behaviours
           DC-LD Level E: Other disorders.

Problem behaviours are given proportionally more emphasis and more detailed subdivisions than in ICD-10 or DSM-IV, reflecting the importance of these issues in determining presentation to psychiatric services, placement difficulties and increased risk profiles.

Axis III Level D is further subdivided as follows:

IIID1.2:   Verbally aggressive behaviour
IIID1.3:   Physically aggressive behaviours
IIID1.4:   Destructive behaviour
IIID1.5:   Self-injurious behaviour
IIID1.6:   Sexually inappropriate behaviour
IIID1.7:   Oppositional behaviour
IIID1.8:   Demanding behaviour
IIID1.9:   Wandering behaviour
IIID1.10:   Mixed problem behaviours
IIID1.11:   Other problem behaviours
IIID1.12:   Mixed other problem behaviours
IIID2.1:   Problem behaviours due to pervasive developmental disorder
IIID2.2:   Problem behaviours due to psychiatric illness (type/s)
IIID2.3:   Problem behaviours due to personality disorder (type/s)
IIID2.4:   Problem behaviours due to physical illness/disorder (type/s).

PSYCHIATRIC ILLNESS AND LD

Prevalence of psychiatric morbidity is 4 to 10 times that in the general population. Overall, 20–40% suffer from a concurrent psychiatric illness excluding behavioural problems. This may be due to:

- higher rates in families giving genetic predisposition
- higher prevalence of LD and mental illness in lower socio-economic groups
- vulnerable population
- increased exposure to abuse
- multiple traumatic life experiences
- lack of ego-strengthening early experiences eg lack of consistent primary-care giver
- lack of protective life experiences eg employment, close confiding relationships
- neurochemical abnormalities associated with organic brain abnormalities

- increased rates of other risk factors for mental illness eg epilepsy, sensory impairments
- syndrome specific psychiatric risk associated with genetic phenotype eg obsessive-compulsive disorder associated with Down's syndrome.

BEHAVIOURAL PHENOTYPES

A behavioural phenotype occurs when a known disorder (generally chromosomal) is associated with patterns of behaviour, psychiatric symptoms or personality characteristics that occur frequently enough to be considered a direct manifestation of the underlying disorder. A controversial concept, there is debate as to whether they represent a stereotyped view of the disorder ascribed to the condition or the result of shared life experiences of sufferers.

Furthermore, the concept may not predict or prevent behaviours and may blind clinicians to other potential problems through selective attention. Nevertheless, the evidence base is steadily growing and, providing they are used with caution, behavioural phenotypes may help both the understanding and management of the individual patient and, in a much broader sense, facilitate understanding of the complex inter-relationship between genetics and final expression of personality, behaviours, choices and preferences.

Table 19.6 (on page 394) builds on information given in Tables 19.2 and 19.3.

COMMUNICATING

Thirty per cent of people with LD also have impairments in communication and/or sensory deficits. Sensory and communication problems become more common as the severity of the LD increases. Psychiatric problems also become more frequent as the level of LD increases but the diagnosis becomes more difficult and may be more easily missed or put down to the LD rather than recognised as psychopathology.

The clinician may have to rely wholly on psychiatric signs as symptoms and often requires verbal reports for definitive confirmation and may need to infer symptoms from behaviour because they cannot be elicited by direct questioning. The clinician will often be reliant on second or third hand information. The need for accurate recording of information by carers is crucially important. Wherever possible, symptoms and signs should be verified by direct observation or objective tests (eg antecedent behaviour checklists, daily diaries, sleep charts, etc).

Communication can take a variety of direct and indirect forms and should be tailored to match the abilities of the patient, maximising the validity of the information required to achieve an accurate diagnosis. Families and carers are important but their reports are affected by expectations, personal needs and previous experience of problem behaviours. Professional carers are more likely to report aggressive behaviour than withdrawn or apathetic behaviours. Sleep disruption is a critical factor in avoiding family placement

Disorder	Prevalence	Risk factors	Presentation	Management
Schizophrenia	2–6% in mild/moderate.	Sensory impairment and epilepsy, Velocardiofacial and Prader Willi syndromes.	Verbal reporting of delusions and hallucinations may be impaired and have to be inferred.	Responds to antipsychotics. Often more resistant. Follow NICE guidelines. Non-drug treatment also possible. Avoid polypharmacy.
Anxiety disorders	27%	Major life events, mild LD.	Aggression, agitation, self-mutilation, obsessive fears, ritualistic behaviours, insomnia.	Anxiety associated with autism may respond to low-dose antipsychotic agents. Avoid benzodiazepines. Modified anxiety management on 1 : 1 basis (designed for the individual). SSRI. Daily diaries and information.
Bipolar affective disorder	3–8% bipolar	Family history, impaired bonding.	Hypomania often presents with irritability increased verbal skills and volume, insomnia, disinhibition.	Exclude episodic pain (eg UTI, gastric ulcer). Primary mood stabiliser with atypical antipsychotic for acute mania.
Depression	5–10% Under-diagnosed in severe/profound LD.	Family history. Low self-esteem. Multiple life events.	Atypical symptoms more common. Biological features may be only guide. Anhedonia or loss of skills often present. In severe LD may present with self-harm or increased irritability.	Antidepressant, sedation more with older drugs. Use sedating antidepressant (eg mirtazepine) if sleep disturbed (common). Ensure adequate dose but start low. Non-pharmacological interventions also important including grief work, psychotherapy, etc.
Challenging Behaviour: Includes aggression and self-injurious behaviour (SIB).	10–15% usually accepted. Most common reason for psychiatric referral.	Autistic spectrum, impairment of verbal communication. Syndromes (Autism, Lesch-Nyhan, Retts).	'Culturally abnormal behaviour of such intensity, frequency or duration that the physical safety of the person or others is likely to be placed in serious jeopardy'.	Exclude physical problem (pain, infection, etc). Improve communication opportunities. Manipulate environment to minimise triggers. Exclude psychiatric illness. Only then consider drug treatment: Low-dose antipsychotics, antidepressants, tranquillisers. Naltrexone for SIB. May need to consider physical restraints (eg arm splints) for SIB.
Dementia	Neuropathic changes seen in all people with	Age. Down's syndrome. Any brain damage.	Loss of skills and language, memory problems, new onset epilepsy.	Exclude pseudo-dementia, anaemia, hypothyroidism, depression. EEG/CT-scan.

Disorder	Prevalence	Associations	Clinical features	Management
Down's aged over 40. Clinical symptoms in 30% by age 50. Mean age of onset 54. Increasing prevalence as average life expectancy increases.		Epilepsy.	Assess using psychiatric screening tools, specific dementia tests for LD (Dementia in Mental Retardation (DMR)). Functional skills tests (Assessment of Motor and Processing skills (AMPS)).	Responds to acetyl cholinesterase inhibitors. Treat co-morbid epilepsy with newer anti-convulsants to reduce further cognitive impairment. Sleep disturbance may respond to melatonin.
Personality disorders. Diagnosis with personality assessment schedule or other standard instruments is more difficult if it requires self-reporting.	25–30%	Organic brain injury, some syndromes, impoverished early life experiences, childhood abuse.	Emotionally unstable commonest, but all seen. Tendency to avoid labelling and to ascribe all behaviours to the LD but personality disordered presentations are clearly seen in a subgroup of LD.	Identify and treat associated mental illness, maximise quality of life. Individual, group or family therapy may help. Safe boundaries, consistent approach, staff debriefing to minimise splitting. Low-dose antipsychotics to minimise background anxiety and over-arousal. Therapeutic communities of limited value and only appropriate for the most able subgroup.
Pervasive developmental disorders (PDD). Autism: 'Wing triad' – impairments in reciprocal social interaction, language and imagination.	Includes autism, Asperger's and Retts syndromes. Prevalence rising possibly due to increased awareness and better diagnosis.	Family history. Affective disorder in 1st degree relative. M : F = 15 : 1 (mild), 2 : 1 (severe). Controversial and unproven link to MMR vaccine and bowel disease. Neurodevelopmental disorder. Associated with some syndromes (fragile X, tuberose sclerosis, Down's).	Period of apparently near-normal development followed by arrested skills with deterioration. Absence of 'theory of mind' (empathy, understanding other's point of view). Sensory gating deficits common. Literal in comprehension, struggle with humour.	Incurable neurodevelopmental disorder; impact on function can be minimised. 'Autistic-friendly environment'. Single or conjoint therapy with low-dose anti psychotic plus SSRI for autistic anxiety. Place of intensive early interventions pioneered in the USA is controversial. Support and information for parents available through National Autistic Society.

Table 19.5 Psychiatric disorders in LD

Syndrome	Behavioural phenotype
Aicardi syndrome	Lethargy, self-injury, aggression, sleep problems.
Angelman syndrome	Inappropriate bouts of laughter, cheerful and excitable temperament, cope poorly with change.
Cornelia de Lange syndrome	Guttural tone of voice, self-injurious behaviour, autistic-like behaviour.
Down's syndrome	Increased rates of autism, OCD and dementia. ADHD common (especially males). Typical stereotype: friendly, placid, musical.
Fetal alcohol syndrome	Disinhibition with aggression and ADHD. Mood disorders common in childhood.
Fragile X syndrome	Social anxiety, gaze avoidance, poor concentration, increased autism risk.
Klinefelter's syndrome	Childhood passivity and introversion, adolescent insecurity and anxiety with social fearfulness, controversial links to psychopathy and aggression in adulthood.
Lesch-Nyhan syndrome	Severe, compulsive self-injurious behaviour that the individual seems to want to stop.
Noonan syndrome	Stubborn repetitive behaviour and poor social skills and integration.
Phenylketonuria (PKU)	Poor concentration, disinhibition, irritability, odd mannerisms, anxiety and poor social skills.
Prader-Willi syndrome	Overeating with abnormal satiation, sleep abnormalities, skin picking. Frequent and severe temper outbursts, lability of mood and increased risks of affective disorders and schizophrenia.
Smith-Magenis syndrome	Altered pain tolerance with severe self-injurious behaviour especially head banging, hand biting and pulling fingernails and toenails.
Sotos syndrome	Large people who tend to show aggression and emotional immaturity. Controversial whether this is inherent or learned because of the frightened response it often elicits.
Tuberose sclerosis	Poor concentration, explosive temper outbursts, disinhibition, poor social interactions.
Turner syndrome	Poor concentration, difficulty making friends, eating disorders and increased risk of depression.
Velocardiofacial syndrome	Increased risks of many psychiatric disorders notably including schizophrenia, affective disorders and autism.
Williams syndrome	Social skills deficits but overfriendly and disinhibited along with 'cocktail party' speech. Hypersensitive to noise, over-empathic, prone to emotional upsets at odds with otherwise friendly superficial appearance. At high risk of abuse.

Table 19.6 Behavioural phenotypes

breakdown and is very likely to result in presentation to services but the expectations of elderly parent carers as to a 'normal' length of sleep varies greatly. It is not uncommon for parents to complain of sleep disturbance with early morning waking only to discover that their adult offspring with a LD is being put to bed very early and waking an appropriate eight hours later.

If the adult patient with LD can communicate, they remain the most important source of information and all efforts should be made (including seeking assistance from speech and language therapists) to ensure they can be heard.

COMMUNICATION TIPS

- Keep language simple.
- Avoid long sentences.
- Avoid jargon.
- Avoid negatives.
- Keep examples concrete.
- Avoid abstract concepts.
- Be aware of literal meanings.
- Use humour cautiously as it may be misunderstood or taken literally.
- Check whether there are any 'special' words which should be avoided because they are upsetting to the patient.
- Use sign language or pictures if patient uses these.
- Check comprehension back by getting patient to repeat what they have understood.
- Use a sign language 'translator' if you're not fluent.

CAPACITY AND CONSENT

Issues relating to capacity and consent are covered in Chapter 10.

In relation to LD it is worth reiterating that under English law it is illegal for anyone to give consent on behalf of another adult regardless of whether or not that adult has capacity. A doctor cannot accept consent from a third party nor omit treatment because the individual cannot give valid consent. Capacity should be assessed every time a treatment decision is considered and appropriate action taken. An individual's capacity may vary with the complexity of the decision.

FORENSIC ISSUES

Epidemiology

Accurate figures for offending by people with LD are even more difficult to obtain than for the general population. Many minimise their disability and try to pass for 'normal' as part of their survival tactics in a world which takes advantage of, and victimises, those who are different. They may not be recognised by the police or court systems as having an LD and may not identify themselves as such. Studies indicate that lawyers are most likely to identify people correctly as having an LD but also that people who have LD are least likely to have legal representation.

- Prison studies indicate a prevalence of 9.5% (IQ below 70) in the USA with a 1.6% below 55 (total 11.1% against expected maximum 3%). An Australian study found 13% below 70 while in the UK LD was not over-represented in prison populations.
- Five per cent of people detained by UK police attended special schooling and a further 10% attended emotional and behavioural disorders schooling.
- Out of the people attending court in Australia 14.2% had an IQ below 70 and 18.8% a borderline IQ (70–80). Both groups were less likely to have legal representation than defendants with higher IQs.

Offence analysis

- Public order offences/misdemeanours most common.
- Sexual offending five times the general population:
  - more likely to commit minor or nuisance offences than serious offences
  - physical violence is rare
  - less likely to target specific victims (by age or sex)
  - opportunistic and impulsive rather than premeditated
  - majority are 'developmental' offences – inappropriate sexual expression because of a lack of opportunity for legitimate sexual activity or a lack of skills in understanding and responding to socially acceptable behaviour.
- Arson also over-represented and predominantly a developmental disorder with enjoyment of fire and a lack of true understanding of the risks rather than planned arson for secondary gain.
- Serious crime statistics (murder) are often misleading as these cases attract far greater in-depth study, trials last longer and low IQ is more likely to be identified.

Causes

- Low socio-economic status.
- Gullible and more likely to be drawn into offending by others.
- Less likely to conceal offending behaviour.
- 'True' increased risk of offending behaviours associated with:
  - history of traumatic brain injury (particularly frontal lobe)
  - epilepsy
  - any syndrome associated with impaired social skills, increased aggressive behaviour or impaired empathy.

People who truly lack the ability to understand that their actions may cause harm or distress to others, for example, in severe cases of autism, generally lack a guilty mind or *mens rea* and therefore concepts of guilt and punishment may be of limited value.

People with LD as victims

This is more common than offending behaviour but is significantly under-reported. The Seattle Rape Relief Project found that 75% of people with LD had survived at least one sexual assault with 10% knowing their assailant. Assaults within residential homes by fellow residents are rarely reported to the police and indeed are often not acted upon at all.

Crimes against people with LD tend to be minimised by the use of euphemisms such as abuse or neglect or mercy killings rather than rape or assault or murder. People with LD have difficulty reporting crimes, difficulties being believed, difficulties coping with the court systems and risk double victimisation. Recent changes in legislation offers improved protection through the vulnerable witness procedures and the use of 'special measures' such as video interviews.

People with LD are more likely to:

- have impaired judgement in making safe choices
- lack basic knowledge in self-protection or protection in the home
- have deficits in adaptive behaviour to escape from risky situations
- have accompanying physical or sensory impairments making them 'easy targets'
- live in high-risk environments
- have contact with potentially unscrupulous 'benefactors'
- be targeted by abusers
- look and act like victims, behaviour known to increase risk of becoming a victim.

SERVICES FOR PEOPLE WITH LD

Service models

The re-development of LD Services has, until recently, paralleled those of Mental Health Services with a shift from institutional to community-based services. The thrust of recent legislation appears to move the provision of mental health care for people with LD towards generic primary and secondary services with facilitation from specialist LD Services as outlined in Figure 19.1. Current provision is a mixture of delivery models, and the pace of change and degree of inclusion varied.

- People with LD tend to experience difficulties in:
  - advocating for themselves
  - accessing appropriate services
  - receptive and expressive sensory impairments.
- Providing support for their health needs including mental health is complicated by:
  - communication difficulties
  - multiple pathologies (Complexity)
  - modified presentation of symptoms and signs
  - fear bred from alienation or lack of experience
  - vulnerability
  - intolerance.

- These factors affect both the client (patient) and the health professional.
- The function of any specialist health service for people with LD should be to overcome these barriers to access equality of health care outcomes, while maintaining equality of access to health care process.

Mental Health Services

In providing Mental Health Services it is reasonable to expect access to:

- CMHT
- assertive outreach
- crisis intervention
- rehabilitation
- substance misuse
- forensic
- psychiatry of old age
- CAMHS, etc

but to be supported, where, appropriate and only to access entirely alternative provision where there is:

- risk to others
- vulnerability
- complexity that precludes this
- communication or social ability that is significantly compromised.

Valuing People (DoH, 2001) describes a model of provision in which:

- services develop in response to 'Person Centred Plans'
- local authorities commission in partnership with LD-appropriate support for housing
- occupation and activity provision is supported by the local authority including further education and mainstreamed increasingly in the workplace and colleges/schools
- health care is mainstreamed with targeted specialist input.

Alternative models exist which either:

- deny the need for any alternative provision
- reinforce exclusion by the over-provision of specialist input and over-ownership of responsibility for direct patient contact within such services.

Neither of these service models is consistent with the prevailing philosophy of care or legislative framework.

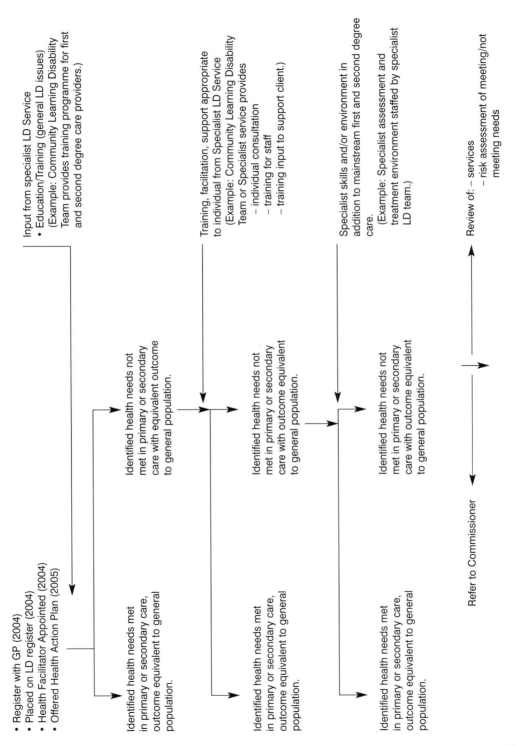

Figure 19.1 Proposed model of service provision for people with LD

Chapter 20

Liaison Psychiatry

Peter Aitken

CONTENTS

Liaison Psychiatry

BASIC SCIENCE

Bio-psycho-social model

This is a holistic model for understanding:

- physical (biomedical)
- psychological and
- social components to a health problem.

For each of these three areas four groups of factors are identified:

- predisposing factors to the health problem
- precipitants to the health problem
- factors maintaining the person in the unwell state
- protective factors which if removed or disturbed may in themselves be contributing to the unwell state.

The model links well with clinical services, in the main doctors, pharmacists and nurses contribute to the bio-medical assessment and treatment; nurses and psychologists contribute to the psychological assessment and treatment; occupational therapists and social workers contribute to the social assessment and treatment.

Stress coping paradigm

This is a model of coping; individuals have coping resources that are:

- **internal**: emotive or cognitive
- **external**: behavioural.

In response to stress the individual utilises their resources in coping strategies in an effort to neutralise the unpleasant experience of anxiety.

Adaptive coping involves normative strategies drawing on healthy resources with healthy resolution of the anxiety.

Maladaptive coping strategies result in incomplete resolution of the anxiety by failing to neutralise the provoking stimulus in a healthy manner.

Stress performance curve

Yerkes–Dodson. At rest, a modest baseline catecholamine release is sufficient to maintain cardio-respiratory function. On waking, physiological performance increases in response to stress, experienced as arousal, up to a peak. At this peak, performance is maximised. If stress drives arousal further, the additional catecholamine released is experienced by the individual as anxiety. Further stress-driven increases in catecholamine release induce panic.

Illness behaviour

People seek help for disorganised symptoms which they make sense of by attributing them to a number of existing internal models for illness that they may have:

- experienced
- witnessed in others
- acquired through the media.

According to the Goldberg and Huxley–Filter Model, they usually seek help from (in order):

- relatives or friends
- health professionals
- primary care
- specialist care.

Patients occupy the 'sick role'; their responsibility is to get well. This is the basis for the usual 'contract of care' between a patient and a health professional.

Health professional advice and treatment in the majority of people leads to a resolution of their anxiety about the symptom and a return to health.

For some people the emotional–cognitive reward of meeting with health care becomes a reason in itself to consult. For some this is conscious and understood, for others it is conscious and not understood and for the majority it is unconscious and not understood.

The term 'abnormal illness behaviour' suggests a patient seeking help from health professionals to meet unmet emotional needs in the absence of discoverable organic pathology.

Antidepressants

Antidepressants are indicated in depression and anxiety; their off-licence use is in sleep disorder, pain, atypical pain, post-traumatic stress disorder, and organic mood disorder.

Antipsychotics

The key acute role of antipsychotics is in sedation and rapid tranquillisation. They are indicated for schizophrenia, bipolar mania and other psychoses; off-licence use includes organic delirium, Parkinson's disease, Huntington's chorea, delusional disorder, delusional parasitosis.

Anticonvulsants

Anticonvulsants are indicated in epilepsy and bipolar mood disorder; off-licence use is in trigeminal neuralgia, atypical pain, and organic mood disorder.

Hypnotics

Benzodiazepines are indicated for the short-term treatment of anxiety disorders and initial insomnia. They are useful in the general hospital inpatient setting where the circumstance and the environment may be the precipitants. Short-term use limits the risk of tolerance and dependency. They are increasingly regarded as the first line in the management of acute behavioural agitation as part of rapid tranquillisation regimens.

CLINICAL PRACTICE

Referral practice

Referrers to liaison psychiatry should identify the specific issues on which they wish for advice:

- diagnosis
- behavioural disturbance
- cognitive functioning
- abscond risk
- compliance risk
- capacity and consent
- nursing management
- pharmacotherapy
- psychotherapy
- psychiatric admission
- psychiatric follow-up
- alcohol or drug detoxification
- self-harm assessment.

They should identify:

- themselves
- their unit
- best time and location for the patient to be seen.

They should obtain consent from the patient for the referral and where consent is absent they should inform the liaison psychiatry service of the difficulty.

Liaison psychiatrists should:

- see patients on time
- write clear, concise management plans in the medical notes

- keep their own full assessment records in the mental health notes and
- write concise letters to the general practitioner in a style and with content that can be copied to the patient.

The Emergency Department

This is the commonest place for self-harm to present, also behavioural disturbance, intoxication and head injury. The majority of mental health presentations occur out of hours. There are variable mental health practice skills and variable appropriate environments for mental health assessments and security arrangements. This department may be the local place of safety for Mental Health Act assessments. There should be senior involvement in a local self-harm management committee.

The medical ward

Timeframes on the medical ward are minutes to hours, in contrast to psychiatry where the timeframes are days to weeks. The medical ward lacks safe space for confidential history taking. There is a lack of mental health expertise among the nursing and medical staff. There is a need for psycho-education of both staff and patients to counteract the fear and stigma.

Communication

For communication with the patient:

- maximise possibility of successful communication by selecting a safe environment, free from interruption, by arrangement, and with consent
- identify the preferred language
- use interpreters if necessary
- enable hearing and vision
- check meaning
- check narrative consistency
- check with informant history.

For communication with health professionals:

- speak to professionals face to face and on the phone
- record meetings in the notes with times and dates
- write a concise, actionable care plan in the medical notes
- write a full assessment in the mental health notes
- sign, date and time entries
- dictate a concise letter to the general practitioner using style and language which can be copied to the patient.

History

When taking the history, concentrate on the illness experience. Ask about models of illness in family members, history of childhood illnesses and prolonged hospital admissions. Also obtain a history of peer illnesses and illness behaviour and peer influences, including television soap operas and other influences.

Mental State Examination

Place the emphasis on appearance and behaviour, describe perfusion, blood pressure, pulse, temperature, best level of psychomotor functioning. Also perform the Mini Mental State Examination and frontal lobe testing, and bedside neurological testing for apraxia and aphasia.

Environmental safety

Ask yourself the following questions.

- Where am I seeing this patient?
- Why am I seeing seeing this patient now?
- What is my role?
- Can I make the setting safer?

Remove any risk items. Remove other people who might be at risk. Recruit staff who are trained in breakaway, control and restraint. Identify escape routes. Make sure medication is available and that there are staff to deliver it.

Risk assessment

Risk is issue-specific, contextual and exists within a given timeframe. Common risks assessed for:

- risk of suicide
- risk of self-harm
- risk of harm to others
- risk of harm to children
- risk of absconding
- risk of treatment non-adherence
- risk of neglect and exploitation.

Methods of risk assessment include:

- **actuarial estimate**: based on populations
- **individual estimate**: based on history of previous behaviours.

Acute behavioural disturbance

The causes of acute behavioural disturbance are **biological**, **psychological** and **social**. Assessment and management of acute behavioural disturbance is holistic.

Take the **environment** into consideration by looking at:

- context
- precipitants
- perpetuating factors
- risks to patient, carers and other patients.

Make the environment safe.

Find and **consult**:

- previous histories
- notes
- databases
- informant information from staff
- other people who know the patient
- other agencies.

Medical and surgical assessment should be made of cardiorespiratory function, metabolic disturbance, intoxication, poisoning; head injury, fractures and blood loss.

Psychiatric assessment should include accurate alcohol history, behavioural assessment, mental state examination, (and Mini Mental State Examination), frontal lobe testing.

In **management** of the patient you should:

- create a safe environment (eg well lit), remove unnecessary stimuli
- orientate
- de-escalate
- break away
- control and restrain
- employ adequate trained people
- perform medical and surgical assessments
- manage identified causes
- manage behaviour with benzodiazepines with respiratory monitoring and flumenazil available, have atypical antispsychotics as adjunct; use oral or orodispersible routes for preference, then intramuscular, then intravenous; review and document
- explain to the patient what happened when they have recovered.

Insomnia

Sleep disorders are common, and are very common in general hospitals. Causes vary but include:

- environment
- disease
- pain
- hunger
- depression
- anxiety

- substance withdrawal
- drug treatment
- drug side-effects
- delirium
- dementia.

Assessment of the patient should include:

- timing of the problem, early, mid and late insomnia
- history of duration, predisposing and alleviating factors
- treatment history
- compare subjective insomnia with objective observer report, frequency and duration.

Management of insomnia can be by:

- sleep hygiene and education, effects of caffeine, some people find caffeine promotes sleep
- management of the ward environment
- management of precipitating factors
- for initial insomnia a short course of a hypnotic sedative can be used
- for late insomnia, consider antidepressants
- for those with a history of long-term benzodiazepine use or significant alcohol history continue benzodiazepines.

Bereavement

Bereavement is a common, normal human experience following a significant loss. It may involve fluctuating periods of intense sadness with associated anxiety and tearfulness, also feelings of anger, guilt, despair, hopelessness, identification with the loss, fear, loneliness, and thoughts of death and suicide. The experience is most intense in the immediate aftermath of significant loss and attenuates with the passing of time. The memories of the bereavement remain and are triggered by emotionally congruent cues or triggers, for example anniversaries. These can be environmental or internal, emotive or cognitive. Depressed states and physical illness can reactivate the intensity of a previous bereavement. Accommodation to bereavement requires the healthy acquisition of coping resources as protective factors.

Bereavement may be described as pathological when accommodation is insufficient to enable the person to return to their best previous level of social functioning.

Adjustment

Adjustment is a normative response to a stressful 'life event'. It involves the development of adaptive coping responses. It draws on internal emotive–cognitive and external behavioural resources.

Self-harm

Injury to self, a behaviour, a final common path: a deliberate act, often to relieve distressing emotional content, or in response to crisis as a coping strategy, a means of meeting unmet emotional need, or part of a journey toward suicide.

- 1% of new self-harm presentations are dead through suicide within 1 year.
- Rates fall in areas where there are self-harm services.
- Self-harm repetition is a predictor of suicide.
- Brief interventions, such as problem solving, are shown to reduce symptoms of depression and anxiety and to reduce the frequency of self-harm episodes.

Management includes:

- improving the patient's engagement with mental health, social and non-statutory services
- conducting psychosocial assessments of all persons presenting
- managing co-morbid mental illness, alcohol and substance misuse and personality disorder.

Suicide

- UK rate is 10 per 100,000 per year.
- Target is to reduce this by 20% by 2010.
- Highly prevalent in people with severe mental illness, in whom lifetime rates are 10–15%.
- Also highly prevalent in self-harm populations.
- Also in eating disorder populations, 60% of people with anorexia nervosa in contact with specialist inpatient services by the age of 35.

Somatisation

Somatisation is a chronic condition, characterised by numerous unexplained medical symptoms before the age of 30. Symptoms often have a basis in prior experience, memory, or a model of the disease or in cognitive distortions arising from the physiological consequences of anxiety and arousal.

The fourth revision of the Diagnostic and Statistical Manual of Mental Disorders (DSM-IV) states that this disorder occurs when all of the following are present:

- four pain symptoms, including four separate sites or systems
- one pseudo-neurological symptom
- one sexual symptom
- two gastrointestinal symptoms.

These are unexplained by medical investigation and not intentionally produced or feigned.

Management involves treatment of the associated depression, cognitive behavioural therapy and cognitive reattribution.

Factitious disorder

This is the intentional production of medical, surgical, or gynaecological symptoms, with limited, or no, conscious appreciation by the patient of the reason. Patients:

- are usually female
- have a good relationship with health-care staff
- are often in caring professional roles, including nursing and baby sitting
- tend to be loyal to one hospital
- often seek powerful care figures.

Management should focus towards mental health or social care options.

- The patient should be identified to the care team when admitted to the general hospital.
- Multi-agency care plans should be clearly written.
- The patient should be included on a register in the general hospital.

Patients risk undergoing inadvertent invasive investigations or surgical procedures and having to endure their complications. Hospitals risk the consequences of conducting these procedures on patients with no organic pathology and patients having prolonged hospitalisation.

Munchausen syndrome

This is a subtype of factitious disorder. It is the intentional production of medical or surgical symptoms with limited or no conscious appreciation by the patient of the reason. Patients:

- are usually male
- have an itinerant lifestyle
- are not known to the hospital.

Management is by confrontation or challenge, which results in the patient moving on. Details are often held in a register and shared with neighbouring hospitals. The aim is to reduce unnecessary invasive investigations or surgical interventions, thereby reducing the risk of medical accidents and the use of acute-bed days.

Alcohol dependency

The main clinical problem is alcohol withdrawal following medical admission. Of male admissions, 25% have an alcohol-use disorder.

It is necessary to take a history of the units of alcohol consumed in a typical week.

- Safe limits are 14 units in women and 21 units in men for a week.
- Heavy use would be 21 units for women and 28 units for men.
- Use CAGE or AUDIT–C to identify problem use.
- Consider MCV and Gamma GT.

The World Health Organisation states that a dependency syndrome should include three of:

- compulsion to drink
- difficulty controlling alcohol use
- withdrawal
- tolerance
- continued use in the face of harm
- also rapid reinstatement after abstinence, narrowing of repertoire and salience.

The **withdrawal syndrome** spectrum ranges from sweating and anxiety to withdrawal seizures.

- **Mild withdrawal** can be managed by adequate nutrition and hydration.
- **Moderate withdrawal** can be managed with benzodiazepines, oral thiamine and vitamin C in supervised outpatient setting.
- **Severe or complicated withdrawal** should be handled as a medical inpatient.

Oral chlordiazepoxide is the recommended **management**, the initial dose being titrated against severity within a range of 5–40 mg four times daily (British National Formulary section 4.10.) Parenteral vitamin B is recommended, especially if delirium tremens, ataxia, ophthalmoplegia, confusion, memory disturbance, hypothermia, hypotension, or unconsciousness are present.

The differential diagnosis of confusion includes Wernicke's encephalopathy and hepatic encephalopathy.

Opiate dependency

The main medical problems of opiate dependency are:

- hepatitis B and C
- human immune deficiency virus (HIV) -related disorders
- infective endocarditis.

The main surgical problems are:

- abscesses
- fractures
- sinuses
- vascular thrombosis.

There are high rates of co-morbidity for self-harm, alcohol-use disorders and affective disorders, and personality disorder. Rates of primary psychotic illness are lower, relatively. Poly-substance misuse with stimulants carries the additional risk of psychosis. This group are at high-risk for suicide.

Physician needs to establish:

- history of use
- dependency
- routes of administration
- complications.

Clinical management may include methadone substitution. Addictions specialists should be engaged and legislation, eg Misuse of Drugs Act, Health and Safety at Work, Mental Health Act, should be taken into account.

Depression

Depression is common.

- It occurs in 14% of medical inpatients.
- 7% are detected.
- 2% receive treatment.

Sleep disturbance and loss of energy are confounded by physical disorder and inpatient environments. Core symptoms should be present most of the time for at least two weeks and include:

- low mood
- loss of energy
- loss of pleasure.

The diagnosis of depression should be made on the basis of a clinical interview. Progress can be monitored by self-report questionnaire. Validated instruments include:

- General Health Questionnaire
- Hospital Anxiety and Depression Scale
- Beck Depression Inventory.

Anxiety

Anxiety is a common response to threat, medical investigation, results and diagnosis, especially following bad or uncertain news. It is a state of high arousal. Symptoms of anxiety include:

- tremor
- sweating
- palpitations
- 'butterflies in the stomach'
- urinary hesitancy
- breathlessness
- pain.

Management is by psychological education, cognitive behavioural therapy and short-term use of benzodiazepines. Some selective serotonin reuptake inhibitors and SNRI antidepressants have indications for the treatment of anxiety.

Stress

Stress is a precipitating factor for physiological arousal becoming anxiety. It can be internal or external to the person.

Delirium (see Chapter 16)

There are two subtypes:

- **Excited delirium**, elevated behaviours, agitation. Patient is characteristically disorientated with hallucinations, paranoid ideation, thought disorder and other features of psychosis. Mood incongruent delusions may emerge. Symptoms fluctuate, they are worse in low light levels at night and can remit completely during the day.
- **Retarded delirium**, is seen in the quietly confused patient sitting unnoticed by nursing staff. They are equally confused, at high-risk of inadvertent neglect, they refuse or leave meals and fluids. They have a higher risk of mortality.

Delirium is rarely treated under the Mental Health Act because of the common law provision for immediately necessary care required to prevent irreversible deterioration or death in patients lacking the capacity to consent.

Dementia

General hospital admission often follows an acute decline in social functioning following a bio-psycho-social event.

- Dementia can be distinguished from delirium on the basis of a longer history and the relative absence of concomitant medical or surgical events. The decline is global.
- Dementia of Alzheimer's type is typically a slow decline with short-term memory loss preceding autobiographical memory loss, and physical decline.
- Dementia with a vascular basis tends to progress in stepwise decline and may well be associated with a medical event. The presentation reflects the area of brain most affected. At each decline the clinical picture may resemble delirium.
- Lewy Body dementia is associated with Parkinson's disease and haloperidol should be avoided.

Organic mood disorder

Depressive states occur commonly in response to ill health and threat to life. Organic mood disorder can also be part of:

- endocrine disorder, especially thyroid disease and diabetes
- the para-neoplastic syndrome (manic states occur with cerebral disease, metastases, para-neoplastic syndrome, tuberculosis, stroke and treatment with steroids).

Dissociative disorder

Dissociative disorder is divided into disorders of:

- memory awareness and identity
- movement and sensation.

Establish inconsistency between the patient's history and the clinical observation. **Management** is by engagement and psycho-education on the role of stress on bodily function. Physiotherapists and occupational therapists use behavioural strategies to overcome the disability.

Eating disorder

Eating disorders have a high mortality. Severe anorexia nervosa, with a body mass index below 15, is associated with cognitive deterioration. It can require acute medical admission for urgent medical support, or as part of a re-feeding strategy. Renal and hepatic dysfunction, electrocardiogram abnormalities, with risk of sudden cardiac death, and overwhelming septicaemia are serious problems. Other eating disorders not otherwise specified are common, especially as part of chronic illness. They require multidisciplinary dietary and nutritional assessment. The Mental Health Act may be required and medico-legal input is advised.

Severe mental illness

Patients with schizophrenia or bipolar mood disorder may be admitted to general hospitals for medical and surgical co-morbidity. Communicate clearly with the care co-ordinators in the sector or with the specialist mental health teams and primary care. A consultant liaison psychiatrist can usefully assume clinical and RMO responsibility for the patient's mental health care during the episode. Admissions require planning around environment and provision of mental health nursing.

Sexual dysfunction

Sexual dysfunction is widespread in general hospital populations as part of organic diseases such as:

- hypertension
- prostatic hypertrophy
- diabetes mellitus
- thyroid disorder
- side-effects of commonly prescribed drugs, antihypertensives, antidepressants, diuretics, antipsychotics and sex hormones.

Bancroft (1989) suggests a model for understanding sexual dysfunction within the context of physical illness by recognising:

- the direct physical effects of the condition
- the psychological effects of the condition
- the effect of drugs and other physical conditions on sexuality.

Treatments include:

- treatment of underlying causes
- review of medication

- advice
- use of lubricants
- use of aids
- use of the Masters and Johnson sensate focus technique for treating psychological sexual dysfunction, and treatment of depression or anxiety
- pharmacotherapy.

Pain

Pain is the commonest presentation in medicine. It is an individual subjective experience and a common presentation of psychiatric disorders, including anxiety, depression, somatoform disorder and hypochondriasis. In **somatoform pain disorder**:

- there is a preoccupation with pain
- the pain causes significant distress or impairment
- psychological factors are judged to have an important role in the onset and maintenance
- pain is not feigned
- pain is not better accounted for by a mood, anxiety or psychotic disorder.

Management is multidisciplinary, with a pain team. Underlying medical and psychiatric conditions should be treated. There is a role for analgesics, antidepressants and mood stabilisers, as well as cognitive behavioural and behavioural therapies.

Post-traumatic stress disorder

This follows six months after an episode of acute trauma.

- There is frequent and distressing re-experience of a traumatic event.
- The event is usually significant and regarded as life-threatening to the patient or a loved one.
- There is associated avoidance of triggers and numbing.
- There may be secondary phobic anxiety.

Management is with cognitive behavioural therapy or antidepressants. Counselling and debriefing after acute events have not been found to be protective. Post-traumatic amnesia and early use of benzodiazepines may modify the risk.

Unexplained medical symptoms

These should be investigated in a specialist centre.

- Motor symptoms that remain unexplained following medical investigation are common but the emergence of a subsequent organic explanation for these symptoms is rare.
- The prevalence of co-existent affective and anxiety disorders is high, many patients have personality disorder.

- Shorter duration of symptoms and co-existent anxiety or depression are associated with better outcome.
- Reinvestigation is expensive and potentially dangerous; it should be avoided where no clear clinical indication exists.

BRIEF INTERVENTIONS

Cognitive behavioural therapy

Cognitive behavioural therapy, also cognitive therapy and cognitive reattribution model, model mental functioning in terms of affects, behaviours and cognitions with associated arousal. It is formally conducted over ten 1-hour sessions with a trained therapist, using a diary for work in between. The therapist helps the client identify automatic negative thoughts and constructs a hierarchy for challenging them. It is effective in anxiety and depression, somatoform disorders and health anxiety.

Interpersonal therapy

Interpersonal therapy is useful in depression and anxiety. It can also be used in irritable bowel syndrome.

Dialectical behavioural therapy

Dialectical behavioural therapy involves both individual and group work. It is effective in some personality disorders, especially emotionally unstable/borderline type.

Problem solving

Problem solving is a brief intervention focused on facilitating the client to:

- identify the main problems contributing to their symptoms
- rank the problems in order of severity
- rank the problems in order of solubility
- work to solve the problems they can solve.

It usually takes three to five sessions. It reduces the symptoms of depression and anxiety, and may reduce the frequency of self-harm.

SERVICE MODELS

In reach model

This involves mental health assessment from a community mental health team. It is less likely to understand the issues for a general hospital and less likely to have formed the informal working relationships necessary to bridge cultural differences.

Self-harm team

The self-harm team is often nurse-led, although it can be entirely social-work-based. The requirement is to:

- conduct a psychosocial assessment
- engage the client
- offer a brief, solution-focused intervention.

Consultation-Liaison psychiatry

This comprises dedicated consultant psychiatrists with speciality training in liaison psychiatry serving the mental health needs of the general hospital. They offer:

- consultation and advice on treatment
- direct care
- development of policy, training and education.

Dedicated services are multidisciplinary and form good professional working relationships alongside general hospital colleagues. The focus of the work is largely inpatient and emergency departments. Some services are exclusively outpatient and leave emergency psychiatry and self-harm assessments to crisis services. Services near academic centres are often termed Departments of Psychological Medicine.

MEDICO-LEGAL ISSUES

(See Chapter 10 in particular.)

Mental Health Act 1983 England and Wales

- Section 5(2): the Act can apply on general hospital inpatient wards. Emergency Departments are not regarded as inpatient areas.
- Section 4: has power of conveyance, it can apply to a general hospital.
- In general, a medical disorder cannot be treated under the Mental Health Act.

Common Law

Common Law comprises the Case Law built up over time as a series of legal judgements, modified through appellate courts, ultimately the House of Lords. It establishes the legal principles of:

- **Medical duty of care**.
- **Medical negligence**: Bolam, House of Lords.
- **Best interests**: applies to patients lacking the capacity to give informed consent. The doctor should seek to: improve capacity, consult appropriately, take account of advance directives, and act to reduce the risk of death or irretrievable harm. The greater the time from the need to make a life-saving clinical decision, the more the requirement to consult and work to improve capacity.

Capacity

The role of the liaison psychiatrist is to assess the mental state and advise on what impact it has on the capacity for the specific clinical issue.

Consent

See Chapter 19.

FURTHER READING

Bancroft, J. 1989. *Human sexuality and its problems*. Edinburgh: Churchill Livingstone.

Guthrie, X.X. & Creed, X.X. 1996. *Seminars in liaison psychiatry*. Xxxx, Gaskell.

RCPsych 2003. *The psychological care of medical patients – A practical guide*. Xxxx, RCPsych CR108.

Chapter 21

Forensic Psychiatry

Tim Amos and Arden Tomison

CONTENTS

Forensic Psychiatry

FORENSIC PSYCHIATRY

Forensic psychiatry

Forensic, (ie pertaining to the law), **psychiatry** covers the interface and interaction between psychiatry and the law in all its aspects. It embraces the assessment and treatment of mentally disordered offenders.

Development of forensic psychiatry

Forensic psychiatry developed during the 1970s but can trace its origin back through the centuries. The relationship between crime and mental disorder has long excited public imagination. Perennial themes include:

- punishment versus humane care
- individual responsibility
- the role of mental disorder in criminal behaviour
- public safety versus individuals' rights.

Role of forensic psychiatrist

The forensic psychiatrist works within a number of spheres, primarily the health and criminal justice systems. The emphasis is on multidisciplinary and multi-agency working within:

- services including **health** primary care, secondary mental health care, substance misuse, learning disabilities, neuropsychiatry and head injury, and social services
- **the legal system** involving the police, prisons, probation, courts, solicitors, and the Home Office.

Forensic psychiatry services

Most secure services work to the guiding principles of the **Reed Report**, which outlined that the care of mentally disordered offenders should be:

- by health and social services
- with regard to the needs of the individual
- as far as possible in the community
- under security no greater than is justified by the degree of danger
- in such a way as to maximise rehabilitation
- as near as possible to their own families or homes.

Practically, at present, specialist forensic services are organised around hospitals with different levels of physical security ranging from high-security hospitals (eg Broadmoor) through medium-secure units to low-secure provision offering short- or long-term treatments. Some units have special expertise (eg female patients, learning disabilities, personality disorders, head injuries, autistic spectrum disorders).

CRIME AND PSYCHIATRIC ISSUES RELATED TO OFFENDING

The causes of crime

The causes of crime include the following:

- Genetic factors
  - greater concordance in monozygotic than dyzgotic twins
  - adoption studies confirm the genetic influence
  - possibly linked via personality factors (eg hyperactivity, impulsivity)
- Physiological factors
  - abnormal measurements (electroencephalograms, skin conductance)
  - failure in arousal and/or autonomic system leads to inability to condition normally
  - organic disorders especially brain damage
- Psychological factors
  - hyperactivity
  - cognitive impairment (decreased IQ) with deficits in executive functions and planning skills being important
  - poor academic performance
  - personality traits, eg impulsivity, sensation seeking, lack of control
  - distorted style of social information processing (misinterpreting others)
  - mental disorders
- Social factors
  - Family factors
    - low income/poverty
    - ineffective, inconsistent parenting
    - marital disharmony and broken homes
    - criminal behaviour within the family
    - parental mental disorder, especially depression
  - Broader factors
    - peer group (especially if delinquent)
    - local drug use and availability
    - city location
    - schooling
    - unemployment
    - exposure to violence (local, including home, and visual media)
    - labelling (caught juveniles go on to offend more).

Crime data

There are two main types of crime, those against the person and those against property.

- Crimes against the person (ie 'violent crime') include homicide, wounding and assault, sexual offences and robbery.
- Crimes against property (far more common) include burglary, theft and handling stolen goods, fraud and forgery, arson and criminal damage.

The most common crimes are those involving the use of drugs and motoring offences.

There are about five million notifiable offences each year in England and Wales. These recorded crime figures only provide a partial picture of crime committed because

- not all crimes are reported to the police
- not all those that are reported are recorded.

Less serious offences are particularly under-represented in this way. Attempts to measure the levels of crime more accurately include population and victim surveys such as the British Crime Survey. This suggests that the amount of crime may be four times higher than that recorded by the police.

Most offending is committed by young men. Half of all indictable offences (those carrying at least three months imprisonment) are committed by those aged under 21 years. Men offend four times as commonly as women, who have an earlier peak age of offending (16 years). About 30% of men have a conviction by the age of 30, compared to 7% of women. Around 7% of men account for about 60% of all convictions. The earlier the onset of criminal behaviour, the longer the career and the higher the frequency of crimes.

Violent crime

There are over 500,000 violent crimes each year, about 5% of all recorded crime; mostly minor assaults and wounding. Violent offenders have a peak age of around 18 years and are much more likely to be male. Around half of violent offences are either in the home or in public houses with alcohol being a major factor. In up to one-third of cases the victim has been actively involved.

There are about 700 **homicides** in England and Wales, the majority being either the murder of a family member or the result of aggression between young men, with alcohol use common in both the offender and the victim. In about 75% of offences the victim is known to the perpetrator. The most common methods are the use of an instrument and punching/kicking. Guns are rarely used in the UK (in contrast to the USA). Infants are most at risk, two-thirds being killed by their mother.

Sexual crime

Sexual offences comprise less than 1% of all indictable offences and most are committed by men.

Rape

Offenders tend to be young men who are sexually inexperienced and frustrated, often with a criminal record.

- one-third are relatives or long-term acquaintances of their victims
- one-third are brief acquaintances
- one-third are strangers.

Reconviction rate is low (10%) but 15–20% are reconvicted of sexual assault and similar percentages are reconvicted of a violent offence.

Victims are mostly women but a few are men. Many suffer post-traumatic stress disorder (or anxiety/depression) and in a significant minority (20%) these symptoms persist.

Indecent assault

Indecent assault covers various behaviours, some of which may be linked to poor social skills.

Paedophilia and child sexual abuse

Paedophilia is sexual offending by adults against children.

Child sexual abuse is the involvement of children in sexual activities which they do not fully comprehend and to which they cannot give informed consent.

Epidemiology is difficult; between 10 and 50% of women recall some experience of abuse.

Sexual activity is usually fondling, with vaginal or anal intercourse being rare. The majority of cases do not involve violence, more usually there are persuasion and coercion.

The offender is usually male (up to 10% may be female) and commonly a family member, particularly stepfathers. Alcohol is often a factor. Recidivism occurs in about one-third (higher in homosexual paedophiles) and a minority progress to become violent sexual offenders.

Most victims are known to the offender and up to one-half are related. Girls are twice as likely to be victims.

Effects on victims can be divided into early and long-term.

- Early effects
  - inappropriate sexual behaviour
  - physical symptoms in urogenital or anal area
  - emotional symptoms – anxiety, depression, anger, guilt.
- Long-term effects
  - chronic mood disorders
  - low self-esteem
  - self-harm
  - difficulties in relationships.

The extent of the effects depends on the extent of the abuse, disclosure of abuse, formal proceedings, other problems in the family environment and individual psychological processing.

Incest is most common between brother and sister but is most commonly reported between father and daughter.

Psychiatric issues of sexual offending

There is rarely major mental illness involved, but learning disability may be a factor. Offenders are often sexually inexperienced with poor social skills.

Assessment of the likelihood of any further sexual or violent offending can be difficult.

Treatment can include:

- rarely, diagnosis and management of psychiatric disorder
- group therapy
- behavioural therapy
- improvement of social functioning
- anti-libidinal treatment (may help in some cases).

Arson

Arson is defined as fire setting to property which may endanger lives (1000 die annually by fire in England and Wales). The majority of offenders are under 18 years old, 25% are under 13. Legally, arson is regarded as very serious and perpetrators can receive life imprisonment.

Profitable	insurance fraud; to cover other offences
Revenge	against society (ie burns police station), employers, or jealous
Political	terrorists
Accidental	difference between accident and recklessness can be difficult to establish
Pleasure and excitement	• hero fire-setters • firebugs – obtain intense satisfaction or relief from fire setting • erotic/sexual excitement
Psychotic/organic	about 10%: schizophrenia, learning disabled, personality disordered, alcohol disorders, organic disorders
Pyromania	motiveless, impulsive fire setting
Suicide by fire	

Table 21.1 Classification of arson offenders

Arsonists are not a homogeneous group. Any mental disorder that is found should be treated. However, in the majority of cases, there is no mental disorder and behaviour is often impulsive or acting out of emotional distress, especially in women.

Acquisitive crime

This is the most common type of non-motoring crime. It involves depriving others of their property and includes shoplifting (legally: theft). It is almost always for simple gain, often on a small scale. Commonly associated with substance misuse, it is used to finance the purchase of drugs.

Some rare associations with syndromes include:

- kleptomania (compulsive stealing) = impulse control disorder
- secondary grandiose delusions ('own everything')
- affective states (forgetfulness or disinhibition)
- organic states (brain damage or dementia).

CRIME AND MENTAL DISORDER

Associations between crime and mental disorder

Crime is very common (over 5 million offences a year) and mental disorder is also very common (up to 50% of the population) so there is likely to be an overlap. However, most people with a mental disorder do not commit crimes and most criminals do not suffer from a mental disorder. The mentally ill account for a very small proportion of all violence.

There is an association between mental disorder and crime. Evidence comes from birth cohort studies and from prison and psychiatric population studies. Crime studies have shown that individuals with mental disorder are more likely to have been arrested, with substance abuse being the best predictor. People with mental disorder may be:

- less likely to be aware of the consequences of their actions
- more likely to be detected/caught
- more likely to be remanded
- more likely to be noticed in prison
- more likely to come from lower socio-economic backgrounds (a characteristic shared with criminal population).

Finally, prison may precipitate mental disorder or mental disorder may pre-dispose to criminality (especially drugs).

Schizophrenia

The absolute risk of offending is very low. Offences are mostly trivial and related to poor social skills. Criminal careers start later in those with schizophrenia compared with those in general population.

There is evidence of higher rates of violent offending than in the general population. Individuals with schizophrenia have been shown:

- in community studies, to have a rate of violent behaviour up to four times that of a non-mentally disordered group
- in case register studies, to have violent convictions up to four times the rate of the general population and twice the rate of other mentally disordered groups
- in prison studies, to make up 5% of remand prisoners
- in homicide studies, to have than overrepresented in the general population.

The risk of violent offending increases markedly if combined with substance misuse.

acute psychosis	
delusions	• systematised paranoid delusions • held with great conviction • when accompanied by strong affect (fear, anger, jealousy, anxiety, sadness) • which lead to loss of self control
hallucinations	• command auditory • olfactory or gustatory
thought disorder	
high level of arousal	

Table 21.2 Symptoms of schizophrenia associated with violence

Deterioration in personality and social functioning usually lead to more minor offending.

Affective disorders

The risk of criminal behaviour is hard to estimate because of

- range of disorders
- difficulty distinguishing between affective and other disorders
- making the diagnosis (rarely done).

Depression

- **Minor violence** can be the result of the general mood state, eg irritability and frustration.
- **Major violence** is rare, it is often the result of depressive cognitions/thoughts (guilt, self-blame, failure, feeling that the world is too dreadful). Most victims are family, eg infanticide or whole family killings with suicide of perpetrator.
- Other crimes may be the result of impaired concentration (**shoplifting**), or the side-effects of medication (**driving offences**).
- Crime/legal process may lead to depression/suicidal acts.
- Ideas of guilt and unworthiness may lead to false confessions.

Mania/hypomania

- seldom linked with serious violence
- more commonly linked to public-order offences (via irritability, alcohol)
- excessive spending
- fraud may be associated with grandiose delusions.

Substance misuse

Substance misuse is very commonly associated with antisocial behaviour and acquisitive offending.

It is associated with other mental illness, especially schizophrenia, affective disorders and personality disorders (increased risk of criminal behaviour).

Alcohol

Alcohol consumption has been reported prior to offending in:

- up to 60% of homicides/assaults (many victims as well)
- 50% of rapes
- 40% of property offences
- significant number of driving offences.

Drugs

The category of the drug and the nature of its use make for major differences.

- There is little evidence for criminal behaviour being higher in cannabis users (except possession).
- 80% of opiate users have at least one conviction.
- US figures suggest that up to 50% of offenders have used opiates.

Relationship between misuse and crime

- Acute intoxication can lead to impaired judgement.
- Intoxication reduces inhibitions.
- Neuropsychiatric complications can occur (especially with alcohol).
- Illegal activity is linked to drugs.
- Crime is used in financing the use/habit (especially drugs).
- Reduction in employment opportunities has financial implications.
- Social network and moral inhibitions are lacking.

Personality disorders

These are common in offenders. There is no strong link between any specific disorder and specific offences, although dissocial personality disorder is strongly associated with violence.

Many offenders have more than more type of personality disorder with the most common being dissocial (or antisocial) and emotionally unstable (both impulsive and borderline types) while paranoid features, if not the disorder, can also be apparent.

Other psychiatric symptoms and disorders, particularly alcohol or drug disorders, are often associated and tend to increase the risk of offending.

'Psychopathic disorder' is used in a number of ways:

- as another term for antisocial disorder (best avoided)
- as a legal term within the 1983 Mental Health Act, where it can cover a number of personality and other disorders
- as a variant on 'psychopathy', now often defined using the assessment tool – the Psychopathy Checklist, revised version (PCL-R) (see page 449).

Organic disorders

Organic disorders, particularly affecting the frontal lobes, can lead to disinhibited behaviour which can become criminal.

Epilepsy

- There are limited data on a specific association with criminal acts but traditionally considered to be significantly associated.
- There are suggestions of increased violence and offending but these are rarely related directly to seizures, fewer than 50 cases in the literature. Peri-ictal states may contribute more.
- The relationship is a complex one:
  - people with epilepsy are over-represented in all institutions
  - epileptic syndrome is an epiphenomenon of brain dysfunction which may cause other problems
  - low self-esteem, related to social rejection, can be a precursor to antisocial behaviour
  - there is increased co-morbidity for major psychiatric disorders.

Head injury

- There are difficulties in categorising brain trauma.
- Prison populations suggest a high level of head injury (culture, high prevalence of alcohol and drugs).
- There is a possible link with subsequent violent behaviour, including homicide.

Special syndromes

It can be difficult to distinguish between pathological reactions and more extreme variants of normal. There may be distinct syndromes or associations with other mental disorders, eg schizophrenia, depression, personality disorder, alcohol or drug (especially cocaine) dependence and organic disorders. For more details see Chapter 12.

Pathological (morbid) jealousy – Othello syndrome

- This is more common in men (most victims are women).
- Partners are intimidated, controlled, threatened and pressed for confessions.
- It is a common cause of violence ('wife battering').
- Jealousy motivates a significant proportion of serious violence.

Erotomania – De Clérambault syndrome

- There is a possible conflict with law, eg injunctions.
- It is probably more common in women (sampling difficulties).

CRIMINAL LAW AND PROCEEDINGS

This section refers to the law in England and Wales. Other countries have different processes.

Criminal law is that part of the law which is concerned with crimes, ie acts which are considered to be offences against society and which are punishable by the State.

Civil law is concerned with the rights and obligations of individuals to one another; it includes **family law**, **contract law** and the **law of tort**. A tort is a civil wrong, such as negligence, nuisance, defamation, or trepass, for which the remedy is a common law action for damages.

Common law is law derived from previous cases and therefore by precedent ('case law').

Other laws are **statutes**, which come from Acts of Parliament.

Offence

Most offences, particularly minor ones, never come to the attention of the police. In many reported cases the police are unable to identify a suspect.

Arrest

The legal process for criminal behaviour starts with the apprehension of the suspect, usually by the police. It is therefore the police officer who makes the first decision about whether to take action and if so what action to take. If the police believe an offence has been committed a suspect can receive a caution (minor offences), a fixed penalty (eg speeding fine), or be prosecuted.

Interview

The statutory requirements and codes of practice which the police must follow during the interview process are governed by the Police and Criminal Evidence Act 1984. To the long-standing rights to be cautioned and have access to a lawyer were added the tape (and video) recording of all interviews and the role of the Appropriate Adult for interviews with juveniles, those with learning difficulties and those with mental disorder.

Detainees must be 'fit to be interviewed' according to three broad criteria:

- ability to comprehend police caution
- fully orientated for time, person and place
- able to give answers which are not likely to be misconstrued.

Prosecution

The decision to prosecute is taken by the Crown Prosecution Service (CPS) who work alongside the police but are an independent agency headed by the Director of Public Prosecution (DPP).

Remand

Once charged, there is a court hearing (the defendant does not always have to appear) for the magistrates to determine if there is a case to answer. If a final decision on the case cannot be made at the first hearing, the defendant will be remanded on bail (ie in the community, sometimes with restrictions) or in custody (in a remand prison).

The courts

The courts are a hierarchical system.

Magistrates' Court

Over 95% of all criminal prosecutions are dealt with in magistrates' courts. Magistrates may be lay (that is not a professional lawyer), in which case usually three sit, together with a legally trained clerk for legal advice. There are also legally trained stipendiary magistrates who tend to sit alone.

Magistrates' courts function as trial courts for minor offences or courts of preliminary investigation for more serious offences, where the prosecution have to establish a *prima facie* case. The nature and seriousness of the offence determine whether it is a:

- **summary offence** – this is minor and is tried in the magistrates' court
- **indictable offence** – this is serious, has to be tried in the Crown Court and carries at least three months imprisonment
- **either-way offence** – this is an intermediate offence and can be tried in either court.

Crown Court

The most serious offences (murder, rape, wounding, grievous bodily harm, robbery, burglary) are tried in the Crown Court.

Defendant	accused individual(s)
Lawyers	two sides (adversarial) representing the defendant and the Crown (prosecution). They present the evidence and cross-examine witnesses.
Witnesses	Individuals who give evidence and may be: • witness to fact: say what they saw • professional witness: give testimony in their professional capacity • expert witness: the only witnesses able to give opinions
Jury	twelve drawn from the public to consider the evidence and come to a conclusion (verdict) of guilty or not guilty
Judge	instructs the jury on points of law, sums up and passes sentence

Table 21.3 Crown Court components

Higher courts

Once a case has been heard in the Crown Court, either side can make representations to the High Court and the Court of Appeal where senior judges sit and consider the case. Cases which are viewed as legally important may go to the House of Lords to be heard by the Law Lords, the most senior judges in England and Wales. Some cases are then pursued in the European Courts.

Criminal responsibility

A fundamental principle of English Law is that for an individual to be found guilty of an offence, two elements need to be proved:

- *Actus Reus* or 'guilty act'. An illegal act or omission has occurred and has been carried out by an identified individual.
- *Mens Rea* or 'guilty mind'. The individual had the state of mind necessary to commit the act. Aspects of behaviour contributing to this include intentionality, recklessness, competence and responsibility.

Some offences, eg most traffic offences, only require *actus reus*.

Children under the age of 10 are exempt from criminal responsibility. Since 1998, children above the age of 10 are criminally liable.

Fitness to stand trial

The criteria for fitness to stand trial are usually related to whether the defendant is physically well enough to last the trial.

Fitness to plead

Pleading is the defendant's opportunity to admit or deny the charges.

The criteria for fitness to plead are not laid down within statute but stem from the nineteenth-century case of Pritchard (who was deaf, without speech and unable to communicate) and are that a defendant should be able to:

- understand the charge (indictment) against them
- understand the details of the evidence against them
- follow court proceedings
- challenge a juror
- instruct legal advisors.

Verdict

The verdict is the sole responsibility of the jury who usually retire to a separate room to consider all the evidence.

Sentencing

Sentencing is one of the main roles of the judge, who sentences the defendant according to specific guidelines. The main sentences are custody, community sentences, probation and fines.

Afterwards

A number of procedures can occur after sentencing, including appeals (against conviction or the sentence) and, for those who are imprisoned, consideration for parole and eventual release.

PSYCHIATRY AND THE CRIMINAL JUSTICE SYSTEM

Developments in psychiatry and the law (especially in relation to human rights) have resulted in changes which have brought the two systems closer together and allow for a shared approach to individual cases. Recently, this notion has begun to be extended to those with personality disorder.

Court and police liaison

There is a process for moving individuals from the criminal justice system to the health system. Police may use section 136 (see chapter 10), and can ask for Mental Health Act assessments at a police station. Diversion at the point of arrest (DAPA) allows transfer from the police cells to hospital, or the community where the offence/incident is relatively minor and there is clear evidence of a mental disorder. In such cases the individual can be dealt with under the civil part (section 2 or 3) of the Mental Health Act (1983). This usually results in no charges.

Similar schemes run in some courts, particularly in inner cities, where a mental-health professional (psychiatrist/community psychiatric nurse) assesses referred individuals at the court and produces brief reports to assist deliberations.

Diversion schemes are beneficial provided there is:

- a practical protocol agreed by all agencies
- local enthusiasm for the process in all agencies
- sufficient resourcing, for example personnel and beds.

In court

Fitness to plead and stand trial

Psychiatrists may be asked to assist the court where there is severe mental illness, usually psychosis, or marked learning disability, where a psychologist can often provide useful extra information, eg IQ.

Insanity (McNaughten Rules)

Insanity is a legal term defined by statute. It arose from the case of Daniel McNaughten who, in 1842, shot and killed the prime minister's private secretary. McNaughten had a persecutory delusion system involving the prime minister. After the trial, the McNaughten Rules were established:

> '... that at the time of the committing of the act, the party accused was labouring under such a defect of reason, from disease of the mind, as not to know the nature and quality of the act he was doing, or if he did know it, that he did not know it was wrong.'

Whether a particular condition is a disease of the mind is a legal, not a medical, question. It is a matter for medical or psychiatric experts to testify as to the factual nature of the condition but it is for the jury to say whether that is evidence of a defect of reason from the disease of the mind.

The insanity defence is available for all indictable crimes and if successful leads to a special verdict 'not guilty by reason of insanity'.

Outcome if unfit to plead or found insane

If a defendant is found unfit to plead, there is a 'trial of the facts' that can either result in an acquittal or a conviction. For those found unfit to plead or not guilty by reason of insanity, there are four possible disposals:

- admission order with or without restrictions (equivalent to section 37 with or without section 41 – these are sections of the Mental Health Act – see Chapter XX)
- guardianship order
- supervision and treatment order
- absolute discharge.

Homicide defences

These relate to part of the Homicide Act 1957. The Act defines murder as the 'unlawful killing of a human being with malice aforethought' (ie the intention to kill or to cause grievous bodily harm). Manslaughter is still unlawful killing but the full criteria for murder are not met, possibly because of diminished responsibility where the individual is:

> 'suffering from such abnormality of mind ... as substantially impaired his mental responsibility for his acts.'

Other reasons for a manslaughter verdict are mitigating circumstances such as provocation and killings as part of a suicide pact. Infanticide may be outcome when a woman kills her own child of less than a year.

Intent

Experts are often asked to help with this matter when specific intent, which only applies in certain offences, is a key issue.

Automatism

A complex area where legal definitions do not fit with medical ones. If a person has no control over an act, then there is absence of *mens rea*. Sane automatisms are considered to be one-off events as a result of external causes, such as confusional states, night terrors and hypoglycaemia, and result in an acquittal. Insane automatisms are behaviours which might recur and are said to be the result of an internal cause, such as epilepsy, brain diseases and sleep walking. Sentencing is left to the judge with disposals to either hospital or the community.

Court report

Reports are written for the court and not for either side (defence or prosecution). Remember that court reports tend to be used 'beyond the court' and may find their way into medical notes. Reports should be written in clear concise non-technical language with an unambiguous division between fact and the opinion, which should be based on the evidence as presented in the body of the report.

A typical report might have three main sections:

- **Introduction** – details of charges (and courts), where and when seen, confirmation of explanation to subject about reduced confidentiality, details of sources of background information (eg police summary of case, witness statements, interviews, convictions, previous medical records and psychiatric reports)
- **Body** – family and personal history, medical and psychiatric history, alcohol and substance use, personality, offending and violent behaviour, index offence, current circumstances, mental state examination, any investigations
- **Conclusions** – opinion as to diagnosis, fitness to plead, mental state at time of offence, mental disorder and offending, contribution of mental disorder to risk of re-offending, prognosis and recommendations to court re treatment, management and disposal.

PRISON

Custody

The use of custody, or banishment from society, as a means of punishment has been used for centuries. There have always been arguments about its value in respect of punishment as opposed to rehabilitation, retribution as opposed to prevention, as a deterrent and as a part of justice.

Prison populations

Recent years have seen an enormous increase in the UK prison population from 44,000 in 1993 to over 75,000 in 2004. Critics have argued that the subsequent levels of over-crowding have restricted the opportunities for (re)training and increased the potential for problems within prisons.

There is a high turnover with more than 50% of untried prisoners spending less than one month on remand and 80% of sentenced prisoners released within one year of sentencing.

Prisoners tend to be young men from unstable community circumstances to which they return on release. Over 50% re-offend within two years.

Categories

There are currently about 140 prisons, divided into various categories by security, function, age and gender.

Security

- **Category A**: most secure with imposing physical security and intensive procedural security (searching, X-raying of bags etc)
- **Category B and C**: decreasing levels of security
- **Category D**: open prisons (mainly) for offenders coming to the end of long sentences.

Within prisons, there are designated areas including very secure units ('the block') and segregated units for vulnerable (mainly to attack from other prisoners) prisoners ('rule 45').

Function

Prisons can be:

- local
- remand
- training
- specialist.

Age

Prisons are divided by the age of their inmates:

- juvenile (under 18)
- young offenders (18–21)
- adult.

There is increasing concern about the number of older (over 50) prisoners, particularly with regard to their health, both physical and mental.

Gender

Women remain a minority (5%) but numbers have increased dramatically over the last ten years to almost 4000. The majority of women are in prison for theft, handling and drug offences, with only about 10% in custody for violent offences. There is some evidence that they have higher rates of mental disorder, including psychosis and self-harm than men.

Mental disorder in prisons

Studies looking at the prevalence of mental disorder in prison have given varying figures depending on the prison population (remand/convicted, male/female), study methodology (interview by psychiatrist or non-clinical researcher) and diagnostic criteria:

- psychosis, 2–14%
- neurosis, 6–75%
- substance dependency/misuse, 23–63%
- personality disorder, 10–78%.

One study reported that about 3% of the sentenced prisoners who were seen should have been transferred to psychiatric inpatient care.

Health care in prisons

After two centuries as a separate service, prison health care is now the responsibility of the National Health Service (NHS) and is commissioned in the same way as other health services, aiming to provide care:

- appropriate to need
- comparable to the NHS
- not disrupted by being in prison
- that minimises isolation from the rest of the prison and other health care in the community
- that uses the opportunities of prison to improve health
- that treats those who are hard to engage in the community.

Practically, the emphasis is on:

- reducing the number of prisoners in health care and the time they spend there
- increasing day-care places

- improving wing services
- more appropriate skill mix
- better integration between prison and NHS staff
- quicker transfer for seriously ill patients
- increased collaboration by NHS staff for the severely mentally ill.

Suicide in prison

One major aim of current policy is to reduce prison suicides. Numbers have tripled in the last 20 years to about 90 per year, with higher rates than in matched general population males. Most are by hanging from window bars, often with bedclothes. Those on remand are particularly at risk. All prisons have a suicide prevention strategy which generally includes:

- listeners (samaritan – trained inmates)
- anti-bullying programmes
- changes to physical environment
- staff training
- reception screening
- clear management plans for those with mental illness, substance misuse and self-harm
- periodic reviews, audits and research.

RISK ASSESSMENT AND MANAGEMENT

Risk is part of everyday clinical practice.

Risk management

Risk management plays a major role in the current emphasis on quality in the NHS and is one of the cornerstones of clinical governance. In this context, it is a means of reducing the risks of adverse events occurring in organisations by systematically identifying, assessing, reviewing and seeking ways to prevent the occurrence of adverse events. Risk management is a three-stage process:

- risk recognition
- risk assessment
- risk reduction (containment).

Risk assessment and management have always been crucial aspects of psychiatric care particularly with respect to harm of self or of others, the latter being of greater importance to forensic psychiatrists.

Clinical risk assessment and management

Awareness of potential risks is a prerequisite for a full assessment, which may be informed by the use of various risk tools. Risk assessment is primarily a clinical skill and 'the decision on risk is made when all these strands (of information) come together in what is known as clinical judgement'. Risk assessment must be accompanied by subsequent risk management. Risk should be managed within a clinical team and not by a single individual. Forensic mental health teams are multi-disciplinary and each professional provides input to the risk assessment. The team must also contain anxieties about risk.

Good risk management includes:

- thoroughness: comprehensive history taking with attention to detail and accurate recording
- multidisciplinary teams: involve all members
- interagency working: co-operation with appropriately shared information
- listening to carers/relatives.

Risk assessment scales can be used but any tool is only an aid to the assessment process and not sufficient in itself. Clinical tools include:

- **HCR-20**
  - structured clinical guide designed to assess the risk of future violence
  - checklist of 20 items considered risk factors for violent behaviour
  - includes static historical, present clinical and future risk management variables.
- **PCL-R** – the Psychopathy Checklist (PCL) and the revised version (PCL-R) serve to operationalise the construct of psychopathy.
  - There are items categorising presentation, affective state, lifestyle, personality traits.
  - Psychopathy defines an extreme personality disorder which involves ego-centred impulsive self-gratification and a callous disregard for others.
  - There is significant overlap between psychopathy and dissocial personality disorder.
  - Psychopathy is not used according to the Mental Health Act (1983) definition.
  - Psychopathy has been found in some studies to be a better predictor of violence than either psychiatric diagnosis or substance abuse.
- **MacArthur Risk Assessment Study** – this study assessed a large sample of psychiatric patients on a wide range of variables which had been previously reported as predictors of violence. Four 'domains':
  - dispositional – demographic, personality, psychopathy, cognitive
  - historical – social, psychiatric admissions, supervision compliance, offending, violence
  - contextual – stress, social support, accommodation, means of violence, availability of victim
  - clinical – symptoms, diagnosis, substance misuse, fantasies, functioning, future plans.

Major findings have highlighted the role of clinical factors such as substance misuse and psychopathy in the prediction of violence. The investigators have developed a risk assessment tool called an **Iterative Classification Tree** which aims to categorise individuals as high or low risk.

The Royal College of Psychiatrists has reviewed all the evidence and has produced a list of risk factors which are associated with violence. It has also produced more general guidelines which aim to aid the process of assessment and management.

The National Confidential Inquiry into Suicide and Homicide by People with Mental Illness

This Inquiry aims to collect detailed clinical data on people who die by suicide or commit homicide and who have been in contact with mental-health services, and to make recommendations on clinical practice and policy that will reduce the risk of suicide and homicide by people under mental health care. A list of such recommendations published in 2001 included:

- staff training in the management of risk of suicide and violence (with regular updating)
- all patients with severe mental illness and a history of self-harm or violence to receive the most intensive level of care
- individual care plans to specify action to be taken if patient is non-compliant or fails to attend
- prompt access to services for people in crisis and their families
- assertive outreach teams to prevent loss of contact with vulnerable and high-risk patients
- atypical antipsychotic medication to be available for all patients with severe mental illness who are non-compliant with 'typical' drugs because of side-effects
- strategy for those with dual diagnosis
- local arrangements for information-sharing with criminal justice agencies.

Chapter 22

Old-age Psychiatry

Nicholas Ardagh-Walter

CONTENTS

Old-age Psychiatry

DEMENTIA SYNDROMES

The word 'dementia' is used to denote either a clinical syndrome or a group of specific diseases (Alzheimer's, vascular dementia etc).

Epidemiology and projected population changes

The **prevalence** by age (from EURODEM studies) is:

- 65–69 years, 1%
- 70–74 years, 4%
- 75–79 years, 6%
- 80–84 years, 13%
- 85–89 years, 22%
- 90–94 years, 32%.

Between 1991 and 2040, UK numbers of over-60s are expected to increase from 21 to 26% of the population, with over-85s increasing by 60%. The prevalence of dementia will therefore increase markedly.

Definitions and diagnosis

The **International Classification of Diseases (ICD-10) criteria** include:

- due to disease of the brain
- usually of a chronic or progressive nature
- multiple higher cortical functions impaired, including
  - memory
  - thinking
  - orientation
  - comprehension
  - calculation
  - learning capacity
  - language
  - judgement
- consciousness is not clouded
- deterioration in emotional controls, social behaviour or motivation commonly accompany and occasionally precede the impairments of cognitive function.

Some workers suggest these criteria are excessively slanted towards Alzheimer's type dementias because other conditions, such as fronto-temporal dementia and dementia with Lewy bodies, do not fit this description well.

Behavioural and Psychotic symptoms of Dementia (BPSD) affect most cases and include delusions, hallucinations, apathy, agitation and insomnia.

Differential diagnoses

- **Depressive disorders**. Depression and anxiety can affect attention and motivation, hence their effect on functioning and cognition. Dementia often causes depression and anxiety.
- Patients with a **late-onset depressive disorder** often show mild irreversible cognitive deficits. (These may correlate with white matter changes on computed tomography (CT) or magnetic resonance imaging (MRI) scans.)
- **'Depressive Pseudo-dementia'**. A relatively rapid onset of cognitive impairment, usually with depressive symptoms and often subjective memory complaints. A family or personal history of depression is frequent. On cognitive testing they often complain of not knowing the answer rather than guessing or drawing attention away from their problems. Treatments for depression are effective but many progress to dementia within five years.
- **Delirium**. The main clinical features are identical to dementia. Distinguished on time course and overall clinical picture.

Conditions producing a dementia-like syndrome

The primary degenerative brain diseases are:

- Alzheimer's disease (60% of cases)
- dementia with Lewy bodies (10%)
- fronto-temporal dementias including Pick's disease
- progressive supranuclear palsy
- multisystem atrophy.

Other brain conditions include:

- vascular dementias (10–30%)
- tumours (primary and secondary)
- chronic subdural haematoma
- normal pressure hydrocephalus
- epilepsy
- post head injury
- multiple sclerosis.

Infective conditions include:

- neurosyphilis
- post encephalitis
- acquired immune deficiency syndrome (AIDS)
- Creuzfeldt–Jakob disease.

Toxic/metabolic include:

- hypothyroidism
- Korsakoff's syndrome

- B$_{12}$ deficiency
- hypoglycaemia
- hepatic or renal failure
- drug toxicity (eg benzodiazepines).

Other conditions which can mimic dementias are:

- depression; depressive pseudodementia
- schizophrenia
- delirium
- mild cognitive impairment (age-related cognitive decline).

General management of dementias

Management of dementias must include:

- giving a diagnosis to patient and perhaps to the carer/family member
- education
- professional support to enable adjustment to the diagnosis
- links with statutory services and self-help organisations (eg Alzheimer's Society)
- legal and financial considerations:
  - driving licensing
  - enduring power of attorney
  - making a will
  - benefits.
- assessing the carer's stress levels and needs
- setting up of services (day-care/home-care) if needed.

ALZHEIMER'S DISEASE

Alzheimer's disease is the most common cause of dementia.

Diagnosis

The diagnosis given in the fourth revision of the Diagnostic and Statistical Manual for Mental Disorders (DSM-IV) is classified as follows:

- A. Memory impairment plus one of: aphasia, apraxia, agnosia or impaired executive function
- B. Impairment in social or occupational functioning
- C. Gradual onset and decline
- D. Not due to
  - (i) other central nervous system conditions (eg cerebrovascular disease)
  - (ii) systemic conditions known to cause dementia
  - (iii) substance-induced conditions
- E. Not exclusively during a delirium
- F. Not better accounted for by another axis 1 disorder, eg depression.

Natural history

The **median survival** is six years from diagnosis.

Rate of decline on Mini Mental State Examination (Folstein – MMSE) averages 2.5 points annually in the moderate stage.

Predictors of faster decline are:

- younger age at onset
- more severe disease
- use of antipsychotic drugs
- possibly extrapyramidal features and psychosis.

Pre-dementia covers a period of up to five years preceding symptoms when there may be subtle cognitive impairments, mainly in acquiring new memory. Depressive symptoms often precede any clear cognitive decline.

In **mild disease**:

- there is impaired new learning/short-term memory
- there are mild language deficits, ie word finding; reduced vocabulary; some circumstantial speech
- dyspraxia is demonstrated on drawing tasks
- visuospatial impairment often impairs driving
- reduced motivation and depression are common
- patients can usually live in the community but may require support, and ability to carry out Activities of Daily Living may be impaired
- insight is variable between patients
- there are usually no focal neurological signs.

In **moderate disease**:

- there is marked short-term memory loss; long-term memory is often affected
- there is more severe dysphasia
- behavioural disturbance (restlessness, apathy, insomnia, frustration) emerges
- psychotic phenomena are frequent (persecutory delusions, hallucinations)
- the patient is either unable to live outside an institution or requires intensive support.

In **severe disease**:

- speech becomes minimal
- marked behavioural disturbance is common
- fleeting/changing psychotic phenomena occur
- there is incontinence
- there is motor deterioration with weight loss
- there is reduced mobility
- involuntary movements occur
- occasionally there may be seizures.

Investigations

No test gives a satisfactorily specific or sensitive finding.

- **Standard CT** shows increased cortical atrophy with enlarged ventricles and widened sulci but this is not a sensitive or specific finding.
- **Temporal lobe orientated CT and MRI** may show atrophy of the hippocampus and other medial temporal lobe structures early in the disease.
- **Single photon emission CT** (SPECT) shows temporoparietal hypoperfusion.
- **Electroencephalogram** (EEG) is usually abnormal; decreased alpha and increased theta and delta.

Aetiology

The aetiology of Alzheimer's disease is mostly unknown although its neurobiology is well-investigated.

The following are **risk factors** for Alzheimer's disease:

- increasing age (incidence may level off in extreme old age)
- family history: relative risk is 3.5 for a first-degree relative; less if onset is in very old age
- apolipoprotein E: e4 allele homozygosity carries higher risk
- Down's syndrome
- depression
- hypertension
- for a few early-onset cases: presenelin-1 and -2 and amyloid precursor protein mutations.

Others risk factors being investigated include:

- other genetic factors: ie α2–macroglobulin gene
- intelligence/education
- history of head injury (eg boxers and, possibly, footballers)
- aluminium intake
- dietary homocysteine intake
- female gender
- high alcohol consumption, although it is not clear that these cases are Alzheimer's disease.

Possible **protective factors** include:

- oestrogen therapy
- non-steroidal anti-inflammatory drugs
- antioxidant intake
- moderate alcohol consumption.

Neurobiology

Alzheimer's disease can present with any of the following signs.

- senile/neuritic plaques: amyloid core, halo of distorted neurites with associated tau
- neurofibrillary tangles: neuronal inclusions, composed of abnormal intracellular components
- both of the above are found in smaller numbers in normal ageing
- granulovacuolar degeneration
- Hirano bodies
- neuronal loss (cholinergic neurones)
- amyloid: widespread deposition
- mutations of the gene for amyloid precursor protein cause familial Alzheimer's disease
- vascular: amyloid angiopathy.

Specific management

Management of Alzheimer's disease involves the following:

- Cholinesterase inhibitors are found in mild to moderate disease (generally MMSE > 12)
- Consider memantine in moderately severe disease
- Control vascular risk factors
- Gingko biloba extract and Vitamin E are used without strong evidence.

VASCULAR DEMENTIAS

The vascular dementias are a clinically and pathologically heterogeneous group overlapping with other dementias.

Diagnosis

The NINDS-AIREN (International Work Group) diagnostic criteria are:

- 1 Dementia
- 2 Cerebrovascular disease: with clinical and CT/MRI evidence
- 3 Dementia within three months of a stroke **or** abrupt onset or stepwise course.

Clinical features are variable but include:

- abrupt onset
- stepwise deterioration
- fluctuating course
- focal neurological deficits
- history of stroke
- deficits in executive function rather than short-term memory or language
- preservation of personality
- patchy preservation of some cortical functions.

Multifocal disease presents with:

- gait disorders
- urinary incontinence
- rigidity
- bradyphrenia.

Major features are found in the Hachinski Ischaemic Score but this score does not differentiate well between vascular dementia and Alzheimer's disease.

Prognosis

Median survival from diagnosis is slightly better for vascular dementia than for Alzheimer's disease.

Investigations

Investigations used in the diagnosis of vascular dementia are:

- **CT and MRI**: multiple, bilateral, dominant hemisphere vascular pathologies, especially involving limbic system
- **SPECT**: patchy, asymmetrical lesions
- **EEG**: normal or focal abnormality.

Aetiology

This type of dementia can be caused by various vascular problems.

- Large vessel occlusion
  - thrombosis
  - artery-to-artery embolism
  - cardiac embolism
- Small vessel disease
  - lacunae
  - ischaemic white matter lesions (eg subacute arteriosclerotic encephalopathy or Binswanger's disease)
- congophilic angiopathy (cerebrovascular amyloid)
- haemodynamic factors: hypoxic encephalopathy
- haemorrhage: intracerebral or subarachnoid
- single strategic infarct, eg thalamic
- genetic, eg Cerebral Autosomal Dominant Arteriopathy with subcortical infarcts and leucoencephalopathy (CADASIL)
- conditions associated with cerebrovascular pathology:
  - subacute lupus erythematosus
  - polycythaemia rubra vera

Treatment

Treatment of vascular dementia requires:

- control of vascular risk factors
  - hypertension (NB hypotension is also undesirable)
  - smoking cessation
  - control of lipid and glucose levels
- investigation and treatment of sources of emboli where appropriate
- acetylcholinesterase inhibitors: one positive trial of galantamine has been published
- under investigation are the uses of nimodipine, memantine and gingko.

DEMENTIA WITH LEWY BODIES

This type of dementia comprises 12–20% of cases of dementia.

Consensus criteria for dementia with Lewy bodies

The consensus criteria for this type of dementia are:

- A – Progressive cognitive decline
- B – Two of the following:
  - fluctuating cognition
  - recurrent visual hallucinations
  - spontaneous parkinsonism
- C – Features supportive of diagnosis are:
  - repeated falls
  - transient loss of consciousness
  - neuroleptic sensitivity
  - systematised delusions
  - hallucinations in other modalities.

The early features of dementia with Lewy bodies are different from those of Alzheimer's disease: namely, short-term memory and language loss are less marked. There is visuospatial dysfunction and fluctuating loss of attention over a 24-hour period.

Investigations

Investigations used in the diagnosis of dementia with Lewy bodies include:

- **CT and MRI**: medial temporal lobes preserved, compared to Alzheimer's disease
- **SPECT**: differences from Alzheimer's disease are not well established but a dopamine ligand has shown nigrostriatal degeneration early in dementia with Lewy bodies
- **EEG**: diffuse slowing, with focal delta transients in temporal lobes in 50% of cases.

Neurobiology

- **Lewy bodies**: these are intracellular inclusions which stain for ubiquitin and α-synuclein in the cortex and in some brainstem nuclei. (They are also found in Parkinson's disease, but mainly in the substantia nigra; smaller numbers are found in the cortex.)
- Range of pathologies is similar to Alzheimer's disease and vascular dementia.
- Cholinergic deficit is more marked than in Alzheimer's disease.

Treatment

Treatment of this type of dementia is with:

- Acetylcholinesterase inhibitors: such as rivastigmine
- Atypical antipsychotics for delusions and hallucinations, but these carry a high risk of adverse events
- L-dopa: some benefit but delirium is not uncommon.

FRONTO-TEMPORAL DEMENTIA

This is the most common of the dementias caused by fronto-temporal lobar degeneration – variants including Pick's disease and a motor neurone disease type.

- Onset is usually between the ages of 45 and 65 years, mean duration is eight years.
- There is a family history of disease in 50% of cases.
- frequency 24–60 per 100,000
- It constitutes 12% of presenile dementias.

Main clinical features

Fronto-temporal dementia has an insidious onset and a gradual progression. **Behavioural features** include:

- an early decline in social conduct
- disinhibition, impulsivity, apathy
- perseveration
- utilisation behaviour
- hyperorality.

Affective features include:

- an early instability
- subsequent blunting and unconcern.

Other features of fronto-temporal dementia are:

- early loss of insight
- speech output becomes reduced
- memory is not consistently impaired.

Investigations

The investigative results in this type of dementia are:

- **EEG**: is usually normal
- **CT**: usually shows non-specific atrophy
- **MRI**: shows frontal atrophy
- **SPECT**: shows frontal deficits.

SEMANTIC DEMENTIA

This is a form of fronto-temporal lobar degeneration that affects the anterior temporal lobes.

- Onset is between 50 and 65 years.
- It is sporadic.

Clinically, speech is fluent and grammatically correct but relatively empty of meaning. The following are impaired:

- comprehension of the meanings of words
- object recognition
- face recognition
- behaviour (egocentricity, rituals, narrowed repertoire).

While the preserved functions are:

- recent memory
- motor skills.

OTHER DEMENTIAS

Normal pressure hydrocephalus

- This comprises 1–2% of cases of dementia
- 80% of patients are over 70 years old
- It presents with fluctuating cognitive impairment, incontinence, gait disturbance
- There are many psychiatric/behavioural features (depression, agitation, aggression, apathy and hallucinations)
- **Investigations** include:
  - ○ **CT**: periventricular hypodensities and ventricular dilatation with small sulci
  - ○ **MRI**: the above and signs relating to cerebrospinal fluid movement
  - ○ **lumbar puncture**: various procedures are used, interpretation is not straightforward
- Treatment is by shunting to divert the cerebrospinal fluid; preselection of cases is necessary.

Human immunodeficiency virus (HIV) type 1-associated dementia

- This dementia occurs in < 1% of otherwise asymptomatic cases of HIV infection, and in 7–10% of symptomatic cases. The use of antiretrovirals has reduced its prevalence.
- Widespread cognitive impairment occurs with mental slowing.
- Broad range of behavioural changes occur.
- Motor features appear (from clumsiness to paraplegia and incontinence).
- **MRI** indicates atrophy, usually ventricular, with white matter hyperintensities on T2 images.
- Cerebrospinal fluid investigation is useful to exclude secondary infections and to confirm typical HIV findings, ie pleocytosis, antibodies and range of protein markers.

Prion diseases

Prion diseases are rare. They entail spongiform vacuolation, astrocytic proliferation and neuronal loss. There is accumulation of abnormal prion protein (from gene *PRNP*).

Creutzfeldt–Jakob disease

- This can be inherited, sporadic or acquired (by transmission or iatrogenic).
- 30% of patients have prodrome (insomnia, depression, aches, weight loss).
- It is a rapidly progressive dementia, often with:
  - myoclonus
  - cerebellar ataxia
  - extrapyramidal/pyramidal signs
  - cortical blindness
  - akinetic mutism.
- Cerebrospinal fluid is generally normal (some markers are being investigated).
- **CT/MRI** scans have no diagnostic features.
- **EEG** show characteristic sharp waves in 70% of cases.
- Progresses to death in < 6 months.

Kuru

Kuru is a rare disease found in the cannibals of Papua New Guinea that is now disappearing.

Variant Creutzfeldt–Jakob disease

- This disease appeared in 1995 in young people in the UK.
- It was thought to be the result of eating infected beef.
- Age range of patients is 16–48 years.
- **Clinical features**: depression, anxiety, withdrawal, behavioural change, delusions, visual and auditory hallucinations, aggression, insomnia, emotional lability, persistent dysaesthesiae, progressive cerebellar signs, dementia, myoclonus, chorea.
- **Prognosis**: median length of time to death is 14 months.

- Investigations used for diagnosis are:
  - **CT and MRI**: normal or mild atrophy
  - **EEG**: shows generalised slow wave
  - **Tonsillar biopsy**: abnormal prion deposits are demonstrable.
- This variant is histologically distinct from Creutzfeldt–Jakob disease.
- It involves a different strain of abnormal prion protein.

Gerstmann–Sträussler syndrome (Gerstmann–Sträussler–Scheinker disease)

This is a familial disorder with chronic cerebellar ataxia and pyramidal signs leading to dementia.

Multiple system atrophy

These are uncommon disorders showing:

- symmetrical parkinsonian syndrome
- pyramidal signs
- autonomic failure
- cerebellar ataxia.

It may progress to a dementia.

Progressive supranuclear palsy (Steele–Richardson–Olsiewski syndrome)

The main features are:

- symmetrical parkinsonian syndrome
- downward and upward gaze paralysis
- truncal ataxia; early falling
- dementia.

Huntington's disease and Wilson's disease

These diseases are covered in Chapter 16.

DEPRESSIVE DISORDER IN OLD AGE

Epidemiology

- The prevalence of depressive disorders in the elderly is 5% (3–13%).
- Subsyndromal depression is more common.

- The prevalence of depressive disorder is consistent between the ages of 65 and 100 years but there is some decline in extreme old age.

Higher levels are found in:

- those who attend general practitioners, 15–20%
- care home residents, 15–20%
- general hospital inpatients, around 20%.

Presentation

Typical depressive symptoms occur but commonly there are:

- agitation
- somatic preoccupations
- endogenous features
- delusions.

The main differential diagnoses are:

- dementia (producing low mood, apathy, agitation or delusions)
- anxiety disorders
- alcohol misuse disorders
- delirium.

Drugs	beta-blockers, antipsychotics
Metabolic	anaemia, hypothyroidism, B_{12} or folate deficiency, occult carcinoma
Infective	urinary tract infection
Inflammatory	temporal arteritis
Intracranial	post stroke, post head injury, subdural haematoma, Parkinson's disease, delirium

Table 22.1 Other conditions commonly presenting with depression in the elderly

Investigations

A subgroup shows ventricular dilatation on **CT** and also periventricular and deep white matter changes on **MRI**. This group shows more cognitive impairment and has a worse response to treatment.

SPECT may show frontal and paralimbic hypoperfusion.

Prognosis

Statistics vary depending on the patient setting and, probably, treatment adequacy.

For inpatients: at two years, 60% have intermittent or continuous periods of being well but 20% develop chronic symptoms.

Risk factors

The following are risk factors for depressive disorders in the elderly:

- chronic ill health
- handicap
- social isolation (including that caused by sensory impairment)
- lack of a confidante
- family history: a weaker association for late onset than in early onset cases
- female gender; widowed/divorced
- genetic: a smaller contribution than in the young
- life events, especially those involving loss or threat of loss, bereavement
- subtle brain disease (identified on CT and MRI scans as white matter changes)
- specific medical illnesses causing depression (eg Parkinson's disease)
- being a carer (shown in carers of people with dementia).

Management

Management of these disorders involves:

- provision of education and diagnosis
- addressing of any concomitant medical illnesses
- social management where needed to reduce isolation and ensure adequate care, companionship and nutrition.
- assessment of risks, including self-neglect and suicide
- specific treatments.

Antidepressant medication is usually a mainstay of management.

- Selective serotonin reuptake inhibitors (SSRIs) are usually the first-line treatment.
- There is a risk of postural hypotension with tricyclics and monoamine oxidase inhibitors (MAOIs).
- The central anticholinergic effects of tricyclics are undesirable in case there is a subclinical dementing process, although lofepramine is frequently used.
- High doses are used less, augmentation with low-dose lithium is frequent.

Psychotherapies can also be used.

- Cognitive behavioural therapy (CBT) and interpersonal therapy are both supported by evidence.
- Individual or group therapy.
- Problem solving in primary health care.
- Focal grief work.

Electroconvulsive therapy (ECT) is the most effective treatment for severe depression, and is well tolerated in the elderly.

- Delusions, melancholy and marked agitation predict a good response.

- ECT should be considered especially where there is inadequate diet/fluid intake, suicidal risk, severe retardation or non-response to other treatments.
- Relative contraindications to ECT:
  - cerebrovascular accident or myocardial infarction within previous three months
  - cerebral or aortic aneurism
  - severe respiratory or cardiac disease
  - dementia is not a contraindication to ECT but its presence increases the risk of post-treatment delirium.

Suicide

Suicide rates in the elderly have fallen significantly in the last decade but are still higher than in other age groups.

Risk factors include:

- mental illness, usually depressive disorder
- physical illness
- male gender
- single/separated/divorced/widowed
- bereavement
- alcohol misuse
- anankastic and anxious personality traits.

Prevention strategies are similar to those needed for younger people. Fifty per cent of suicide victims contact their general practitioner in the month before the suicide, lending support to attempts to improve the general practitioner's recognition of depression, although this approach is not backed by evidence of success.

ANXIETY

Both prevalence and incidence of most anxiety disorders seem lower in old age, but there may be presentation/referral bias.

In patients over 65 the prevalence is:

- social phobia, 1%
- simple phobia, 4%
- generalised anxiety disorder, 4%
- obsessive-compulsive disorder, 0.1–0.8%
- agoraphobia, 1.4–7.9%.

Panic disorder is unusual in old age.

Anxiety is common as a symptom of dementia.

The clinical features, aetiologies and treatments vary little as compared to those used in younger adults, although some experiences, such as physical illness and bereavement, are more common in old age.

Differential diagnosis is necessary from depression and dementia (also delirium).

Treatment is as for younger patients:

- CBT is the most widely used psychological treatment.
- Tricyclics and benzodiazepines are more likely to give rise to adverse events than other drugs.

DELUSIONAL DISORDERS AND SCHIZOPHRENIA OF LATE ONSET

Terminology and classification

These are a heterogeneous group of disorders falling under various categories. 'Late paraphrenia' is not in ICD-10 or DSM-IV and there are no separate codings for late-onset disorders; in ICD-10, schizophrenia and delusional disorder are used.

Terms also in use include:

- 'late onset schizophrenia' (onset 40–59 years)
- 'very late onset schizophrenia-like psychosis' (> 60 years)
- neither are in ICD-10 or DSM.

There is debate over the continuity of the diagnosis of schizophrenia over varying ages of onset.

Epidemiology

Incidence is 17–24 per 100,000 per year; females outnumber males.

Clinical features

There are differences from young onset schizophrenia.

- Persecutory delusions predominate, although other delusions commonly arise.
- Partition delusions are common (ie delusions involving the belief that something/some person can pass through what would normally be a barrier).
- First-rank symptoms are less common.
- Affective features are common.
- Personality is better preserved, there are fewer 'negative' symptoms.
- Cognitive deficits are very mild, and progression is slow over time.

Aetiology

The aetiology can be:

- Genetic:
  - risk in first-degree relatives is reduced compared to early onset schizophrenia
  - no genetic markers have been found.

- Deafness (particularly early onset and bilateral)
- Visual impairment (associated with visual hallucinations)
- Schizoid and paranoid personalities.

Prognosis

There is a poorer response to antipsychotic treatment: 50–75% of patients have a partial or no response.

The disease is chronic unless treatment is successful and compliance is good.

Management

Given the lower success rate of antipsychotic treatment, a good therapeutic engagement becomes more important. Antipsychotic treatment requires lower doses (eg 1–2 mg per day of risperidone). Low-dose depot antipsychotics can be very successful when accepted. CBT may be used, but there is no evidence for its use in this age group.

DELIRIUM IN THE ELDERLY (see also Chapter 16)

Epidemiology

Prevalence varies depending on situation:

- in elderly medical admissions 10–16%
- in nursing homes 5–15%
- postoperative incidence is 37% (higher with hip fractures).

Differential diagnosis

Delirium must be differentiated from **dementia**. All of the main features of both conditions are shared. The time course and symptom pattern should be weighed up, bearing in mind the typically fluctuating and shorter term history of delirium.

Anxiety states and depressive disorders with apathy should also be considered.

Prognosis

If the underlying cause is addressed then some improvement is usual but of elderly general hospital patients at six months, up to 40% are still cognitively impaired.

Mortality, dependency, length of hospital stay and discharge to institutions are all more common.

Risk factors

Risk factors for delirium include:

- increasing age
- structural brain disease
- visual impairment
- pain
- polypharmacy.

There are **medicolegal considerations**. A patient incapacitated by delirium and actively objecting to treatment in a general hospital is usually best treated under common law. Although 'mental illness' is not defined by the Mental Health Act 1983, not all psychiatrists would agree that delirium falls under this category.

ALCOHOL MISUSE

Prevalence of alcohol misuse in the USA:

- community prevalence is 2–3% in males, 1% in females
- among medical inpatients the prevalence is 6–18%
- higher prevalence in males, the socially isolated, and those who are single/separated/divorced.

Presentation is with:

- falls
- drowsiness
- delirium
- depression
- poor control of co-morbid conditions, such as hypertension or diabetes.

CAGE has been validated in the elderly but gross under-detection is usual because:

- patient is less likely to disclose
- clinicians are less likely to suspect elderly than young patients
- clinicians are prone to believing it understandable: therapeutic nihilism.

Older people are more vulnerable to the effects of alcohol because higher blood levels are generated per amount consumed (because of changed body composition) and there is more psychological impairment at a given blood level.

Treatment

- **Medical**: admission is usually indicated for detoxification. Increased caution is needed with benzodiazepine use.
- **Psychological**: the same treatment approaches should be used as in the young. Some evidence exists that results are better if these are delivered within a group of similar ages.

'Alcoholic dementia' (see Chapter 23)

Whether this exists as a pure diagnosis is controversial.

- Cognitive impairment is common among chronic heavy drinkers but most of this may be the result of Korsakoff's psychosis, co-existing other forms of dementia (eg vascular), sequelae of head injuries and chronic social disorganisation.
- Evidence of cortical atrophy is seen on MRI or CT scans in 50–70% of chronic severe alcoholics. This is partially reversible on abstinence.

EARLY ONSET SEVERE MENTAL ILLNESS IN OLD AGE: 'GRADUATES'

This is a patient group who have had a long history of care by psychiatric services, often long-stay hospital patients. The main diagnostic group is those with schizophrenia.

- **Cognitive impairment**:
  - ○ 75% of hospitalised patients with schizophrenia show cognitive impairment, but whether this progresses is controversial
  - ○ outcomes are diverse, with some declining slowly into a dementia but others remaining stable.
- **Symptoms**: some studies report an improvement in old age.
- **Physical health**: very poor, patients often become frail.
  - ○ tend to be heavy smokers
  - ○ almost half suffer from urinary and/or faecal incontinence
  - ○ iatrogenic problems are common, including tardive dyskinesia, dental decay worsened by anticholinergic therapies, and consequences of weight gain and poor diet
  - ○ mortality is increased.
- **Social disabilities**: are severe, arising from the illness as well as institutionalisation.

PSYCHOPHARMACOLOGY IN OLD AGE

Changes in body function occuring with ageing.

- Absorption is altered as a result of reduced gastric acidity and a thinner gut wall (diazepam levels rise more slowly).
- Protein binding is variable (bound fraction of drugs such as diazepam is reduced).
- Fat content is increased (higher relative blood alcohol levels).
- Hepatic oxidation of drugs is reduced (blood levels of antipsychotics are increased).
- Renal excretion is reduced (raised levels of lithium and desipramine metabolites).

There is an increased frequency of adverse drug reactions because of:

- polypharmacy
- co-existent pathology

- altered pharmacodynamics
- altered pharmacokinetics.

Age-related changes in specific drug groups

Antipsychotics

Lower doses are required in the elderly because of the increased risk of adverse effects.

- anticholinergics: increased risk of delirium, constipation, urinary retention
- antiadrenergic: increased risk of postural hypotension producing falls
- dopaminergic blockade: increased risk of parkinsonian effects, tardive dyskinesia but decreased risk of acute dyskinesia and oculogyric crises
- histaminergic: probable increased risk of sedation.

Antidepressants

Lower doses are required and responses to treatment are slower: 6–8 weeks are therefore needed for adequate trial of treatment.

Tricyclics	SSRIs	MAOIs	Other
• increased plasma levels	• few cardiovascular effects	• moclobemide has few cardiovascular effects and is supported by trials in the elderly	• Venlafaxine: little dose adjustment required for age
• anticholinergic/ antiadrenergic as antipsychotics	• no anticholinergic effects, so chosen for Alzheimer's		
• older tricyclics seldom used as first line because of side-effect profile	• better tolerated than tricyclics	• non-selective MAOIs cause significant postural hypotension/ sedation and lower doses are needed	

Table 22.2 Effect of antidepressants in old age

Mood stabilisers

- **Lithium**: doses are halved; initiate with caution because of renal function, usually at 200–400 mg daily. Generally well tolerated, although non-toxic side-effects (polydipsia, polyuria, tremor) are common.
- **Carbamazepine**: increased risk of delirium and falls.
- **Valproate**: commonly used for aggression in dementia; risk of sedation and falls.
- **Benzodiazepines**: increased risk of falls, memory loss and delirium.

Anti-dementia drugs

The cholinesterase inhibitors (donepezil, rivastigmine, galantamine) have UK licences for use in mild to moderate Alzheimer's disease:

- they correct cortical cholinergic deficits
- randomised controlled trials demonstrate their benefit in dementia with Lewy bodies and vascular dementia
- cautions in asthma, active peptic ulceration, cardiac conduction disorders and prostatism
- onset of action is 4–6 weeks.
- adherence should be considered before prescribing.

Trials indicate a modest improvement or stabilisation of cognitive function. Only a few trials extend as far as two years. Other domains, such as BPSD, are often more important than cognition.

Memantine enhances glutaminergic transmission and is licensed for moderately severe dementia.

PSYCHOTHERAPIES IN OLD AGE

Freud thought that people beyond late middle age could not use psychoanalysis. Reasons given have included mental rigidity and an insufficient life expectancy to benefit but this view has changed in the last 20–30 years. Older people often reflect well and their aware-ness of a finite life span can improve motivation. The amounts of formal psychotherapy given to older people in the National Health Service (NHS) are very small, for historical and societal reasons.

There are few additional contraindications in the elderly, but cognitive impairment suffi-cient to hinder learning and integration is a contraindication for some therapies such as individual psychodynamic therapy and CBT – although systemic family therapy is used for patients with dementia. Common practical problems to be overcome include transport, a suitable setting and hearing loss.

Dynamic psychotherapy

This usually involves one session per week from six weeks (eg focused grief work) to 18 months.

Indications are similar to those for younger people, namely:

- recurrent interpersonal problems
- neurotic symptoms (CBT/medication more often used)
- to promote personal integration/maturation
- secondary prevention after mental illness.

Common problems are found in psychotherapy.

- Several different 'generational' transferences are possible (eg parental).

465

- Older clients may place demands/needs onto the therapist that younger therapists find difficult.
- Common issues include losses and threats of losses.
- Aims of therapy include containment of anxiety, processing of past traumas, renegotiation of past stages of life (Erikson, 1966: seven stages of man) and integration of life story (Erikson's last stage: integrity versus despair).
- Story-telling is especially important for aiding integration and the generation of meaning. This is an argument for Reminiscence Therapy.

Cognitive behavioural therapy (CBT)

Usually used for depressive and anxiety disorders, there is substantial evidence supporting its use.

- CBT is not normally used as sole treatment for severe depression.
- Applied in individual or group settings: some practitioners believe the latter is more effective in this age group.
- Memory and ability to comprehend the therapy are needed but mild memory disturbance and inability to read and write are relative, not absolute, barriers (audio tapes can be used instead of paper recording).
- Adequate introduction, preparation and setting of expectations are required (especially if not well accultured to psychological therapies).
- May need more help in staying focused on the therapy model.
- Shorter sessions if concentration is limited.
- Scheduling of activities demands appreciation of real physical limitations.

Interpersonal therapy

Interpersonal therapy is well suited to the elderly. It was developed for use in depression but is used in a broad range of other situations.

Identifies four common themes in depression, all of which are common in old age:

- grief (eg bereavements)
- role transition (eg retirement, onset of dependency because of ill health)
- role dispute (eg changing roles within marriage)
- interpersonal deficits (recurrent interpersonal problems): may re-emerge as options become restricted.

Cognitive analytic therapy

This therapy needs little or no adaptation for the elderly.

It can be used for depression or anxiety but is more used for recurrent personality problems, eg borderline or narcissistic traits. These may re-emerge in old age, and memories of early traumatic experiences can reappear. Therapy for long established patterns of behaviour and thinking/feeling (ie personality) can often be successful but large, rapid shifts are not the norm.

This therapy may be used for professional and family carers of people with dementia, to provide a framework in difficult cases and to help avoid or dispel 'malignant social processes'.

Systemic therapy

Treats people by treating the systems within which they live, usually involving the family, but others such as neighbours or even care-home staff can be involved.

Most family therapy teams use an eclectic mix of approaches but there are several major approaches:

- structural
- strategic
- Milan systemic
- solution-focused
- social constructionist.

Applicable to the elderly, even when the index patient is significantly demented. Systemic therapy has a good track record although the number of services in the UK is small. In this age group, the family is usually a powerful influence and older people occupy a variety of roles – not just dependence.

Occasionally, slower pace, shorter sessions or summarising at intervals are needed if cognition is mildly impaired, but usually little adaptation is needed.

Often used as one, single session.

Common themes are:

- changes of role; dependence, illness, care
- conflicts and patterns from early adult life re-emerge in old age
- the older person's capacity to choose and to have responsibility for his or her actions.

Cognitive and behavioural learning strategies in dementia

Used for specific problem behaviours and for more general maintenance of function. Before planning therapy it is helpful to assess the strengths and weaknesses: a cognitive profile.

Reducing cognitive load by:

- reducing the length and complexity of speech to the patient
- supporting the meaning using visual cues
- reducing distractions.

Usually used as a strategy to improve or maintain general functioning, reduce stress and enable participation in pleasurable activities.

Techniques directed at a specific behaviour can be:

- Use of cues and prompts. Often the patient will need training to use these. A favoured technique is cued recall of behaviour with fading cues (ie the patient is reminded of the desired behaviour with decreasing frequency).

- Stimulus control methods: (use of the environment to modify behaviour) eg operant conditioning.
- Modifications required for cognitively impaired subjects.
  - assess and take account of cognitive strengths and weaknesses
  - work on small number (usually one) of learning tasks at a time
  - learning may be slow and incomplete – ie a problem behaviour is usually reduced in frequency but is not abolished.

Reminiscence and other therapies, eg music, multi-sensory rooms, exercise classes for patients with dementia, have been generally thought to enable patients to undertake pleasurable and stimulating activities, improving/maintaining function and wellbeing, and reducing problem behaviours.

MAINTAINING AGEING PEOPLE IN THE COMMUNITY

A major aim of services in the UK in recent decades has been to:

- comply with most people's wishes
- reduce overall dependence on services
- increase quality of life and participation in the community
- reduce long-term care costs.

Agencies involved:

- **Primary care**: general practitioners, nurses, occasionally practice counsellors
- **Specialist mental health services**: CMHTs and Day Hospitals to provide mental health assessment and treatment and some social care (social environments, home assistance etc)
- **Social services**: varying levels of integration with the primary- and secondary-health services (day care, help with tasks in the home).
- **Voluntary agencies** provide sitting services, 'befriending' schemes, home care, self-help groups, advice, information and advocacy.

Person-centred care

- an influential approach to dementia care was founded by Tom Kitwood
- based on establishing humane and healthy social/philosophical stance
- key concept is 'malignant social process' which can magnify the biological effects of dementia
- '**Dementia Care Mapping**' is the standardised audit process of an institution's practice.

LEGAL AND ETHICAL ISSUES

Capacity (competence), consent to medical treatment, testamentary capacity, Court of Protection, Enduring Power of Attorney are covered in Chapter 10.

Issues around admission and incapacity

In **the Bournewood case** the House of Lords overturned the decision of the Court of Appeal and effectively ruled that an incapacitated patient need not necessarily be detained under the Mental Health Act if he or she is not actively objecting to hospital admission. It is, however, good practice actively to discuss such situations with patients and relatives and the Act is sometimes used, as it provides statutory safeguards to the patient.

For delirious patients in general hospitals, use of common law rather than the Mental Health Act is generally recommended.

Guardianship Orders (Mental Health Act, section 7) state that the guardian (usually the local authority or a relative) is empowered to:

- require the patient to reside at a specified place (eg nursing home)
- require the patient to attend for medical treatment, etc
- require access to the patient by a professional or other person.

There is no power to convey the patient to a place of residence, which can cause problems if the patient is not compliant.

Driving

The DVLA requires notification when a driver has a diagnosis of dementia but relatively mild cognitive impairment is not a bar to driving. Older drivers, broadly, have good safety records, and may compensate for cognitive deficits by, for example, not driving at night. When a doctor has concerns about the safety of an older driver in most cases the older driver can be persuaded at least to have their driving assessed; this is done at assessment centres, the most reliable measure being an on-road test. General Medical Council guidance where a patient refuses to notify the DVLA, and more detailed guidance, are covered in Chapter 10.

Advocacy

Advocacy may enable old people to assert their own wishes when dependent on families, carers, professionals and caring institutions.

Living wills (advance directives)

Although guidance exists in case law, the obligation of health professionals to follow them has not been properly tested. In general, the more serious the decision being taken, the greater the degree of mental capacity should be demonstrated by the patient.

Elder abuse

This has only been widely acknowledged in the past 20 years.

ICD-10 categories include:

- neglect or abandonment
- physical abuse
- sexual abuse
- psychological abuse.

Financial abuse may arise in relation to a misuse of an Enduring Power of Attorney. Although abuse may be a criminal problem, approaching it as a complex social problem is often more fruitful. Incidents are rarely isolated. A cycle of maladaptive behaviour may operate in which difficult behaviour by a dependent person triggers abusive acts which increase distress, perpetuating the cycle. Carers often lack knowledge of available means of support.

Abuse may occur in care homes and hospitals where poorly trained carers commonly endure high rates of assault and abuse by residents.

Interventions include:

- continued monitoring
- organising home care, day care and respite to provide relief for the carer
- psychotherapeutic work (marital therapy, individual therapy, family therapy)
- management of physical and psychiatric illnesses
- legal approaches
- multi-agency co-ordination.

ORGANISATIONAL ISSUES

Interface with other services

Primary care

Education and training of workers will enable appropriate management within primary care or referral of others (eg early referral of suspected dementia). Community psychiatric nurses may be attached to groups of practices, telephone consultations can be facilitated etc.

Medicine for the elderly

There are **consultation services**, in which specific patients are referred from one service to another for advice, and **liaison services**, which have mental-health workers based in the general hospital, working with/alongside the medical team. The latter should provide multidisciplinary team resources. There should be joint wards for patients with mental and physical health needs.

Social Services

Closer working can be promoted through:

- joint Trusts incorporating the necessary parts of both organisations
- joint NHS and Social Services community teams
- pooled budgets.

Consequences of inadequate organisational arrangements include poor communication and perverse incentives. Social Services charges for some provisions but NHS services are free.

Housing

Planning is needed for appropriate provision for their elderly client groups. Innovative ventures are possible only with commitment from specialist services to provide ongoing support, eg regular visiting from a community psychiatric nurse to a housing scheme.

Voluntary organisations

These can provide a range of services: information, written and verbal, support groups, advocacy services and, at a national level, support for research and representation to policy makers. The Alzheimer's Society provides resources for patients with dementia and their carers. Some organisations are providers of care.

Respite and continuing care

Long-term institutional care is funded by the NHS only for particular groups of patients, mainly those fulfilling locally agreed criteria relating to the degree of ongoing specialist management needed. The provision of this care varies. Ideally, long-stay NHS beds allow the concentration of resources on a difficult-to-manage group of patients, but some districts provide through private-sector care-home beds.

The Community Care Act (1993), requires care-home places, funded by the local authority, to be provided for as long as necessary. The provision is predominantly in private-sector care homes and is means-tested. Respite care is similarly organised.

Chapter 23

Substance Misuse (Addiction) Psychiatry

Karen J Williams

CONTENTS

Substance Misuse (Addiction) Psychiatry

DIAGNOSTIC CATEGORIES

Substance misuse is categorised in the International Classification of Diseases (ICD-10), by the type of substance(s):

- alcohol
- opioids
- cocaine
- other stimulants
- cannabinoids.

and the associated disorder:

- acute intoxication
- harmful use
- dependence
- withdrawal states
- psychosis
- behavioural disorders.

It is very important to clarify whether there is dependence or not. Dependence syndrome is a collection of symptoms, three or more of which should have been present in the preceding year, namely:

- strong desire or sense of compulsion to use the substance
- difficulties controlling substance-using behaviour
- physiological withdrawal state on ceasing or reducing the substance, or use of substance to alleviate withdrawal
- evidence of tolerance
- progressive neglect of alternative activities/interests
- persistent use, despite clearly negative consequences.

Dependence can be upon one drug or a class of drugs. Dependence is well described for alcohol, opioids, benzodiazepines and to a lesser degree for cocaine, amphetamine and cannabis, but not LSD or other hallucinogens. Use of a number of substances is very common.

Dual diagnosis

Probably more accurately described as co-morbidity, this is a common feature in both patients presenting with a primary substance-use disorder and those being seen for other mental health issues.

Studies of psychiatric patients have found that 29% experienced substance-misuse disorder at some stage, with one-third of those with affective disorder having co-morbid substance misuse and rates for co-morbid substance use and psychotic disorder being 20–65%.

In addiction populations the prevalence of mental ill health is approximately 40%, with anxiety and affective disorders as the most common diagnoses and co-morbid antisocial personality disorders in approximately 15%. It is widely accepted that many patients with substance-misuse disorder have personality traits of impulsivity and novelty seeking and undoubtedly some patients present as unhappy, non-conformist and aggressive. However, it is often difficult to separate cause from effect of the substance use and premature labelling of patients as having a personality disorder is not recommended.

EPIDEMIOLOGY

Drug and alcohol use

- Fewer females are affected than males.
- Fewer older people than younger ones.
- There is a correlation with deprivation.
- Most of a population's alcohol is consumed by a small number of heavy drinkers.
- The prevalence of drug and alcohol use is increasing.
- There is high prevalence of use in prison populations.

Dependence (Office of National Statistics figures, 2002)

- **Cannabis**: 4.6% male, 1.6% female
- **Stimulants**: 1.7% male, 0.7% female
- **Opiates**: 0.2% male, 0.1% female
- **Alcohol**: 10% male, 3% female.

Hospital population (St. Georges, 2003)

- 23% are smokers
- 14% have alcohol misuse
- 12% have drug misuse
- Many have poly-substance use
- Many cases being missed.

AETIOLOGY

Genetics

- Low alcohol use in Asians with variant of alcohol dehydrogenase.
- Alcohol dependence: region on chromosome 4 confers protection and on 1 and 7 confers susceptibility.
- Adoption studies of alcohol dependence in the male line.
- Recent studies show inheritability of drug dependence, but not usage.

Sociology

- There are links between certain occupations and alcohol.
- Family use of alcohol/drugs has an effect.

There is less evidence for drug use, but effective ways of reducing alcohol consumption in a population include:

- raising prices/taxation
- restricting availability
- minimum age for purchase
- reducing alcohol levels for driving
- sobriety check points.

Cultural aspects

- Different drinking styles exist in different countries, eg north vs south Europeans.
- There is reduced prevalence for misuse of certain substances in certain religions.
- Ethnic minorities are under-represented in treatment populations. Possible causes include poorly developed stimulant services and predominantly White staff and patients.

Females

- Use and misuse are less prevalent in females.
- Females are under-represented in treatment populations, particularly the more structured and intensive treatments, eg inpatient or residential rehabilitation.
- Possible causes include the preponderance of male patients and staff in treatment settings, or reluctance to access treatment because of concerns about child-care/social service issues.

Behavioural and social learning theories of addiction

- Substance-use disorders occur because of the interacting influences of environment and learning processes with the individual's own temperament/biological makeup. Less emphasis is on the genetics.

477

- Environment, particularly peer pressure and parental behaviour, is thought to influence initiation into substance use.
- **Modelling**, **operant conditioning** (reinforcement) and **cognitive mediators** (expectation, thoughts, feelings, self-efficacy) are thought to be important in the early stages of substance use. Personal factors, such as failure to develop alternative coping strategies, or having a thrill-seeking or impulsive personality, may help maintain the substance use.
- With more chronic use, **classical conditioning** comes in to play with the development of conditioned craving and conditioned withdrawal responses in situations where the substance is used.
- In severe dependence the main behavioural drive is to avoid withdrawal symptoms (negative reinforcement), but continued failure of coping strategies, association with peers who are substance users, together with more stereotypical patterns of use are also important factors.

Neurobiological theories

- Alcohol potentiates γ-aminobutyric acid (GABA). Chronic alcohol exposure leads to reduced NMDA (N-methyl-D-aspartate) and glutamate function, and alcohol withdrawal leads to their increase.
- Pleasure and reinforcement are mediated through the mesolimbic dopamine system, which is stimulated in all substance misuse (except benzodiazepines). Dopamine is also important in anticipation and withdrawal.
- GABA is the target for benzodiazepines and γ-hydroxybutyrate.
- The μ opiate receptor is key in opiate addiction, κ stimulation may cause dysphoria and the δ receptor is implicated in reinforcement.

ALCOHOL HISTORY AND EXAMINATION

Recommended screening tests

- AUDIT (Alcohol Use Disorder Identification Test) has very high specificity and sensitivity and is useful in non-specialist settings.
- CAGE: is fast but not as reliable.
- MAST (Michigan Alcohol Screening Test).
- TWEAK (in pregnancy).

Taking an alcohol history

- Start by eliciting the current drinking type, pattern and quantities. Ask the patient to describe a typical day's or week's drinking and to quantify the drinking into units of alcohol.
- The percentage of alcohol gives you the number of units in a litre, eg 1 litre of 40% spirit is 40 units, and a 75 centilitre bottle of 40% spirit contains 30 units.

- Particular attention should be given to early morning drinking, the presence of withdrawal symptoms, drinking to control withdrawal symptoms and craving.

Alcohol withdrawal symptoms and alcohol-related problems are described in Tables 23.1 and 23.2.

	Features and associated conditions	Onset after stopping or reducing alcohol
Common	Nausea, vomiting, hypertension, tremor, sweating, anxiety	6–8 hours
Withdrawal fits	Hypoglycaemia, hypomagnesia, hyponatraemia	48–96 hours
Delirium tremens	Delirium, misperceptions, visual hallucinations, paranoid delusions, fear	48–72 hours

Table 23.1 Alcohol withdrawal symptoms

Alcohol-related problems	Examples
Physical	Black-outs, fits, peripheral neuropathy, gastritis, liver disease
Socio-economic	Job loss, financial and housing problems
Social	Relationship and family problems
Forensic	Drinking and driving, drunk and disorderly, violence
Psychological	Anxiety, depression, sleep disorders

Table 23.2 Alcohol-related problems

- Remember to take a history of when alcohol drinking began and when problems and/or dependence began. Also gather information on previous treatment and help seeking.
- Gauge the attitude of the patient to their drinking by eliciting their own beliefs about the positive and negative aspects of their drinking.

Mental state examination

An examination of the patient's mental state should investigate:

- withdrawal symptoms, intoxication
- mood disorders, suicidal ideation
- psychosis (alcoholic hallucinosis, delirium tremens)
- signs of delirium (delirium tremens, Wernicke's syndrome)

- cognitive function: specific memory disorder in Korsakoff syndrome; global intellectual deterioration in dementia.

Physical examination

A physical examination of the patient should investigate:

- signs of liver disease
- cardiovascular complications: hypertension, cardiomyopathy
- central nervous system signs, exclude space-occupying lesions and elicit specific neurological syndromes such as those of Wernicke and Korsakoff.

Investigations

The following investigations should be performed:

- mean corpuscular volume
- γ-glutamyl transferase
- urea and electrolytes
- liver function test
- glucose
- blood alcohol/breath alcohol can easily be measured, this may help with determining dependence and tolerance, as well as assessing compliance.

COMPLICATIONS OF ALCOHOL MISUSE

Wernicke–Korsakoff syndrome

- Caused by thiamine (Vitamin B$_1$) deficiency.
- Many alcohol patients are thiamine deficient because of diet and reduced absorption in the presence of alcohol.
- Alcohol withdrawal causes further thiamine depletion.

Wernicke syndrome

Features of the syndrome are:

- ophthalmoplegia with nystagmus on lateral gaze
- ataxia with wide-based gait
- acute delirium.

It should be noted that this 'Classic Triad' is only seen in a minority of patients with significant thiamine deficiency.

There should be a high index of suspicion for all cases with neurological signs, especially those with unexplained hypoglycaemia/hypothermia.

Pathology shows symmetrical changes in:

- third ventricle
- floor of fourth ventricle
- periaqueductal system
- central thalamic nuclei
- mamillary bodies
- the brainstem
- the cerebellum
- terminal portions of the fornices.

Treatment is with high dose parenteral B vitamins, six hourly for three days.

Korsakoff's psychosis

This is not a psychosis but a chronic memory disorder. Classically, but not always, it is preceded by Wernicke's encephalopathy.

Features of Korsakoff's psychosis are:

- recent memory loss, but unimpaired working memory
- disorientation in time and place
- confabulation
- personality changes, eg apathy and lack of insight.

Pathology of Korsakoff's psychosis shows:

- variety of sub-cortical lesions and cortical atrophy
- impaired frontal cortical blood flow.

Treatment (although the psychosis is largely irreversible) involves:

- psychological help with memory training and aids
- anticholinesterase inhibitors may be of some use.

Alcoholic dementia

This type of dementia is probably caused by the neurotoxic effects of alcohol.

The following functions are impaired:

- short- and long-term memory
- visuospatial organisation
- maintenance of cognitive set and impulse control
- visuo-perceptual abstraction.

Pathology of alcoholic dementia:

- cortical shrinkage, especially the frontal lobe
- mild ventricular enlargement
- may be reversible with abstinence
- may affect psychological therapy and prognosis.

Alcoholic hallucinosis

- This usually has an acute onset in the absence of impaired consciousness.
- It can last several months.
- Other causes must be excluded.
- Neuroleptics may help.

MANAGEMENT OF ALCOHOL WITHDRAWAL

Aims

The aims when managing alcohol withdrawal are:

- To eliminate serious alcohol withdrawal symptoms (fits and delirium tremens) in dependent individuals
- prevent Wernicke–Korsakoff's syndrome
- reduce mild withdrawal symptoms.

Setting

Most patients can be detoxified in the community. Preferably with community psychiatric nursing support and monitoring.

People with previous serious complications on alcohol withdrawal (eg fits and delirium tremens), those in unsuitable living accommodation and those with poor physical and/or nutritional status should be detoxified, if possible, in hospital.

Medical/nursing management

- A reducing regime over seven days of Chlordiazepoxide or Diazepam. Oxazepam is the prefered benzodiazepine in severe liver disease.
- Parenteral vitamins, ie Pabrinex, should be given.
- Carbamazepine may be used to prevent fits and/or control withdrawal symptoms.
- Fluids, glucose, urea and electrolytes, and mental state should be monitored.
- Provide good nursing care and monitoring of withdrawal symptoms with titration of doses as necessary.

Complications

Delirium tremens is a medical emergency which carries a significant mortality. Treatment should include:

- increasing the dose of benzodiazepine, maximum 200 mg chlordiazepoxide per day
- full Pabrinex treatment as for Wernicke–Korsakoff syndrome
- use of neuroleptics with care

- monitor fluid, glucose and electrolytes
- exclude other cause for delirium
- appropriate nursing care as for patients with delirium
- use of Mental Health Act may need to be considered.

If **alcohol withdrawal fits** appear:

- exclude other causes
- monitor urea and electrolytes and glucose
- use medication to treat the fits.

MEDICATION IN THE PREVENTION OF RELAPSE

- **Disulfiram** (Antabuse): an aversive medication which causes unpleasant and potentially harmful effects when taken with alcohol. Its effects last for seven days and its use should be supervised, often this is by a family member.
- **Acamprosate**: GABA analogue, it is an anti-craving drug, can improve abstinence and reduce the length and severity of binges. Very safe and few contraindications.
- **Naltrexone**: may reduce the euphoria associated with drinking by blocking the opioids and increasing aversive effects, eg nausea. Safe and with few side-effects except for patients on opioids.
- Underlying psychiatric illness should be treated.

PSYCHOLOGICAL THERAPIES USED IN ADDICTION

Most research has been performed on alcohol patients eg project MATCH which found the twelve-step approach, cognitive behavioural therapy and motivational interviewing equally efficacious.

Motivational interviewing

This therapy uses the Prochaska and di Clemente 'stages of change model' of addiction. The stages are:

- precontemplation
- contemplation
- preparation
- action
- maintenance.

The patient may move around the stages many times before they achieve maintenance. Motivational interviewing works with the ambivalence inherent in addiction and targets appropriate therapy for each stage. It incorporates many features of client-centred counselling, with therapist and patient working together on the problem, by using open-ended questions and reflective listening.

In non-specialist areas brief motivational enhancement using FRAMES has been successful, ie:

- **F**eedback
- **R**esponsibility
- **A**dvice
- **M**enu (for change)
- **E**mpathy
- (enhancing) **S**elf-efficacy.

Cognitive behavioural therapy

Cognitive behavioural therapy addresses drink as the underlying problem. It can be used with or without associated techniques, eg social skills, problem solving.

Twelve-step approach

- This is used in Alcoholics Anonymous, Narcotics Anonymous, the support groups for affected family members, Al-anon (alcohol) and Families Anonymous (drugs), and in the Minnesota model rehabilitation centres.
- 'Twelve-steps' encapsulates the basic philosophy of the disease model of addiction.
- Abstinence from substance misuse is the goal.
- Alcoholics Anonymous was founded in the USA by two alcoholics, it is now world-wide, although more established and widely used in the USA. It is a free service, consisting of open and closed meetings, also sponsors are allocated for individual support.

Relapse prevention techniques

This therapy includes identification of high-risk situations (eg certain places/situations), emotional changes and/or interpersonal stress that put the individual at risk of relapse. Having identified these factors the therapist and patient work on developing coping and planning strategies to reduce the risk. They also use techniques to prevent a lapse becoming a full-blown relapse into dependence.

Marital and family therapy

This addresses the relationship problems arising from or maintaining the problem. Behavioural marital therapy improves couple communication and problem-solving techniques and reduces relapse.

Psychodynamic psychotherapy and counselling

These may be beneficial for the many patients with underlying psychological issues such as child abuse, bereavement and post-traumatic stress disorder.

Group work

Group work is used in addiction centres in inpatient, outpatient and day-patient settings. Many have a psycho-educational and cognitive behavioural therapy approach.

Residential rehabilitation

- Private or charity-run establishments.
- Usually take patients following detoxification.
- Safe environment for therapies and for learning of new skills.
- Approaches may be 12-step, Christian, practical.
- Rural and urban.
- Single sex/mixed settings.
- Usually alcohol and drug clients.
- Self-funded or by social services.

DRUG MISUSE

Screening tests

- Schedules for assessment in neuropsychiatry (SCAN).
- Composite international diagnostic interview (CIDI).
- Alcohol use disorders and associated disabilities interview schedule-alcohol/drug revised (AUDADIS-ADR).

All are reliable for screening for alcohol and drug dependence but are less reliable for harmful use and abuse.

Taking a drug history

When taking a drug history the following points should be covered:

- Ascertain amount in money (£), weight (g) and bags of all substances used, including alcohol and over-the-counter medicines. (If these are not the same each day record usage over a week.)
- Confirm dependence by asking about withdrawal symptoms, tolerance and craving.
- Ask about route of administration: intravenous, intramuscular, oral, smoked, inhaled or 'chased'.
- If an intravenous user, ask about sites of injection, sharing needles and equipment, complications associated with injection, eg abscess, deep vein thromboses, sub acute bacterial endocarditis.
- If smoked or inhaled, ask about lung symptoms.
- Ask about human immunodeficiency virus (HIV) and hepatitis testing, and any immunisation.

- Ask about drug-related problems with work, family, the law and finances.
- Ask about previous seeking of help or treatment.
- Ask about previous overdoses.
- Find out what they want to do about the problem.

Physical examination

A physical examination should investigate:

- signs of injecting
- complications of injecting (abscess, deep vein thrombosis)
- cardiovascular and respiratory system
- signs of acute hepatitis
- pupil size.

Mental state

When investigating the mental state look for:

- state of alertness
- stereotypies and other movement disorders (stimulants)
- affective/anxiety disorder
- co-morbid psychiatric illness.

Investigations

- Urine dip-stick testing is routinely used, often on an observed sample. This will detect use in the last 3–5 days, except for cannabis and benzodiazepines where the window of detection is longer.
- Saliva testing is currently being developed.
- Blood testing for liver function and, with consent, for HIV, and hepatitis viruses B and C.

OPIATES/OPIOIDS

These users are less prevalent in the general population, but are the most prevalent patients in drug treatment services. They use:

- heroin (aka Brown, smack, H, horse, gear)
- morphine
- codeine and dihydrocodeine
- codeine-based cough mixtures are sometimes misused
- over-the-counter opioid/paracetamol combinations are often abused. A particular concern here is inadvertent paracetamol poisoning.

Treatment aims for opiate dependence

- Stabilise the patient on a pharmacologically pure, legal, substitute.
- Significantly reduce and, if possible, eliminate illicit drug use and the associated health, legal, financial and social problems.
- Engage in treatment to look at underlying or co-morbid problems with physical, psychological or social functioning.
- Treat and screen for high-risk conditions, eg hepatitis.
- Reduce health risks by immunisation (against hepatitis B virus) and health education.
- Many patients will need relatively long periods in treatment (two years or more).
- Maintenance doses should be adequate to minimise any additional illicit use.
- Detoxification should not be considered lightly because of the reduced opiate tolerance and consequent risk of overdose following detoxification.

Opiate withdrawal syndrome

- This is mainly caused by 'noradrenergic storm' on opiate withdrawal.
- Onset is around time of next due dose in opiate-dependent individuals.
- It comprises flu-like symptoms; aches and pains, feeling cold and shivery, pilo-erection, nausea, vomiting, diarrhoea, dysphoria, irritability, craving, dilated pupils.
- Sleep disturbance can last for several weeks post detoxification, other symptoms remit in days.
- It is not dangerous but it is unpleasant.

Drugs used in opiate dependence

Methadone

This is the most commonly used substitute for stabilisation programmes.

- It is a long-acting synthetic opioid.
- Usually given by oral route but intramuscular or intravenous administration may be used for chronic non-responders to oral treatment.
- Duration of action is 24–30 hours.
- Started at a safe dose < 40 ml daily and dose is titrated upwards.
- Stabilisation dose is usually 50–100 ml daily.
- Given at supervised consumption clinics at treatment centres or via community pharmacies for first 3–6 months of treatment, to reduce leakage onto the streets, and to enable adequate doses to be reached early in treatment.
- Safe in pregnancy.

Subutex (Buprenorphine)

- It is a partial opiate agonist.
- At high doses it blocks other opiates.
- It has less overdose potential.
- It has less severe withdrawal symptoms.

- Safety in pregnancy is not tested.
- It can be used in substitute prescribing or detoxification.
- Consumption must be supervised in a clinic initially.

Lofexidine

- This is used in opiate detoxification.
- It is an α2 agonist.
- It is not addictive.
- It blocks noradrenaline release and treats most withdrawal symptoms.
- Side-effects include dry mouth and nose and postural hypotension.

Non-steroidal anti-inflammatory drugs

- These are used in withdrawal for hyperalgesia, aches and pains.
- They are contraindicated in pregnancy, allergy and some asthmatics.
- Care should be taken in gastrointestinal disorders.

Benzodiazepines/sedatives

- These can be a useful adjunct in acute opiate withdrawal.
- Their use should only be short-term, because of the risk of dependence.
- Caution should be exercised when used in conjunction with other sedative medication.

Buscopan/loperamide

- Anti-spasmodics/anti-diarrhoeal treatment may be useful.
- Loperamide, although an opiate, does not cross the blood–brain barrier.

Naltrexone

- This is an opiate blocker.
- It is usually used after detoxification and after a naloxone challenge.
- Duration of action is 72 hours when given orally.
- Observed consumption improves success rates.
- It blocks opiates or may provoke withdrawal in the presence of opiates.
- It can be used in pregnancy if the benefits outweigh the risks.
- Side-effects are generally mild and self-limiting, eg headache, gastrointestinal symptoms.
- Liver function tests should be monitored.

STIMULANTS

The following are 'stimulants':

- crack (cocaine base)
- cocaine hydrochloride (coke, Charlie, C)

- amphetamines (speed, whiz)
- ecstasy (MDMA), has stimulant and hallucinogenic properties.

The compounds listed above:

- stimulate the reuptake of central amines, amphetamines also provoke their release
- produce a less specific withdrawal syndrome
- produce psychological craving that is very marked and powerfully reinforced
- may be used in binges over several days interspersed with days of abstinance rather than daily.

Complications

- Intravenous use (cocaine and amphetamine) carries the risk of blood-borne viruses, clots, abscesses.
- Intranasal use (cocaine) can cause damage to the nasal septum.
- Crack use can cause respiratory conditions, eg crack lung and pulmonary oedema.
- Other complications are:
  - hypertension
  - cardiac arrhythmias and myocardial infarction
  - acute paranoia
  - depression
  - longer term psychotic states.
- They are not safe in pregnancy.
- Hyper-pyrexia can occur in Ecstasy use.

Management

Management of stimulant use involves:

- assessment and treatment of co-morbid psychiatric symptoms/other substance misuse
- cognitive behavioural therapy, psycho-education about drug effects, relapse prevention
- drug diaries, self-monitoring and urinalysis
- addressing of housing/social/financial issues
- family interventions
- symptomatic treatment of insomnia and depression (no evidence for medication otherwise)
- ear acupuncture
- Dexamphetamine sulphate replacement is used for heavy long-term intravenous amphetamine users. Replacement is short-term with regular psychiatric and physical reviews.
- Cocaine replacement therapy is not used.

BENZODIAZEPINES

Signs of intoxication

The following are signs of intoxication:

- drowsiness
- ataxia
- slurred speech
- blurred vision
- paradoxical excitement.

Withdrawal symptoms

- Dependence can occur after three weeks continuous use.
- Withdrawal symptoms can occur 1–3 weeks after reducing/stopping.
- They are not inevitable.
- They include: tremor, insomnia, tinnitus, visual disturbance and weight change.

Principles of management of benzodiazepine dependence

- Assessment should be made of underlying mental health issues/other substance use and motivation as before.
- Convert to a long-acting benzodiazepine.
- Short-term use should be reduced to zero over six weeks.
- For long-term usage, reduce the dose by 1/8th every two weeks.
- Treat insomnia and anxiety.

OTHER SUBSTANCES

Cannabis

- This is the most widely illegally used drug.
- It is smoked or taken orally.
- It impairs reaction times.
- It can cause anxiety, paranoia and insomnia.
- It is an important prognostic factor in schizophrenia.
- Physical complications from smoking are as for cigarettes.

Hallucinogens

- These include: LSD, magic mushrooms, etc.
- There is no physical dependence.
- Acute anxiety and long-term flashbacks can be problematic.

Solvents

- These include: petrol, toluene, butane, glues and aerosol propellants.
- They can be inhaled directly from the container, or poured onto cloth or into bags.
- Complications include confusion, ataxia, cardiac arrest, and they are hepato-toxic.
- There is no dependence.

Tobacco

- Tobacco is a commonly used substance.
- It produces both physical and psychological dependence.
- It has well-documented effects on physical health.
- Its use is more prevalent in deprived populations, eg the homeless, prisoners and the long-term mentally ill.
- Treatment with nicotine replacement patches, inhalers, gums and bupropion with support and education, are generally delivered in primary care.

PSYCHOSEXUAL ISSUES

- Alcohol use stimulates sexual desire.
- Alcohol is associated with unplanned pregnancies and sexual dysfunction.
- Opiates inhibit sexual desire and may cause impotence.
- Heroin inhibits follicle-stimulating hormone and luteinising hormone and may lead to menstrual cycle disturbances and reduced, but not absent, fertility.
- Most female heroin addicts do not work in the sex industry.

Substance misuse and parenting

- Substance misuse in pregnancy is managed by good protocols, liaison and close working between the substance-misuse and obstetric services.
- A significant number of people presenting for substance misuse have children.
- Not all substance misusers are bad parents.
- An assessment of parenting would include how much the children are involved in the substance using lifestyle (scoring drugs, dealing) and the extent to which they witness the substance use.
- Children of problem drinkers are mostly well adjusted. They may experience adjustment problems around adolescence. They are more likely to be early starters of substance use but are also more likely to be abstainers or light drinkers.
- The more relevant risks for such children are linked to marital and domestic violence.

GENERAL MEDICINE ISSUES

Hepatitis B virus, hepatitis C virus and HIV

- These are all blood-borne viruses.
- They are transmitted by sharing needles and other injecting equipment, via unsafe sex and by vertical transmission to babies.
- Hepatitis C prevalence is 40–60% of intravenous drug users.
- HIV prevalence is less than 1% for intravenous drug users, (slightly more for those in London and Edinburgh).
- Hepatitis B and C virus infection may lead to carrier states and to chronic active hepatitis, also to an increased risk of heptocellular carcinoma.
- Both passive and active immunisation is available for hepatitis B.
- Prevention programmes include needle and syringe exchange schemes, education on the risks of sharing equipment and the active immunisation of high-risk groups.

Important drug interactions

- Cannabis is an enzyme inductor and reduces serum levels of atypical antipsychotics.
- Enzyme inductors, eg rifampicin and HIV medication, will lower methadone.
- Antipsychotics will reduce the effects of substances of abuse through dopamine blockade, this may result in increased substance misuse.
- Antidepressants may increase plasma levels of methadone.
- Alcohol often renders psychiatric medication ineffective, older antidepressants will further impair psychomotor retardation.
- Smoking reduces the levels of antipsychotics.

Pain management

- Opiate-dependent individuals may need additional analgesia when in acute pain.
- Use non-opiate medication wherever possible.
- Opioid/opiate medication should be avoided if possible in patients on methadone, subutex and naltrexone. Where necessary potent opiates can be used but weak opiates are best avoided.
- Opioid withdrawal states lead to hyperalgesia.

TREATMENT SERVICES

- There has been recent investment in drugs services, particularly in the criminal justice arena.
- Treatment is overseen by the National Treatment Agency.
- Government policy is in four main areas: treatment, safer communities, availability and young people.

- Local services work together to provide a variety of treatment and harm reduction interventions.
- Statutory National Health Service substance-misuse teams provide medical and nursing treatment and specialist counselling. Most of the work is community based. Some services have specialist wards for detoxification and stabilisation.
- Non-statutory drug and alcohol teams offer more open access provision, needle-exchange schemes, advice and support to families, counselling.
- A multi-agency/professional service for under 18-year-olds.
- Larger cities may have specific services for crack users, with more open access and services which provide outreach to hard-to-reach patients, eg those in the sex industry.
- Shared care with general practitioners.
- Arrest referral schemes.
- A criminal justice team who treat patients on Drug Treatment and Testing Orders.
- Liaison between services and prisons, for aftercare on release. Prisons have their own counselling and advice services 'CARATs'.
- Liaison with general hospitals and for the management of pregnant drug/alcohol users.
- Co-working and consultation for dual diagnosis cases.
- Access to structured day programme, residential rehabilitation, re-integration, training and education opportunities.
- Dual diagnosis services are being developed. Treatment is to be delivered through the general psychiatric services with substance-misuse services inputting for training and consultation.

LEGAL ASPECTS

Prescription

- The Misuse of Drugs Regulations 2001 define who may possess and supply such drugs. Drugs are classified in Schedules 1–5.
- The misuse of Drugs Act 1971 prohibits the supply and possession of certain drugs which are classified to class A, B, or C depending on their dangerousness.
- Special licences are required for prescribing heroin, dipipanone and cocaine for addicts.
- All medical practitioners can prescribe other drugs to addicts.
- Schedule 2 and 3 drugs must be prescribed, in own handwriting, stating the form and strength, and the total quantity of the prescription should be written in words and figures.

Substance misuse and the Mental Health Act (1983)

- There is no provision for treatment purely for substance misuse.
- Substance misuse does not preclude use of the Mental Health Act where other conditions apply.

Chapter 24

Social and Rehabilitation Psychiatry

Rob Macpherson

CONTENTS

Social and Rehabilitation Psychiatry

DEFINITIONS

Rehabilitation is defined as 'Promoting an optimal level of social adaptation both by therapeutic interventions aimed at maximising the individual's social function and by providing appropriately supportive environments' (Shepherd, 1991); the individual is helped to their best adaptation, but not necessarily through re-settlement. Rehabilitation moves away from illness/treatment paradigms. In rehabilitation, symptoms are distinguished from functioning, and interventions are focused on the latter.

WHO (1980) give the following definitions:

- **Disability** is the loss of functional ability consequent upon an impairment.
- **Handicap** is the social disadvantage consequent upon disability.
- **Impairment** is any loss or abnormality of function.

New Long Stay Patient (Mann & Cree, 1978): inpatients 1–5 years who cannot be discharged because of challenging behaviour. These are associated with multiple impairments, social disadvantage and poor occupational skills. Lelliot found high levels of new long-stay patients still within the psychiatric hospital system in the 1990s: mean prevalence was 15–20 per 100,000.

Normalisation (Wolfensberger, 1983) is a concept developed in LD services. Social messages affect the individual. Disadvantaged groups (SMI) need to have access to high-status social activities to normalise and avoid ghettoisation. Individuals should be thought of as 'people' first, and schizophrenic/patients second. Links to recovery model (Rethink); encouragement of a positive attitude and philosophy, even when working with chronically disabled individuals.

HISTORY OF REHABILITATION

Policy background

- **Pre-18th century**: 'Pauper lunatics' were cared for by families, begging or in workhouse. A few institutions existed for the insane poor, including Bethlem Royal Hospital, London.
- **1774 Mad Houses Act**: encouraged treatment and allowed for inspection of asylums.
- **19th century**: moral treatment appeared with higher staff to patient ratios, inmates were encouraged to develop social skills. Role of superintendent was key factor in care.

497

- **1879 Mental Aftercare Association** was founded, providing homes for discharged patients.
- **1930 Mental Treatment Act** allowed voluntary admission, encouraged aftercare and outpatient services.
- **1959 Mental Health Act** sanctioned a medical approach, formal admission was taken out of the legal arena. Informal admissions were the norm.
- **1962 NHS Hospital Plan** started the hospital closure programme, promoted development of the DGH acute unit.
- **De-Institutionalisation** began in the 1950s. Between 1960 and 1985 there was a 50% reduction in beds in UK mental hospitals. The first large hospitals closed in the 1980s. This was associated with the introduction of antipsychotics and with improved attitudes to the mentally ill.

- Two key papers:

  - Goffman (1968) on **Institutionalisation**. This articulated the potentially negative and dehumanising aspects of incarceration in any institution (prison or mental asylum).
  - Wing & Brown (1970) carried out the '**Three Hospitals Study**'. This demonstrated the adverse effect of poor social environment on negative symptoms. Enriched social settings, with increased meaningful activity, led to improvements.

- **1975 White Paper** 'Better Services for the Mentally Ill'. Minimal progress in community provision, psychiatric hospitals dealing with a high turnover with no immediate prospect of abolition. Local authorities provided 28% of minimum requirement.
- **1981 Care in the Community Act** passed responsibility for residential care from the regional to the local health authority.
- **1990 NHS & Community Care Act** enabled/encouraged non-statutory agencies to operate residential care.
- **1996 Spectrum of care** promoted the provision of a range of supported accommodation for people with mental health problems in each district.
- **1999 National Service Framework for Mental Health** set out a framework for service provision targeting those with severe mental illness, including a range of supported accommodation provision. Services are organised through the Care Programme Approach, based on thorough needs assessment.
- **2001 Supporting People** created a single locality budget for residential care, enables clearer assessment of need, sufficient funding is ring-fenced.

Studies of the hospital closure programme

Team for the assessment of psychiatric services (TAPS, Leff) studied the closure of Friern Hospital (Barnet north London), re-provided to a range of community placements with the aid of a 'dowry' of finances ring-fenced for each patient.

Patients moved from long-stay wards to (one year later) independent living 12%; hostels 49%; staffed group homes 6% and unstaffed group homes 4%. Fifteen per cent remained in inpatient provision.

Resettled patients had improved social networks, lower negative symptoms and expressed higher satisfaction with their living situation. Total costs were slightly higher following community re-provision. Very few patients were lost to follow-up.

Studies in other settings (Borge *et al.*, 1999) have shown that patients can be largely successfully discharged from asylums to less dependent and more 'normal' environments.

Although carefully planned and managed re-provision has demonstrated success, concerns in many areas remain, about the lack of supported accommodation and 24-hr nursed care (Holloway, 1998)

REHABILITATION ASSESSMENT

Assessment for rehabilitation is time-consuming, complex and multifaceted.

There are five key components (Wing & Morris, 1981) and assessment must ideally be carried out in the setting where treatment will be given.

- Assess the severity of physical and mental disability.
- Assess talents and interests.
- Develop short- and long-term objectives, establish plans to achieve these.
- Seek appropriate professional/voluntary/family help to achieve the objectives.
- Monitor regularly and modify plans accordingly.

Assessment is a gradual accumulation of information and not a single administration of a test. Potential is determined by trying out new approaches and evaluating the outcome. Persistence is key – relapse and failure to engage should be expected and should not lead to discharge.

Crucially, this is a multidisciplinary approach, key tasks relate to specific staff groups.

- Symptoms/relapse indicators: psychiatrist/nurse.
- Behavioural analysis of problems: psychologists, occupational therapist, nurse.
- Living skills: occupational therapist.
- Occupational skills: work assessment, occupational therapist.
- Social skills/relationships: all.

PSYCHOSOCIAL FACTORS AND SCHIZOPHRENIA

Models

- **Stress-diathesis model of schizophrenia** (Birchwood) states that the individual has a diathesis (genes and/or perinatal trauma) towards schizophrenia which becomes manifest when under stress (mainly psychological and social).
- **Life Events model:** Brown & Burly found greater levels of independent life events in weeks before relapse among schizophrenic patients, compared with controls.

- **Expressed emotion model** is a concept developed by Vaughan & Leff (1974). Its components are critical comments, over-involvement, warmth, positive remarks; it is rated on the Camberwell Family Inventory (score of six critical comments or three out of five on over-involvement indicates high expressed emotion).

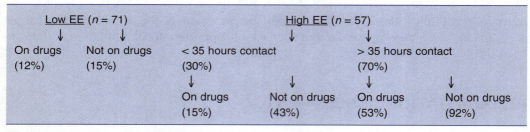

Figure 24.1 Relapse rates of 128 schizophrenics over 9 months.

High Expressed Emotion Carers report more subjective burden of caring and less perceived effective coping. They use avoidance as a coping strategy more.

Professional Carers: one-third of therapists of patients with acute schizophrenia rated high expressed emotion attitudes towards them. Coping styles in staff are important; good factors include setting limits effectively, coping with slow speed of change, ability to be warm about some aspect of a patient (Kuipers).

Poorer outcome and poorer quality of life are associated with high expressed emotion/Critical staff.

Supported accommodation

Maslow's hierarchy (see Figure 24.2) places shelter and physiological needs at the base of a pyramid.

The UK Department of Health 'Spectrum of Care' (1996) states that in every UK district, SMI patients should have access to: independent, normal housing; unstaffed group homes; adult placement schemes; residential care schemes; psychiatric nursing homes; 24-hr nursed National Health Service accommodation; open and secure inpatient beds.

- Provision is, in fact, patchy and variable. It depends on historical pattern of re-provision and de-institutionalisation.
- Group homes (several patients share a home, with regular input from social services/psychiatric team) are increasingly unpopular.
- In the last 10 years, core and cluster, or supported flats have become increasingly popular. Patients prefer the privacy and security, and feel more 'normal'.

'Supporting people' initiative (2002) co-ordinates and ring-fences funding for supported accommodation in each locality, allowing potentially allowing greater awareness of unmet need in the locality.

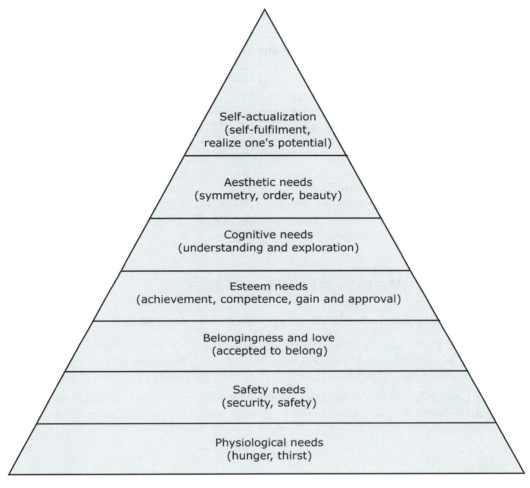

Figure 24.2 Maslow's hierarchy

Twenty-four-hour nursed care

Also termed hospital hostels/wards in the community these are the most researched aspect of supported accommodation. Three pioneering units: 111 Denmark Hill (Maudsley), Cranbury Terrace (Southampton) and Douglas House (Manchester).

RATING SCALES USED IN REHABILITATION SERVICES

- **Scale for the assessment of negative and positive symptoms (SANS & SAPS)**
  - Training is required.
  - Generally reliability is high, weighted towards rating of social functioning.
- **Global assessment scale** (GAS, Endicott *et al.*, 1976).
  - A global rating, with anchor points and a 1–100 score; rates overall clinical status, decreased scores associated with re-hospitalisation.
- **Health of the Nation outcome scale** (Wing *et al.*, 1996).
  - Promoted by the Department of Health, widely used; it has 12 domains and five-point ratings with clear anchor points. It is of limited sensitivity.
- **Camberwell Assessment of Need**
  - Twenty social/health domains. Need (problem area): score can be absent (0), met by services (1) or unmet (2). Also available in a short form (**CANSAS**). It may be used to help care planning.

ATTITUDES TOWARDS MENTAL ILLNESS

Attitudes can be broken up into three components – affective, cognitive and behavioural.

Negative public attitudes to mental illness are widespread (Bhuagra). Rated by 'Star Case Vignettes': show reluctance to be seen by a psychiatrist. Mental hospital may still be seen as a prison. Males are more likely to object to the development of a local hostel.

Need for both public and local education, including clinical settings, to dispel myths and give realistic views of what can be done. Repeated consistent education is needed to change attitudes.

FURTHER READING

Brenner, H. & Boeker, W. 2001. *The treatment of schizophrenia – status and emerging trends*. Kirkland: Hogrere and Huber.

Department of Health – 1991. *Residential needs for severely disabled psychiatric patients: The case for hospital hostels*. London: Department of Health.

—— 1998. *Partnerships in action – new opportunities for joint working between health and social services. A discussion document*. London: HMSO.

Mann, S. A. & Cree, W. 1976. '"New" long stay psychiatric patients: A national sample survey of 15 mental hospitals in England and Wales 1972/3.' *Psychological Medicines*, 6, 603.

Mueser, K. T. & Tarrier, N. 1998. *Social functioning and schizophrenia*. New York: Allyn Bacon.

Shepherd, G. 1998. 'System failure? The problems of reductions in long stay beds in the UK.' *Epidemiology and social functioning*, 7, 127–134.

Thornicroft, G. & Strathdee. 1996. *Commissioning mental health services*. London: HMSO.

Watts, F. N. & Bennett, D. H. 1991. *Theory and practice of psychiatric rehabilitation*. John Wiley & Sons.

Wing, J. K. & Brown 1976. *Institutionalism and schizophrenia*. Cambridge University Press.

Wing, J. K. & Morris, B. 1981. *Handbook of psychiatric rehabilitation practice*. Oxford University Press.

Wykes, T., Tarrier, N. & Lewis, S. 1999. *Outcome and innovation in psychological treatment of schizophrenia*. John Wiley & Sons.

Chapter 25

Psychotherapy

Andrew Clark

CONTENTS

Psychotherapy

PSYCHOLOGICAL DEVELOPMENT THROUGH THE LIFE CYCLE

There are a number of models of thinking about psychological development across the life cycle. These include:

- Freud's stages of psychosexual development
- Erikson's stages of psychosocial development
- attachment theory.

These stages are best thought of as 'developmental lines' which may be re-activated throughout life at times of stress.

Freud's stages of psychosexual development

Freud suggested that psychological development takes place in a series of developmental stages which correspond to the physical stages of children's development. He observed that the child is most aroused or excited by different parts of its body at different developmental times and that this in part shapes the way the child makes sense of the world. He believed that a child could get stuck or fixated at one of these stages resulting in the development of certain pathological character traits.

- **Oral stage** (0–1 year)
  - Child's preferred mode of relating to the world is through its mouth.
  - Pleasure is from sucking and tasting.
  - Fixation at this stage → excessive dependency/greediness.
- **Anal stage** (1–3 years)
  - Child learns sphincter control.
  - Learns to crawl and walk.
  - Fixation at this stage → anxieties about control and obsessional behaviour.
- **Genital stage** (3–5 years)
  - Child becomes aware of his or her own and other people's gender.
  - Child becomes aware of his or her genitals, which become a source of pleasure.
  - Child becomes aware of parents' relationship and may feel excluded from this.
  - Child may develop feelings of rivalry towards the parent of the same gender (Oedipus complex).
  - Fixation at this stage → histrionic traits.
- **Latency** (6 years to puberty)
  - Psychosexual development is relatively quiescent.
- **Puberty and adolescence**
  - Reworking of issues from genital stage in context of emerging adult sexuality.

Erikson's stages of psychosocial development

Erikson's developmental model highlights the main issues that an individual grapples with at different phases of his or her life. These are listed below in Table 25.1 alongside the associated favourable outcome if things go well.

Trust vs mistrust (0–1 year)	Trust and sense of security
Autonomy vs self-doubt (1–2 years)	Self-control and self-efficacy
Initiative vs guilt (3–5 years)	Confidence in own ability to act
Competence vs inferiority (6–12 years)	Competence in social and intellectual skills
Identity vs confusion (adolescence)	Development of self-identity
Intimacy vs isolation	Commitment to others, career etc
Generativity vs stagnation	Concern beyond self to family, society, future
Integrity vs despair	Sense of satisfaction and completion

Table 25.1 Erikson's stages of psychosocial development

Attachment theory

This theory was developed by John Bowlby to describe an individual's lifelong innate need for human relationships. Without this an infant would not survive. Attachment behaviour is defined as any form of behaviour that results in a person attaining or retaining proximity to some other differentiated and preferred individual. Attachment behaviour emerges as follows:

- early weeks: infant predisposed to seek proximity to others
- 3rd month: attachment remains indiscriminate and transient
- 6th month: preferred attachment figure(s) established (monotropy)
- 1 year: attachment pattern established, fear of strangers, secure base effect, separation protest
- 3 years: substitute attachment figures accepted
- later childhood: attachment patterns remain relatively stable.

Effect of severe deprivation

Work has been carried out on non-human primates showing that severe deprivation has a profound effect on the immature nervous system. Infant monkeys who are separated from their mother from birth to six months, have lower levels of central nervous system noradrenaline and thinning of the dendritic branches in the cortex and cerebellum compared with mother-reared monkeys. The deprived monkeys develop post-synaptic hypersensitivity leading to an over-reaction to stress. While parallels with human infant development need to be made with caution, it is plausible to assume that early environmental deprivation will have a significant effect on the developing infant brain and mind.

Attachment patterns/Internal working models

During the first two years of life, the infant develops neurally encoded mental representations or internal working models of itself in relation to others and associated affects. These inform the growing infant's expectations and experience of relationships with others, what Bowlby called attachment patterns.

At one year of age an infant's attachment pattern can be measured experimentally using the 'Strange situation', a carefully choreographed sequence of separations and reunion with preferred attachment figure developed by Mary Ainsworth. Observation of the infant's response to separation and reunion has enabled researchers to differentiate four types of attachment patterns:

- **Secure**
  - ○ not distressed by separation
  - ○ greets parent on reunion
  - ○ continues with contented play.
- **Insecure–avoidant**
  - ○ not visibly distressed by separation
  - ○ ignores mother on reunion
  - ○ inhibited play.
- **Insecure–ambivalent**
  - ○ highly distressed by separation
  - ○ alternate between anger and clinging on reunion
  - ○ inhibited play.
- **Insecure–disorganised**
  - ○ distressed by separation
  - ○ freezing and stereotype movements on reunion
  - ○ inhibited play.

In Europe and USA, the proportion of 1-year-old infants showing the different attachment styles are:

- secure, 60%
- insecure–avoidant, 20%
- insecure–ambivalent, 15%
- insecure–disorganised, 5%.

Prospective studies have shown that

- mothers of secure infants are responsive to their babies
- mothers of insecure–avoidant infants are unresponsive
- mothers of insecure–ambivalent infants are inconsistently responsive.

Prospective studies have shown that the attachment patterns identified in the 1-year-old are relatively stable. By contrast to children rated as insecurely attached at one year, those rated as securely attached are more socially resilient at six years of age and more able to tell a coherent story of their life at 10 years of age.

Adult attachment interview

Mary Main developed the Adult Attachment Interview to assess an adult's attachment status. The interviews are rated by an independent assessor and the interviewee is assigned to one of four categories which correspond to the four infant attachment categories described above.

- **Autonomous–secure**: open, coherent account of secure childhood
- **Dismissing–detached**: brief, incomplete accounts of idealised childhood
- **Preoccupied–entangled**: inconsistent, rambling account of over-involvement in last conflicts
- **Unresolved–disorganised**: victims of major childhood trauma.

A number of independent studies have shown a 70–80% correlation between parental attachment status on the Adult Attachment Interview and the attachment status of their 1-year-old children.

Loss

Loss of attachment figures in childhood or adulthood, whether by separation or bereavement, leads to a well-recognised sequence of emotional responses.

- **Phase I**: shock and protest – includes numbness, disbelief and acute dysphoria.
- **Phase II**: preoccupation – includes yearning, searching and anger.
- **Phase III**: disorganisation – includes despair and acceptance of loss.
- **Phase IV**: resolution.

Progression through these phases of grief is influenced by one's attachment style. Insecure attachment styles are often associated with pathological grief reactions as follows.

- **Insecure–avoidant**
  - **inhibited grief**: absence of expected grief symptoms at any stage
  - **delayed grief**: avoidance of painful symptoms within two weeks of loss.
- **Insecure–ambivalent**:
  - **chronic grief**: continued significant grief-related symptoms six months after loss.

MODELS OF PSYCHOTHERAPY

Psychotherapy may be defined as a form of treatment based on the systematic use of a relationship between therapist(s) and patient(s) – as opposed to pharmacological or social methods – to produce changes in cognition, feelings and behaviour.

All models of psychotherapy share some common features as follows:

- confiding relationship
- explanation of patient's distress
- offer of a different perspective on patient's problems
- instillation of hope
- facilitate emotional expression.

Research indicates that the single biggest predictor of effective outcome to a course of psychotherapy is the quality of the therapeutic alliance between patient and therapist.

COGNITIVE BEHAVIOUR THERAPY

Development of cognitive behaviour therapy

Cognitive behaviour therapy (CBT) is an integration of behaviour therapy based on learning theory and cognitive therapy developed by Aaron Beck.

Behaviour therapy is based on the theoretical view that neurotic symptoms are examples of maladaptive behaviour based on faulty learning. These learnt behaviours develop as a result of classical or operant conditioning.

Classical conditioning (Pavlov) refers to the pairing of an unconditioned stimulus (eg food) with a conditioned stimulus (eg bell) to produce a conditioned response (eg salivation).

Operant conditioning refers to the alteration of behaviour through the presentation or omission of rewarding or punitive consequences.

Wolpe developed a technique of systematic desensitisation for the treatment of phobias. The patient is taught deep muscle relaxation and then invited to imagine feared situations or stimuli arranged in a hierarchy of increasing anxiety. Marks developed the technique further by graded exposure to the feared object in vivo. Rachmann developed exposure and response prevention as a means of treating obsessional rituals.

Cognitive therapy was developed by Aaron Beck initially for the treatment of depression. Its application has since been extended to the treatment of anxiety disorders, personality disorders and psychosis. The model gives primacy to the way we think about ourselves and our world and that feelings and behaviour follow from this. The cognitive model of depression is as follows:

Early experience → dysfunctional assumptions → negative automatic thoughts → depressive symptoms.

The use of CBT in psychosis is an area of growing interest. This treatment approach draws on two theoretical strands.

- **Stress–vulnerability model**. This approach focuses on:
  o enhancing coping strategies, eg distraction techniques for managing auditory hallucinations
  o identifying and modifying the psychosocial precipitating and maintaining factors for the psychotic symptoms, eg family interventions to modify hostile highly expressed emotion.
- **Cognitive therapy approach**. This focuses on encouraging the individual to weigh the evidence that contradicts the delusions and/or hallucinations.

Practice of CBT

Aims of CBT:

- to help the patient identify thought patterns and behaviour-maintaining symptoms
- to help the patient modify thought patterns and behaviour to relieve symptoms
- to give the patient tools to treat their own problems.

Key elements of CBT:

- collaborative therapeutic alliance
- structured and directive approach
- problem orientated
- process of questioning and 'guided discovery'
- use of inductive methods (patient learns to view thoughts and beliefs as hypotheses that can be tested)
- education
- homework assignments
- exposure to feared stimuli.

Suitability for CBT

The following factors increase the likelihood that someone will benefit from CBT:

- ability to form collaborative alliance
- acceptance of cognitive model
- ease of access to thoughts and feelings
- motivation to change.

Concurrent heavy alcohol or drug use will hinder CBT unless the drug use is addressed first.

Indications for CBT

- mood disorders
- anxiety disorders, especially phobias, panic disorder
- obsessive-compulsive disorders
- eating disorders, especially bulimia nervosa
- post-traumatic stress disorder
- personality disorders
- schizophrenia.

PSYCHODYNAMIC PSYCHOTHERAPY

Development of psychodynamic psychotherapy

Sigmund Freud

Freud's model of the mind went through a number of revisions.

- **Affect–trauma model**: trauma → unbearable affect → neurotic symptom. His early interest in hypnosis and development of psychoanalysis was aimed at 'releasing' the unbearable affect leading to a cure of the neurotic symptom.
- **Topographical model**:
  ○ **Unconscious** consists of feelings, thoughts and memories which have been actively repressed
  ○ **Preconscious** consists of feelings, thoughts and memories not in conscious awareness but that are easily brought to mind
  ○ **Conscious** consists of feelings, thoughts and memories in conscious awareness.

In dream life, unconscious wishes (latent dream content) may be converted into manifest dream content through 'dream work' which includes:

- ○ condensation
- ○ displacement
- ○ formation of images
- ○ secondary revision.

Freud developed the idea of two types of thinking governed by quite different rules:

- ○ **Primary process thinking**: typical of dreaming, fantasy and infantile life; no awareness of time or logic; the pleasure principle dominates
- ○ **Secondary process thinking**: laws of time, space and logic apply; reality principle dominates.

This model was also underpinned by his **instinct theory** which proposed that our behaviour and development are influenced by powerful innate drives (eg sexual and aggressive), which seek expression and gratification.

The **structural model** is as follows:

- **Superego** is the internalised parental and social norms, values and ideals (part conscious and part unconscious). It is particularly involved in experience of guilt, perfectionism and preoccupation with what is right or wrong.
- **Ego** is the rationally thinking part of the mind which strives to balance the demands of the superego, id and external reality.
- **Id** covers the largely unconscious primitive instinctual drives.

$$
\text{External reality} \rightarrow \begin{array}{c} \text{Superego} \\ \downarrow \\ \text{Ego} \\ \uparrow \\ \text{Id} \end{array} \rightarrow \begin{array}{l} \text{Compromise} \\ \text{or} \\ \text{Symptom formation} \end{array}
$$

To cope with these competing demands, Freud suggested that the ego develops defence mechanisms which were subsequently described in detail by his daughter Anna Freud. Splitting and projective identification were described by Melanie Klein.

Defence mechanisms

The main features of defence mechanisms are as follows:

- they can be healthy and adaptive as well as pathological
- they are usually unconscious
- they can be classified into primitive, neurotic or mature
- different defence mechanisms are associated with different pathological states.

Primitive defence mechanisms are features of psychosis and severe personality disorder.

- **Splitting**: division of self and other into 'good' and 'bad'.
- **Projection**: attribution of unwanted feelings to others.
- **Projective identification**: putting unwanted feeling into another with such pressure that the other is forced to experience this feeling for themselves.
- **Idealisation/denigration**: overvaluing/devaluing the other.
- **Denial**: repudiation of external reality.

Neurotic defence mechanisms are seen in mood, anxiety, somatoform and obsessive-compulsive disorders.

- **Repression**: the pushing back of unacceptable wishes from consciousness.
- **Regression**: reverting to an earlier mode of functioning.
- **Reaction formation**: emphasising feelings that are the opposite to one's actual wishes.
- **Displacement**: redirecting feelings for one person on to another, eg turning angry feelings against self.
- **Isolation**: separating idea/memory from its associated affect.
- **Rationalisation**: offering logical and believable explanations for irrational behaviour.
- **Intellectualisation**: using abstract thinking to avoid experiencing painful feeling.

Mature defence mechanisms allow partial expression of underlying wishes in a socially acceptable way.

- **Sublimation**: channelling feeling in modified form to find expression in socially acceptable manner.
- **Humour**: use of amusing comment to express difficult feeling, eg anger or sadness.

Transference

Transference is derived from the Latin words *fere* (carry) and *trans* (over). Freud first used the term in 1895 to describe the patient's feelings towards the analyst. Although he initially thought that these feelings obstructed the progress of analysis, he subsequently realised that transference is the means by which the patient brings the unconscious conflicts underpinning his neurosis into the live relationship with the therapist 'the transference neurosis'. Through the patient's free associations and dreams, the analyst interprets the unconscious conflicts and transference to bring insight and change.

Nowadays the concept of transference is used to describe how an individual transfers onto his therapist or others, attitudes and feelings that he used to experience towards important figures earlier in life.

Countertransference

Like transference, Freud initially regarded countertransference, the analyst's feelings towards the patient, as a hindrance to analysis and a sign that the analyst needed further help. Nowadays, following the work of Heimann and Winnicott, the term counter-transference is used to describe those thoughts and feelings experienced by the therapist which are relevant to the patient's internal world and which may be used by the therapist to understand the meaning of the patient's communications.

Melanie Klein

Klein believed that infants are born with an innate destructive drive. She described two basic 'positions' of mental life which arise out of different ways of dealing with these destructive impulses.

- **Paranoid–schizoid position**: hostile feelings are split off from loving feelings and projected into another who is experienced as persecutory
  - dominates mental life for the first few months of an infant's life
  - characteristic mode of functioning in psychosis and severe personality disorder.
- **Depressive position**: hostile feelings and loving feelings are felt towards the same person resulting in experience of guilt and desire for reparation
  - dominates mental life from second half of first year onwards
  - characteristic mode of functioning in depression.

Object relations theory

The major proponents of object relations theory were Fairbairn, Winnicott and Balint.

Key points were:

- the desire to seek a relationship with others is a primary motivational drive
- internal world is made up of internalised relationships
- emphasis on environmental rather than innate influences on development.

Winnicott went on to develop specific concepts, listed in Table 25.2 below.

Transitional object	an object, eg a security blanket, that may be used to represent the other, eg mother, when she is not present
Good-enough mother	a mother (caregiver) who is sufficiently responsive to allow the infant to be spontaneous and creative
True/false self	a compliant false self develops if the infant feels its world is overly intruded upon by the needs of its carer(s)

Table 25.2 Object relations theory

Carl Jung

Jung developed a body of theory known as **analytical psychology**.

Key points are:

- **Collective unconscious** refers to humanity's shared reservoir of symbols and ideas
- **Archetype** describes the innate ideas about human existence
- **Individuation** is the process whereby an individual achieves integration of the different aspects of his or her personality.

Wilfred Bion

Bion was particularly interested in how individuals develop a capacity for thinking.

Key points are:

- **Container**: an infant's capacity to think develops through the experience of having anxiety and distress soothed and thought about (contained) by the caregiver.
- **Alpha function** the conversion of raw sensory experiences (which Bion called beta elements) to meaningful sensory impressions (alpha elements) which can be stored in memory and used as a basis for thought.

The practice of psychodynamic psychotherapy

Psychodynamic psychotherapy refers to a spectrum of treatments of varying intensity and length.

Psychoanalysis	↔	Long term dynamic psychotherapy	↔	Brief dynamic psychotherapy
4–5 times per week		1–2 times per week		once a week
several years		> 1 year		< 1 year

Aims of psychodynamic psychotherapy

- To provide the patient with an experience of being carefully attended to and thought about.
- To enable the patient to gain as full an understanding as possible of the conscious and unconscious factors underpinning their problems.
- To enable the patient to exercise more informed choice over how they lead their lives.

Key elements of psychodynamic psychotherapy

- **Setting**:
  - consistency of timing and length of session (usually 50 minutes)
  - consistency of venue.
- **Therapeutic attitude**: attentive, receptive and reflective.
- **Interventions**:
  - listening to and psychologically 'holding' patient's distress
  - clarification of patient's experience
  - appropriate confrontation of issues which are being avoided
  - interpretation of patient's feelings or behaviour.

Suitability for psychodynamic psychotherapy

The following are important factors in assessing a patient's capacity to benefit from psychodynamic psychotherapy:

- recognition of problem as psychological
- some sense of responsibility for life situation
- curiosity or psychological mindedness
- capacity to relate to another
- capacity to tolerate a certain degree of emotional distress (ego strength)
- motivation and staying power.

The following patients are less likely to benefit from psychodynamic psychotherapy. Those with:

- current abuse of drugs or alcohol
- repeated impulsive acts of violence towards self or others (may benefit from psychotherapy in specialist unit such as day service or residential setting)
- severe organic brain disease
- acute psychotic illness.

Indications for psychodynamic psychotherapy

The following are indications for psychodynamic therapy:

- adjustment disorders
- mood disorders
- anxiety disorders
- personality disorders
- post-traumatic stress disorder.

GROUP PSYCHOTHERAPY

Development of group psychotherapy

There are three broad therapeutic approaches to groups:

- psychotherapy **in** the group
- psychotherapy **of** the group
- psychotherapy **through** the group.

Psychotherapy in the group

This refers to the delivery of an individually based model of psychotherapy, such as cognitive behavioural or psychodynamic, in a group setting. Examples include:

- anxiety management groups
- social skills groups
- art therapy groups.

Psychotherapy of the group

This refers to an approach in which the group, eg a dysfunctional team, is treated as 'the patient'. One of the main proponents of this approach was Wilfred Bion. He suggested that a group operates in two distinct modes.

- **Work group**: the group addresses its task.
- **Basic assumption group**: the group functions on the basis of assumptions that obstruct the group's task. These assumptions include:
  - ○ **dependency**: one person (usually the group therapist) is identified as the one who will provide the group with all its needs
  - ○ **fight–flight**: the group identifies a shared 'enemy' which they either fight or flee from
  - ○ **pairing**: the group identifies a couple who will give birth to a new member or idea which will rescue the group from its predicament.

This approach is particularly associated with therapeutic work with teams and institutions.

Psychotherapy through the group

This refers to the use of the group as the agent of therapy. This approach is associated with group analysis and therapeutic communities.

Group analysis is a theory and method of treatment developed by S. H. Foulkes following the Second World War. The theory brings together psychoanalysis, systems theory and sociology.

Key points are:

- the individual mind is a nodal point within a social network
- each individual mind is a product of the group of which the individual is a part
- when a therapeutic group meets it develops a group mind or matrix which becomes the medium for therapy.

Therapeutic community is a term first coined by Tom Main in 1948. It is a treatment method which uses the therapeutic power of belonging to a carefully structured community. Main set up the Cassel Hospital in Surrey which combines therapeutic community treatment with individual psychodynamic psychotherapy.

Maxwell Jones founded the Belmont Unit which became the Henderson Hospital in Surrey and provides a pure communal treatment. In his study of the Henderson Hospital, Rapoport (1960) identified the following defining characteristics of a therapeutic community:

- **permissiveness**: expression of feelings is encouraged
- **reality confrontation**: residents are directly confronted with the consequences of their behaviour
- **democracy**: there are a flattened hierarchy and shared decision-making
- **communalism**: there is communal responsibility for running of the community.

Therapeutic communities have developed in the following settings:

- inpatient units
- day settings

- addiction recovery
- prison settings.

More recently, the Department of Health has funded two 'satellites' of the Henderson Hospital in Birmingham and Manchester for the treatment of severe personality disorder.

Practice of group psychotherapy

Therapeutic groups are run in a number of different settings including inpatient, day patient and outpatient facilities.

Groups may be **homogeneous** (designed for patients with a common diagnosis or therapeutic issue, eg addiction, eating disorders, consequences of sexual abuse) or **heterogeneous** (designed for people with a mixture of diagnoses and therapeutic issues).

Groups can vary in length from short-term (< 1 year) to long-term (> 1 year).

Aims of group analytic psychotherapy

Group analytic psychotherapy aims to:

- enable patients to understand the conscious and unconscious relational issues underpinning their difficulties
- provide patients with an opportunity to address these relational issues in the here and now of the group.

Key elements in group psychotherapy

Yalom identified the following therapeutic factors in groups:

- interpersonal learning
- catharsis
- cohesiveness
- self-understanding
- universality
- instillation of hope
- altruism
- family re-enactment
- imparting information
- imitation.

Foulkes identified four therapeutic factors that were specific to group analytic psychotherapy:

- mirroring
- resonance
- exchange
- activation of collective unconscious.

The role of the group therapist is to:

- maintain the boundaries of the group, ie membership, time and space
- facilitate open and honest communication
- enable group members to understand their interactions with each other and how this might link to their own relationship patterns
- promote a sense of belonging to the group through exploration of shared concerns.

Suitability for group analytic psychotherapy

The following are important factors in assessing a patient's capacity to benefit from group analytic psychotherapy:

- recognition of problem as psychological
- some sense of responsibility for life situation
- curiosity or psychological mindedness
- capacity to relate to another
- capacity to tolerate a certain degree of emotional distress (ego strength)
- motivation and staying power
- capacity to tolerate being with other people in a group
- risk of regressive transference in individual psychotherapy
- unable to tolerate dyadic intimacy of individual psychotherapy.

The following patients are less likely to benefit from group analytic psychotherapy but may benefit from homogeneous groups specifically adapted for the relevant diagnostic group:

- current abuse of drugs or alcohol
- repeated impulsive acts of violence towards self or others (may benefit from psychotherapy in specialist unit such as a therapeutic community)
- severe organic brain disease
- acute psychotic illness.

Indications for group analytic psychotherapy

As for psychodynamic psychotherapy (see page 517).

The practice of therapeutic communities

The aims, suitability criteria and indications for treatment within a therapeutic community are similar to those for group analytic psychotherapy except that the level of disturbance that can be tolerated in a therapeutic community is greater. Most therapeutic communities will not treat people subject to detention under the Mental Health Act and insist that patients come off psychotropic medication prior to admission. Therapeutic communities are now one of the treatments of choice for people with severe personality disorder.

FAMILY THERAPY

Development of family therapy

There are three main models of family therapy:

- cognitive behavioural
- psychodynamic
- systemic.

Cognitive behavioural family therapy

The cognitive behavioural model focuses on changing a family's behaviour (eg reduction of critical/hostile expressed emotion of close relative) using:

- psycho-educational strategies
- stress management
- problem solving.

This method has been particularly well researched in the treatment of schizophrenia (eg Falloon, 1988; Tarrier *et al.*, 1988).

Psychodynamic family therapy

This model is based on elucidating the conscious and unconscious factors underlying the family's problem. This will involve exploration of issues such as:

- projection from one family member onto another
- over-identification between parent and child
- inversion of parent–child roles
- re-enactment of parent's early experience
- Oedipal dynamics.

Systemic family therapy

Systemic therapy is based on systems theory (von Bertalanffy, 1950).

Key points of this theory are as follows.

- A system is a set of interacting elements within a boundary of variable permeability.
- The family is viewed as a living system, with subsystems such as parents and siblings.
- One cannot understand one member of the system in isolation from the system as a whole.
- If the system is dysfunctional then this may manifest in the form of mental distress in one family member who becomes the 'identified patient'.

Systemic approaches to mental illness began after the Second World War. A number of clinicians became interested in the idea that schizophrenia was the product of disturbed early family relationships and believed interventions focusing on the family system could be helpful.

- Fromm-Reichmann (1948) developed the notion of the 'schizophrenogenic mother'.
- Bateson (1956) proposed the double-bind hypothesis which suggests that schizophrenia was a response to contradictory messages from immediate family.
- Laing (1964) believed that schizophrenia was a natural protective response to living in a 'mad' environment.

These ideas resulted in many parents of psychotic patients feeling blamed. As a result of this, work with the families of people with schizophrenia in the UK has been slow to enter general clinical practice despite much research on the effectiveness of psycho-educational and cognitive behavioural family interventions (see page 531).

Systemic approaches began to be used in Child Guidance Clinics in the 1950s and are now widespread in Child Psychiatry services.

There are now three main approaches to systemic family therapy:

- **Structural** (Minuchin): focus is on structure of family through differentiating functions of the marital, parental and sibling relationships
- **Strategic** (Haley): focus is on problem solving, including the setting of tasks to be carried out between sessions
- **Milan** (Palazzoli): focus is on developing a formulation of the family system through circular questioning. A hypothesis is then put to the family highlighting the conflict between desire for change and processes opposing change. One specific technique is the 'paradoxical injunction' which involves instructing the patient to continue expressing the problem behaviour because of the useful purpose it serves in the family.

Practice of family therapy

Most practitioners of family therapy draw on a combination of psychodynamic, systemic and cognitive behavioural techniques. Interventions tend to be relatively short, eg 4 to 12 sessions.

Aims of family therapy

Family therapy aims to:

- understand an individual's disorder by understanding the family system within which he/she lives
- treat an individual's disorder by changing the family system within which he/she lives.

Key elements of family therapy

- There is re-framing of the presenting problem in terms of the family system.
- Attendance:
  - some practitioners insist on the presence of all members of immediate family
  - other practitioners are more flexible in working with subsystems of a family.
- Live supervision from a reflecting team (may be sat behind one-way screen or in the therapy room).

- Specific techniques, eg exploring unconscious dynamics, circular questioning, problem solving, paradoxical injunction, homework tasks.

Suitability for family therapy

- Motivation: some family members are reluctant to see themselves as having a role to play in the maintenance or management of an individual's disorder.
- There should be some commitment to stay together; family therapy is unlikely to be helpful if the parties concerned have already decided to separate.

Indications for family therapy

The following are indications for family therapy:

- childhood neurotic and conduct disorders
- anorexia nervosa
- schizophrenia
- other psychiatric disorders in which systemic change could be helpful in management.

COUPLE THERAPY

Development of couple therapy

There are three main models of couple therapy:

- cognitive behavioural
- psychodynamic
- systemic.

Cognitive behavioural couple therapy

The cognitive behavioural model focuses on changing a couple's behaviour using the following techniques:

- **Reciprocity negotiation**: each member of the couple is taught to convert a complaint into a wish and then convert the wish into a homework task. A 'give a bit receive a bit' negotiation is encouraged.
- **Communication training**: the therapist 'umpires' live discussions over seemingly trivial household matters, eg whether the toilet seat is left up or down.

Psychodynamic couple therapy

This model is based on elucidating the conscious and unconscious factors underlying the couple's problem. This will involve exploration of issues such as:

- mutual projection between members of the couple
- re-enactment of early attachment experiences within couple relationship
- Oedipal dynamics.

Systemic couple therapy

Systemic couple therapy is based on systems theory (von Bertalanffy, 1950).

Key points are:

- a system is a set of interacting elements within a boundary of variable permeability
- the couple is viewed as a living system, which itself is a subsystem within a larger system, eg family
- one cannot understand one member of the system in isolation from the system as a whole
- if the couple system is dysfunctional then this may manifest in the form of mental distress in one couple member who becomes the 'identified patient'.

Practice of couple therapy

Most practitioners of couple therapy draw on a combination of psychodynamic, systemic and cognitive behavioural techniques. Interventions tend to be relatively short, eg 4 to 12 sessions.

Aims of couple therapy

The aims of couple therapy are:

- to understand an individual's disorder by understanding the couple relationship
- to treat an individual's disorder by changing the couple relationship.

Key elements of couple therapy

Key elements of couple therapy are:

- re-framing of presenting problem in terms of the couple relationship
- specific techniques, eg exploring unconscious dynamics, circular questioning, problem solving, paradoxical injunction, homework tasks.

Suitability for couple therapy

Suitability for couple therapy requires:

- motivation: the member of the couple who is not the identified patient is often reluctant to attend and considerable care needs to be taken in engaging this member who may be wary of seeing him- or herself as having a role to play in the maintenance or management of an individual's disorder.
- some commitment to stay together; couple therapy is unlikely to be helpful if the parties concerned have already decided to separate.

Indications for couple therapy

Indications for couple therapy are:

- relationship problems contributing to psychiatric disorder in one or both partners
- psychosexual problems

- pathological jealousy
- wellbeing of children is at risk.

OTHER MODELS OF PSYCHOTHERAPY

Interpersonal therapy (IPT)

- Developed by Klerman and Weissman in the USA.
- Brief (16 sessions) structured treatment for depression.
- Focuses on **current interpersonal relationships** and how these have contributed to onset and maintenance of depression.
- Particular focus on grief, interpersonal disputes, relationship deficits, role confusion.
- Use extended to dysthymia, eating disorders, post-traumatic stress disorder and personality disorder.

Cognitive analytic therapy (CAT)

- Developed by Anthony Ryle in the UK.
- Integrates cognitive and psychodynamic theory and practice.
- Brief (usually 16 sessions) structured therapy.
- Makes use of written and diagrammatic reformulation.
- Identifies **target problems** and **reciprocal role procedures** which maintain them.
- Reciprocal role procedures refer to internalised relationship patterns and include:
  - traps: vicious circles that repeatedly reinforce negative beliefs about ourselves
  - dilemmas: choices polarised between two alternatives 'false dichotomisation'
  - snags: inappropriate giving up of personal aims.
- Makes use of goodbye letters from patient to therapist and vice versa.
- Advocated in the treatment of mood disorders, anxiety disorders and personality disorders.

Dialectical behaviour therapy (DBT)

- Developed by Marsha Linehan in the USA as a specific treatment for borderline personality disorder.
- Treatment involves:
  - weekly individual sessions focused on functional analysis of risk behaviours, motivation and problem solving
  - weekly group sessions focused on skills training in interpersonal interactions, emotional regulation, distress tolerance and mindfulness
  - out of hours crisis contact with therapist or therapist substitute.
- Therapy has been adapted recently for use in the treatment of eating disorders.

Supportive psychotherapy

- Not based on any one specific theoretical model.
- Emphasis is on supporting and maintaining existing functioning rather than change.
- Elements include: listening, acceptance, facilitating expression of feeling, education, reassurance, advice, involving other people, reaching shared understanding of problems.

Transactional analysis

- Developed by Eric Berne.
- Based on model of the mind that differentiates 'Parent', 'Adult' and 'Child' aspects of the mind.
- Aim of treatment is to identify psychological 'scripts' which hinder 'Adult' functioning.

Gestalt therapy

- Developed by Frederick Perls.
- Based on model of neurosis as caused by splitting the individual's sense of mind–body unity (Gestalt).
- Focus on 'here and now' experience.
- Dramatisation and games are used to allow the patient to explore and express a fuller awareness of self.

Psychodrama

- Developed by Jacob Moreno.
- Group approach in which one member ('the Protagonist') is encouraged to recreate and enact his or her difficulty using improvised dramatic techniques.

Primal therapy

- Developed by Arthur Janov.
- Based on the belief that neurotic problems arise from early infantile or even pre-natal experience that must be imaginatively re-experienced to achieve resolution.

Psychosynthesis

- Developed by Roberto Assagioli.
- Believed the personality is made up of several sub-personalities that need integrating.
- Particularly interested in spiritual dimension of therapy.

PSYCHOTHERAPEUTIC FORMULATIONS OF PSYCHIATRIC DISORDERS

The following section describes cognitive and psychodynamic models of the major psychiatric disorders. The apparent simplicity of the formulations given below should not be taken to imply simple processes. These are complex processes which will be experienced differently by each patient. Both cognitive and psychodynamic models acknowledge the importance of genetic predisposition and wider social contributions to major psychiatric disorders. It is also important to emphasise that within these broad theoretical frameworks there are a number of different variants (see Further Reading).

Mood disorders

Cognitive model

The cognitive model of depression gives primacy to dysfunctional assumptions and negative automatic thoughts.

Early experience
↓
Formation of dysfunctional assumptions
↓
Critical incident(s)
↓
Assumptions activated
↓
Negative automatic thoughts
↓
Symptoms of **depression**

Psychodynamic model

The psychodynamic model of depression gives primacy to the experience of real or imagined loss. Real losses include loss of relationship, role, job, health. Imagined losses include concern that one's own success or aggression has damaged or destroyed someone else.

Early real or imagined loss
↓
Sensitivity to loss experiences
↓
Recent experience of real or imagined loss
↓
Anger, sadness, guilt, emptiness
↓
Loss of self-esteem
↓
Symptoms of **depression**

The experience of depression may be countered by the use of what Melanie Klein termed 'manic defences' such as denial, omnipotence and idealisation. These mechanisms are commonly seen in manic patients.

Anxiety disorders

Cognitive model

The cognitive model proposes that anxiety states result from an overestimation of the danger inherent in given situations as a result of the activation of dysfunctional assumptions.

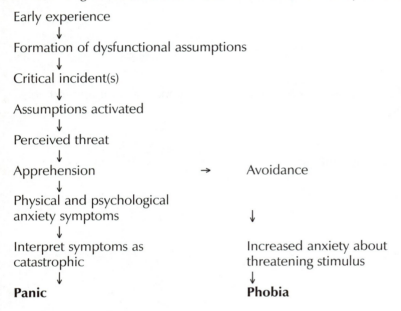

Early experience
↓
Formation of dysfunctional assumptions
↓
Critical incident(s)
↓
Assumptions activated
↓
Perceived threat
↓
Apprehension   →   Avoidance
↓
Physical and psychological
anxiety symptoms   ↓
↓
Interpret symptoms as   Increased anxiety about
catastrophic   threatening stimulus
↓   ↓
Panic   **Phobia**

Psychodynamic model

The psychodynamic model proposes that anxiety that is disproportionate to the level of external threat is generated by the experience of an internal threat to psychic equilibrium. The disproportionate anxiety which is focused on an external threat represents a displacement of an anxiety about an internal threat in the face of disturbing feelings.

Early real or imagined threatening experiences
↓
Internalisation of threatening objects and/or failure to internalise protective objects
↓
Recent perceived threat(s)
↓
Threat of emergence of disturbing feelings → Displaced onto external stimulus
↓   ↓
Anxiety symptoms   **Phobia**

Eating disorders

Both cognitive and psychodynamic models acknowledge the major role of cultural factors in the aetiology of eating disorders. Anorexia nervosa is virtually unknown in countries where thinness is not considered a virtue.

Cognitive model

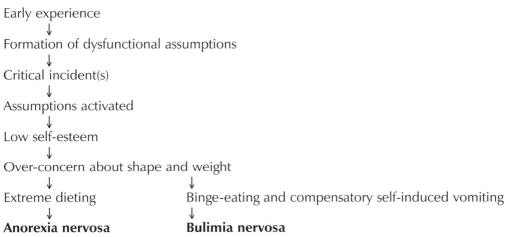

Early experience
↓
Formation of dysfunctional assumptions
↓
Critical incident(s)
↓
Assumptions activated
↓
Low self-esteem
↓
Over-concern about shape and weight
↓   ↓
Extreme dieting   Binge-eating and compensatory self-induced vomiting
↓   ↓
Anorexia nervosa   **Bulimia nervosa**

Psychodynamic model

Early experiences of lack of nurture and emotional/physical intrusion
↓
Emotional hunger and activation of 'no-entry' psychological defences made concrete in relation to food
↓
Denial of adult sexuality (in anorexia)
↓
Bingeing and/or restrictive behaviours
↓
Bulimia and anorexia nervosa

Addictions

Cognitive model

Early life experiences
↓
Formation of dysfunctional assumptions
↓
Exposure to and experimentation with addictive substances
↓
Development of substance-related beliefs
↓
Activating stimuli eg anxiety, depression
↓
Substance use

Psychodynamic model

Early experiences of lack of nurture and/or abuse
↓
Inability to manage difficult feelings
and
inability to tolerate emotional intimacy
↓
Exposure to and experimentation with addictive substances
↓
Use of addictive substance
(to manage intolerable feelings and to act as a substitute for emotional intimacy)

Psychotic disorders

Cognitive model

Enduring vulnerability to psychosis (genetic or neurodevelopmental)
↓
Precipitating stressors (biopsychosocial)
↓
Cognitive distortions and perceptual anomalies
↓
Maintaining stressors (biopsychosocial)
↓
Persistent cognitive distortions and perceptual anomalies

The cognitive model suggests that:

- the psychosocial precipitating and maintaining factors can be modified, eg by family work and psycho-education
- the cognitive and perceptual distortions can be modified by encouraging the individual to weigh evidence that contradicts the delusion or hallucination.

Psychodynamic model

Enduring vulnerability to psychosis (genetic or neurodevelopmental)
↓
Precipitating stressors (biopsychosocial)
↓
Breakdown of the normal perceptual and experiential boundaries between self and external world
↓
Activation of primitive defence mechanisms such as withdrawal from reality, splitting and projection
↓
Psychotic symptoms

RESEARCH IN PSYCHOTHERAPY

History of psychotherapy research

- **1900 onwards**: psychotherapy research based on case study approach.
- **1952**: Eysenck's infamous critique of evidence base for psychotherapy (by psychotherapy he referred to analytic psychotherapy). He suggested that recovery rate from psychotherapy was no better than spontaneous remission.
- **1970s**: controlled trials of psychotherapy emerge.
- **1980**: first meta-analysis of controlled trials in psychotherapy.
- **1980s**: psychotherapy subjected to randomised controlled trials.
- **1996**: authoritative critical review of psychotherapy research published in UK entitled *What Works for Whom?* (Roth and Fonagy).
- **2001**: Department of Health publishes *Treatment Choice Guidelines for Psychological Therapies and Counselling* (Department of Health, 2001), based on up-to-date review of research evidence.

Methodological issues

It is important to distinguish between the efficacy of a therapy (the results it achieves in a research trial) and its clinical effectiveness (the outcome of the therapy in routine practice). Table 25.3 identifies some of the respective methodological issues:

Clinical efficacy	Clinical effectiveness
Research trial	Routine practice
High internal validity	High external validity
Highly selected patients	Routine patients
Randomisation	Patient preference
Extensive monitoring	Routine outcome measures
Use of therapy from a manual	Use of supervised therapy

Table 25.3 Methodological issues in psychotherapy

Other methodological issues include:

- **Measurement techniques and models of therapy**. Different models of therapy target at different psychological changes, for example:
  - CBT – symptomatic relief
  - long-term psychodynamic psychotherapy – personality change
  - family therapy – systemic change
  - outcome measures which are designed to measure those changes targeted by a specific therapy may not be appropriate for a trial comparing the specific therapy with another model, eg Beck Depression Inventory focuses on psychological domains which are the targets of cognitive therapy (developed by Beck).
- **Importance of therapeutic relationship**. Any therapy delivered in a research or clinical setting represents a combination of a therapeutic technique and the personal style of the psychotherapist. An efficacious therapy can be delivered ineffectively.
- The full impact of some therapies may only emerge some time after therapy is completed. However, the longer the **follow-up** period the harder it is to ascribe changes to the therapy itself.
- Significant rates of **attrition** will restrict the conclusions that can be drawn from a controlled trial. In a trial comparing two models of therapy differential attrition rates may reflect differing acceptability of the therapies.

General findings in psychotherapy research

- **Therapeutic relationship**. The quality of the therapeutic alliance between patient and therapist is the single best predictor of benefit and accounts for 25% of the variance in outcome of psychotherapy.
- **Treatment length**. There is some evidence for a dose–response effect (higher dose of therapy leads to greater symptomatic improvement) but this response seems to 'plateau out' after about 20 sessions for neurotic problems uncomplicated by significant personality disturbance. Where there is significant personality disturbance the limited evidence suggests that the therapy needs to be relatively long-term (at least one year).
- **Patient preference**. There is little research evidence on the impact of patient preference. However, the therapeutic alliance is likely to be enhanced by giving appropriate weight to a patient's preference.

Summary of evidence base for treatment of specific disorders

This is summarised in the following publications:

- *What Works for Whom?* (Roth and Fonagy, 1996)
- *Treatment Choice in Psychological Therapies and Counselling* (Department of Health, 2001)
- *NICE Guidelines* for specific disorders as they are published.

These publications and the following summary are based on the following hierarchy of evidence:

- meta-analysis of randomised controlled trials
- > 1 randomised controlled trial
- 1 randomised controlled trial
- non-randomised controlled trials
- descriptive studies
- opinion of respected authority.

The following **cautionary notes** should be recognised:

- **co-morbidity**: many patients in specialist mental health services have more than one psychiatric disorder, which is often an exclusion criterion in research trials. There is little research literature on the impact of co-morbidity on psychological treatments.
- **Biased representation** of theoretical orientations in research literature, eg psychodynamic and systemic therapies are under-represented.
- **Absence of evidence** for the efficacy of a specific treatment for a given disorder does not imply that that treatment is ineffective.

With these cautionary notes in mind, the evidence base for psychotherapeutic treatments of the main psychiatric disorders can be briefly summarised as follows:

- **Depressive disorders**. The best evidence is for CBT and IPT. There is also evidence for the efficacy of brief psychodynamic psychotherapy, group therapy, couple therapy, problem-solving therapy and non-directive counselling in primary care.
- **Schizophrenia**. CBT and family interventions have been shown to be effective in the early post-acute period, in the treatment of chronic psychotic symptoms and in the prevention of relapse.
- **Anxiety disorders** (including panic disorder, agoraphobia, social phobia, obsessive-compulsive disorder, simple phobias and generalised anxiety disorder). The best evidence is for CBT.
- **Post-traumatic stress disorder**. The best evidence is for CBT. There is some evidence for the effectiveness of eye movement desensitisation and reprocessing (EMDR), hypnotherapy and psychodynamic psychotherapy. The efficacy of critical incident debriefing as a preventative intervention is not supported by current research evidence.
- **Eating disorders**. In **bulimia nervosa** the best evidence is for CBT and IPT. In **anorexia nervosa** there is some evidence for the efficacy of family therapy in early onset and eclectic individual therapy in late onset disease.
- **Psychosomatic disorders**.
  - **Chronic fatigue syndrome**. There is some evidence for CBT.
  - **Irritable bowel syndrome and functional dyspepsia**. There is some evidence for brief psychodynamic psychotherapy.
  - **Chronic pain**. There is some evidence for CBT.
- **Personality disorders**. There is some evidence for the efficacy of psychodynamic psychotherapy, dialectical behaviour therapy and therapeutic communities in the treatment of borderline personality disorder.
- **Substance misuse**. There is some evidence for the value of motivational interviewing, CBT and behavioural marital therapy for the prevention of relapse.

FURTHER READING

Barnes, B., Ernst, S. & Hyde, K. 1999. *An introduction to group work – a group analytic perspective*. London: Macmillan.

Bateman, A. & Holmes, J. 1995. *Introduction to psychoanalysis*. London: Routledge.

Bateman, A., Brown, D. & Pedder, J. 2000. *Introduction to psychotherapy*. London: Routledge.

Campling, P. & Haigh, R. 1999. *Therapeutic communities – past, present and future*. London: Jessica Kingsley.

Crowe, M. & Ridley, J. 2000. *Therapy with couples – a behavioural-systems approach*. Cambridge: Blackwell Science.

Falloon, I. 1988. *Handbook of behavioural family therapy*. London: Unwin Hyman.

Hawton, K., Salkovskis, P., Kirk, J. & Clark, D. 2000. *Cognitive behaviour therapy for psychiatric problems – a practical guide*. Oxford: Oxford University Press.

Tarrier, N. *et al.* 1988. 'The community management of schizophrenia: A controlled trial of a behavioural intervention with families to reduce relapse.' *British Journal of Psychiatry*, 153, 532–542.

Chapter 26

Perinatal Psychiatry

Robin Balmer

CONTENTS

Perinatal Psychiatry

PREGNANCY

Mental illness in pregnancy

The first trimester is associated with an increase in minor mental illness (eg mild anxiety symptoms). Pregnancy itself may provoke anxiety (unplanned pregnancy, associated with timing of a previous miscarriage etc).

- The anxiety usually settles with education and reassurance.
- Counselling may be helpful.
- Care should be taken when prescribing during pregnancy (see below).
- Pregnancy is thought to be associated with a decreased rate of major mental illness and suicide.
- Depression in pregnancy is approximately one-third as common as depression starting postnatally.

Studies of the effects of antenatal stress and anxiety have concentrated on obstetric outcome. Women who experienced severe life events in the first trimester of pregnancy had a 50% increase in congenital abnormalities such as cleft palate. There is a strong link between maternal anxiety in the third trimester and behavioural/emotional problems in the resulting children at four years and it is likely that maternal mood has a direct effect on fetal brain development. Reducing maternal anxiety in pregnancy may have protective, preventive effects for children.

Miscarriage

Rate 10–15%, but approximately 5% of couples trying to conceive have two consecutive miscarriages.

O'Hare and Creed (1995) showed that a group of women admitted to hospital had experienced more psychological stress in early pregnancy than women whose pregnancies progressed to labour.

The women who miscarried were:

- more likely to have experienced life events of 'severe short-term threat' in the two weeks beforehand
- more likely to have experienced a 'severe life event' in the three months preceding the miscarriage.

There was an association with:

- childhood maternal separation

- non-UK European origin
- poorer reported relationships with partners
- fewer social contacts.

Stress and immune mediators have been found in the decidual tissue of women who miscarried and who also scored highly on a perceived stress questionnaire.

The miscarriage was often followed by morbidity; depressive reactions were common.

- Friedman and Gath found 48% had depressive illness at one month (four times the expected rate).
- Turner found that 75% experienced a grief reaction that resolved within one month.
- 21% experienced a reaction which had not resolved (there is a strong demand for support and counselling for this group of women).

The rate of suicide is increased after both miscarriage and induced abortion.

Termination of pregnancy

Approximately 10% of women suffer either depression or anxiety after an induced abortion.

Psychiatric sequelae are more likely if:

- there is past psychiatric history
- it is a younger woman
- there is poor social adjustment
- she is multiparous
- she belongs to sociocultural groups antagonistic to abortion.

Drug and alcohol problems in pregnancy

When dealing with drug and/or alcohol problems in pregnancy:

- Begin by taking a thorough drug and alcohol history (see Chapter 23).
- Consider the risk of human immunodeficiency virus infection.
- Ideally, discuss and plan the perinatal care early.
  - A range of management approaches are possible according to local services and the individual circumstances of the case.
  - Co-ordinate management with relevant services.
  - Consider child protection issues.
  - Aim to facilitate engagement with services.
  - Arrange planning meetings both antenatally and postnatally.
- For pain management in labour for opiate users an epidural should be considered (because the opiate receptors are likely to be saturated).

PUERPERAL DISORDERS

Confidential enquiries into maternal deaths in the UK record 'psychological' as the most common cause of maternal deaths from 1997 to 1999. Whether postpartum depressive illness and postpartum psychosis are specific disorders is a matter of debate. Rates of depression after childbirth are higher than in women with young children outside the postnatal period. There may be two groups:

- women who become depressed in relation to motherhood and its demands
- women who show no more likelihood of depression after childhood than at other times.

Classification

The International Classification of Diseases (ICD-10) classifies under specific type of disorder (eg depressive episode). The code 099.3 (mental diseases and diseases of the nervous system complicating the puerperium) from the obstetric section of ICD-10 can be used. If the disorder does not meet these criteria, ICD-10 uses F53 'Mental and behavioural disorders associated with the puerperium, not elsewhere classified'. The problem must commence within six weeks of delivery.

The fourth edition of the Diagnostic and Statistical Manual of Mental Disorders (DSM-IV) uses a 'postpartum onset specifier' which can be added to the diagnosis if it is within four weeks of childbirth. It is acknowledged that, although risk factors, recurrence rates, and symptoms of postpartum onset mood episodes are similar to those of non-postpartum mood episodes, the postpartum period is unique with respect to the degree of neuroendocrine alterations, psychosocial adjustments, the potential impact of breastfeeding on treatment planning and the long-term implications of a history of postpartum mood disorder on subsequent family planning.

Maternity blues ('baby blues')

Maternity blues are common, occurring in 50–70% of women following a normal delivery. They are short-lived, starting on day 3–5 and usually resolving within two weeks.

Onset

- There are symptoms of crying, altered mood, low mood, irritability or elation and insomnia.
- Severe maternity blues may be difficult to distinguish from early postnatal depression or a prelude to puerperal psychosis.

Aetiology

- Aetiology is uncertain.
- Pregnancy and motherhood are times of psychosocial changes and adjustment. Women with maternity blues are more likely to have a history of premenstrual

539

tension, neuroticism, anxiety and depressed mood during pregnancy, fears of labour, and poor social adjustment.
- An increased understanding of the neuroendocrine causes may increase the understanding of postnatal mood disorder.
- Theories advocate a hormonal relationship with the maternity blues and its severity. Progesterone and oestrogen levels drop after delivery and cortisol rises through pregnancy and then falls. Studies are not conclusive in linking these changes with the disorder.

Treatment

- The maternity blues are usually transient and improve within 10 days without treatment.
- Therapy is aimed at being supportive, supplying explanation and reassurance.

Postnatal depression

Aetiology

There is debate as to whether this postnatal disorder differs from psychiatric disorders at other times. Rates of 10–15% within three months of childbirth are similar to non-pregnant samples but are increased compared to the period of pregnancy.

Paykel (1980) found a 20% prevalence of mild clinical depression in a series of women when assessed at six weeks postpartum. The strongest associated factor was occurrence of stressful life events. Previous history of psychiatric disorder, younger age, early postpartum blues and a number of variables reflecting poor marital relationship and absence of social support were also notable. Poor marital support acted as a vulnerability factor, only producing an effect in the presence of stressful life events.

It is also found to have an association with:

- previous history of depressive episode
- marital disharmony
- previous menstrual problems
- severe maternity blues
- Caesarean section
- unwanted pregnancy (both antenatal and postnatal depression).

Recent stressful events are important but there is little evidence for biological factors. There is no association with parity. There have been attempts to link hormonal and biochemical changes in the postnatal period, including levels of thyroid antibodies.

Clinical features

A significant number of women who are vulnerable to postnatal depression do not attend general practitioner or health visitor appointments and barriers to take-up of these services need to be better understood.

Onset is after two weeks postpartum (later onset than postpartum psychosis).

It presents as:

- tiredness, irritability and anxiety, especially around the baby's health
- depressive symptoms, tearfulness and low self-esteem
- sleep disturbance and anorexia
- thoughts of suicide and of harming the baby
- guilt, inadequacy.

It is assessed using the Edinburgh Postnatal Depression Scale (EPDS; see below).

Treatment

Multidisciplinary specialist teams have an important place in the management of perinatal illness and trials have shown the benefit of involving the father in therapy and of interventions promoting interactions between mother and infant. Admission to a mother and baby unit should occur if there is severe depression or a high risk of suicide.

- **Psychological treatment**
  - Psychological treatments, especially counselling, are highly acceptable and efficacious (eg non-directive counselling by health visitor).
  - Cochrane systematic review indicates that professional and/or social support may help in the treatment of postpartum depression.
  - Group-based interventions may be useful but most require one-to-one support initially.
  - Controlled trials have shown the effectiveness of cognitive behavioural therapy and interpersonal psychotherapy in the short-term.
  - Cooper (2003) found that different psychotherapeutic approaches showed little benefit at nine months after birth compared to control. Only psychodynamic therapy reduced depression at 4–5 months.
- **Physical treatments**
  - Selective serotonin reuptake inhibitors (SSRIs)/tricyclics have most data.
  - Fluoxetine is as effective as cognitive behavioural therapy (CBT).
  - There is no advantage in receiving both fluoxetine and CBT.
  - Similar improvements were seen with six sessions of CBT or fluoxetine plus one session of CBT.
  - Electroconvulsive therapy is not contraindicated in pregnancy; any risk is associated with the anaesthetic.
- **Hormonal treatment**
  - Placebo-controlled trial with oestradiol skin patches for two months showed a greater elevation in mood than placebo. Oestrogen therapy may be of modest value at a late stage of severe postnatal depression.

Prognosis

Postnatal depression can have an impact on the cognitive and emotional development of the infant. Children show:

- less interactive behaviour, less concentration and more negative responses
- insecure attachment is more frequent

- behaviour problems, including sleeping and eating problems, and separation difficulties.

Exposure to prolonged severe depression may contribute to a poor outcome. Other factors of importance include social adversity and genetic/constitutional factors involving the infant.

Fathers may become depressed, or at least distressed, when the mother is also distressed. Relationships may fail.

Most episodes resolve by six months postpartum.

Postpartum psychosis

Epidemiology

- Occurs in 2.2 per 1000 births.
- Relative risk of psychosis is elevated in the first month postpartum compared to pregnancy or later in the puerperium.
- Relative risk is approximately 20 times normal risk.
- Increased rate in primigravidae.

Aetiology

- **Psychosocial aetiology**:
  - unmarried
  - first baby
  - Caesarean section
  - perinatal death.
- **Genetic aetiology**:
  - family history of psychosis
  - less genetic loading than in non-puerperal illness
  - familial aggregation of psychiatric (particularly affective) disorder suggesting a major overlap in the familial factors predisposing to postpartum psychosis and bipolar disorder
  - history of affective disorder/bipolar illness. Rates of postpartum psychosis are 20–30% in women with bipolar disorder.
- **Neuroendocrine aetiology**:
  - hormonal factors are unproven despite early onset pointing to them (as with maternity blues)
  - in women with high risk of developing affective psychosis after childbirth, relapse associated with increased sensitivity of dopamine receptors (possible aetiology is a sharp fall in circulating oestrogen levels after delivery).

Clinical picture

- Onset is four days to two weeks post delivery, presenting with
  - confusion, mood changes and insomnia
  - delusions, hallucinations
  - suicidal thoughts.

- Affective picture in the majority (approximately 80%):
  - mania, depression or mixed affective
  - in depressive presentation, often delusions regarding the child.
- Schizoaffective
- Schizophrenia
  - rare
  - mostly in women with previous diagnosis of schizophrenia.
- Acute organic
  - uncommon
  - puerperal sepsis.
- Postpartum psychotic patients had more manic symptoms and 'confusion', while non-postpartum patients had more schizophrenic symptoms.

Treatment

- It is important to assess delusional ideas regarding the child and the risk of harm/suicide.
- Inpatient treatment should keep the mother and baby together unless the risk to self or baby is too great.
- Mother and Baby Units assess:
  - quality of infant–mother relationship
  - practical abilities of mother to look after the infant (eg feeding)
  - psychiatric assessment of mother's illness.
- Antidepressants/lithium can be given.
- Electroconvulsive therapy should be considered for depressive or manic disorders.
- Antipsychotics can be given.

Mothers with schizophrenia are three times more likely to experience a poor outcome than non-schizophrenic mothers, more likely to be separated from their infant at discharge and perceived, by staff, to be at greater risk of harming their infant. There is no evidence, however, that they are more likely to cause actual harm to their infant, or themselves, than non-schizophrenic mothers.

Prognosis

- Most women recover from puerperal psychosis. Affective/schizoaffective disorders are associated with better prognosis.
- There is an increased risk of psychosis after further pregnancy, usually with similar time of onset, duration and diagnostic category.
- Long-term outcome:
  - There is a high risk of non-puerperal recurrences with considerable consistency with index diagnoses.
  - There is some shift to bipolar illness.
  - Further illness is less likely to occur where the index illness occurs with the first child, with onset within one month of delivery, and where the index diagnosis is unipolar depression.

DRUGS AND PREGNANCY

The physiological changes that occur during pregnancy, together with the potential for drugs to affect a developing fetus or neonate, mean that considerable caution needs to be exercised in prescribing. The following pharmacodynamic and pharmacokinetic changes occur in pregnancy:

- delayed gastric emptying
- induced liver metabolism
- increased renal clearance
- increased plasma volume and total body water (especially later in pregnancy)
- reduced levels of albumin (binding) and increased excretion rates mean that it may be necessary to alter the drug dose as pregnancy progresses.

Fetal drug distribution is distinctive.

In addition to prescribed drugs, the picture is complicated by illicit use of drugs and alcohol.

Generic effects of drugs on fetus and child

Drug use causes increased rates of:

- first-trimester abortion
- placental abruption
- intrauterine death
- abnormal presentations.

Cocaine use is linked to increased rates of stillbirth, sudden infant death syndrome and neonatal death.

Opiates

Untreated opiate abuse is associated with a high risk of maternal and fetal complications including increased rates of intrauterine growth retardation and pre-term deliveries. The aim of antenatal mental health care, therefore, is to facilitate engagement with antenatal care and stabilise or reduce drug use. Acute withdrawal syndrome can be prevented by using methadone.

A planning meeting with relevant professionals, including the obstetrician and the maternity and neonatal staff and drug specialists, together with the primary-care team is essential. This allows the parents to identify and clarify issues with professionals, as well as providing an opportunity to consider the need for a child protection case conference.

In the long-term, women who enter methadone programmes have improved pregnancy, childbirth and infant development outcomes, even if use of illicit drugs continues.

When prescribing opiates:

- **Low-dose methadone** maintenance may reduce the severity of neonatal withdrawal and appears to be the best option for ensuring continuity of management of pregnancy and the puerperium.

- **High-dose methadone** may be necessary if the use of illicit opiates continues but it leads to more severe withdrawal in the neonate. If detoxification is contemplated, make gradual incremental reductions in methadone dose, according to the woman's response. Social and psychological support are important. Pharmacodynamic changes in the third trimester may necessitate increasing the dose of methadone.

Cocaine

The woman should be advised to stop as there is no substitute prescription available.

Neonatal withdrawals

Access to skilled neonatal paediatric care is important. Signs of withdrawal range from a high pitched cry, sweats, rapid breathing and poor feeding to convulsions. Withdrawal can be delayed up to 7–10 days where benzodiazepines are involved.

Fetal alcohol syndrome

Incidence of fetal alcohol syndrome is approximately 0.4 per 1000 births.

Alcohol is teratogenic but damage to the fetus probably depends on both amount imbibed and stage of development.

Features of the syndrome are:

- **pre/postnatal growth deficiency**
  - intrauterine growth retardation
  - 'small for dates'.
- **central nervous system effects**
  - intellectual impairment, with mild to moderate mental retardation
  - hearing, visual and behavioural difficulties.
- **physical effects**
  - characteristic abnormal facies: short upturned nose, epicanthal folds, flat maxillary area, reduced palpebral fissures, poorly developed (smooth) philtrum with thin upper lip.

There is no 'safe' level for drinking alcohol in pregnancy (current recommendations are 1–2 units once or twice per week).

- Heavy drinkers are especially at risk, binge drinking may be harmful.
- Attention deficits and behavioural problems occur in infants exposed to moderate levels of alcohol in pregnancy (this is an under-recognised problem).

Fetal alcohol spectrum disorder covers the broad range of categories from milder impairments to full-blown fetal alcohol syndrome.

Reduction in alcohol consumption at any stage of pregnancy is beneficial for the fetus.

Management of the syndrome involves:

- Take a drinking history (see Chapter 23).
- Use a screening tool (CAGE).
- Brief intervention, ie 15–20 minutes, has been shown to be effective. Regular follow-up is required. Consider motivational interviewing in those at greatest risk.
- Note: unsupervised withdrawal from heavy alcohol use may result in withdrawal fits and put the fetus at risk.

Effects of psychotropic and mood-stabilising drugs on the developing fetus and infant

Most psychotropic drugs are lipophilic and therefore cross the placenta.

During the first trimester drugs may produce congenital malformations (teratogenesis). The greatest period of risk is from week 3 to week 11 of pregnancy. All psychotropics should therefore be avoided in the first trimester.

- For a planned pregnancy, counselling and informed consent are needed in deciding whether to continue medication. Only do so if the benefit outweighs the risk to the fetus (continuing prophylactic drugs may be less risky to the mother and fetus than experiencing a relapse).
- Careful screening is needed during pregnancy, including ultrasound to diagnose malformations early.
- Liaise with obstetrician.

Antidepressants	Antipsychotics	Mood stabilisers	Benzodiazepines
Tricyclics (most data) – amitriptyline – imipramine SSRIs – fluoxetine probably safe – discontinuation syndrome in baby (third trimester) MAOIs – avoid (teratogenic in animals)	– most data on chlorpromazine and trifluoperazine – avoid depot – some safety data for olanzapine, risperidone, quetiapine, clozapine	– avoid all in first trimester (teratogenic) Lithium Ebstein's anomaly 10–20-fold higher incidence (1/1000) Carbamazepine and valproate neural tube defects (0.5–1% and 1–5%, respectively) give folic acid	– best avoided – increased risk of cleft lip/palate (first trimester) – floppy baby (third trimester)

MAOI, monoamine oxidase inhibitors.

Table 26.1 Prescribing drugs in pregnancy

Other risks may be to the mother or neonate, and may affect future child development.

In general, only treat with psychotropic drugs when the potential benefits outweigh the risks (for further details see current *British National Formulary* and *Maudsley Prescribing Guidelines*). There are more data available on the teratogenicity of 'older' drugs, but newer drugs may be as safe.

Lithium

Lithium use has been associated with cardiac malformations, including Ebstein's anomaly (inferior displacement of the tricuspid valve into the right ventricle). The risk is probably 10–20 times that in the general population; revised teratogenic risk is 0.05%. The greatest risk to the fetus of cardiovascular defects and cardiac malformations of all types is between weeks 2–6 post-conception.

Neonatal lithium toxicity is also a risk, presenting with hypotonia, cyanosis and poor thermoregulation.

Advice during pregnancy should be as follows.

- Where possible, avoid lithium in the first trimester, being mindful of the risks to mother and fetus of not taking lithium. If lithium is discontinued, this must be done preconception on a gradual basis to minimise the risk of relapse. Relapse rates are up to 50% within six months of discontinuing lithium, with rapid discontinuation associated with increased risk.
- In the third trimester, the maternal glomerular filtration rate increases, producing increased excretion so that the dose needs to be increased (see above) with close monitoring.
- There is evidence that lithium administered in the second and third trimester can reduce the risk of puerperal psychosis.
- At delivery, the glomerular filtration rate rapidly reverts to baseline so that careful monitoring of lithium is needed to avoid toxicity in the mother or neonate. Indeed, lithium should be withdrawn temporarily.

Ultrasound scans and echocardiography are used to monitor fetal progress and the total daily dose can be divided. Lithium levels should be checked monthly and kept towards the lower end of the therapeutic range.

- Be aware of gastrointestinal disturbances and lithium levels.
- Monitor thyroid function.

Sodium valproate and carbamazepine

- Most available data relate to their use in epilepsy. If possible, avoid use in pregnancy. If deemed necessary, use low-dose monotherapy.
- Both drugs are associated with teratogenic effects, particularly neural tube defects (1–2%).
- Folic acid (5 mg) should be taken daily from one month prior to conception up to week 12 of pregnancy to reduce the risk of neural tube defects.

547

- Carbamazepine may cause vitamin K deficiency, increasing the risk of neonatal bleeding (haemorrhagic disease of the newborn). Administer vitamin K to both mother and neonate.

Antidepressants

- Seek the most up-to-date advice.
- If the woman is already on antidepressants and risk of relapse is high, consider continuation.
- Use for depression arising in pregnancy that is unresponsive to psychological treatment: the Avon Longitudinal Study of Parents and Children (Evans, 2001) reported more symptoms of depression (high EPDS scores) during pregnancy than after delivery.
- Older antidepressants (amitriptyline, imipramine, dothiepin) have most evidence available and show no increase in congenital malformations.
- Several prospective studies on SSRIs exist, with most data supporting the safety of fluoxetine. Paroxetine and sertraline, likewise, seem to be comparatively safe.
- There is a possible increase in spontaneous abortion rates.

Benzodiazepines

Benzodiazepines are best avoided in pregnancy.

- They are linked to increased rate of oral cleft if used in early pregnancy.
- Abrupt withdrawal is inappropriate.
- If given in late pregnancy, drug accumulates in the fetus leading to a floppy infant and withdrawal syndrome in the neonate.

Antipsychotics

Conventional antipsychotics are thought to have minimal risk of teratogenicity. Schizophrenia is associated with an increase in pregnancy and birth complications; the risks of remaining untreated are high.

In principle:

- use the lowest possible dosage
- avoid polypharmacy
- regular psychiatric and obstetric monitoring are necessary
- it may be appropriate to switch from atypical to older antipsychotics with more safety data (although reassuring data on atypical drugs are starting to appear).

Lactation and breastfeeding

- All psychotropics are excreted in breast milk.
- Drug concentrations are generally about 1% of those in maternal plasma.

- Little evidence is available about the effects of drugs on the developing child but breastfeeding should be avoided if the baby is not healthy (especially renal or hepatic impairment).
- If mother was taking a drug during pregnancy, continue with same drug as the amount in breast milk is much lower than that in utero.

Specific drugs:

- **Lithium**: opinions vary; avoid.
- **Diazepam**: infant metabolism is slower, leading to accumulation.
- **Fluoxetine**: manufacturer advises avoidance; some links with irritability, and decreased sleep and feeding.

SCREENING SCHEDULES FOR PERINATAL MENTAL HEALTH PROBLEMS

Edinburgh Postnatal Depression Scale

The EPDS is used routinely in primary care.

- It has high sensitivity (86%), specificity (78%) and reliability.
- It is a 10-item self-report questionnaire, devised as a screening test to improve the detection of postnatal depression.
- It has been used antenatally but its predictive value is controversial as many high postnatal scores are picked up prenatally.
- Items are scored 0–3.
- Total of 12 is indicative and triggers further assessment for depression in collaboration with the general practitioner.

Advantages of routine use of the EPDS include:

- raising awareness of postnatal depression among health professionals, women and their families
- helping a woman to recognise and discuss negative feelings
- providing the opportunity for early preventive intervention
- offering the possibility of changing perceptions of what health professionals can offer.

Other screening schedules for postnatal illness are primarily research tools. (For example, the Structured Clinical Interview for DSM-IV Disorders (SCID), a semi-structured diagnostic interview.)

Screening for puerperal psychosis

- Research tools include interview schedules to identify pregnant women who are at high risk.
- It is vital to ask about previous psychiatric history, including previous psychosis.
- Women with a history of postnatal psychosis have a 1 in 4 risk of developing a further psychosis.
- Past history of severe depression, especially bipolar illness, is also important.

Chapter 27

Philosophy and History of Psychiatry

Sandy Robertson

CONTENTS

Philosophy and History of Psychiatry

RELEVANCE OF PHILOSOPHY TO PSYCHIATRY

As a branch of medicine, psychiatry is partly grounded in the natural sciences whose knowledge base is empirical, based on observation and experiment. This leads to the assumption that gaps in our understanding will be bridged by advances in science, particularly the neurosciences, whose achievements in recent decades have been impressive.

On the other hand, psychiatry starts with the **subjective**, with the experiences of individuals in distress, communicated to professionals in words. These experiences are concerned with mood, thought, belief, perception, memory and so forth, that is with the realm of the **mental**. This raises the question of how our inner worlds, to which we have direct 'first-person' access, relate to the shared, outer world of objects which we apprehend in a third-person way.

If our mental states depend on states of our brain and the latter is part of the material world, are we subject to the inexorable causal processes which prevail in that world? If so, what meaning can we give to concepts like desire and intention which seem to play a causal role in our behaviour? Are we in any sense free agents?

Another feature of psychiatry is the frequency of disagreement between professional and patient about what really is the case, particularly with those people diagnosed as psychotic or deluded. The question, explicit or implied, 'Who are you to say that I am wrong?' hangs over many a clinical interview. It is a special instance of a far wider problem: the quest for certain, founded knowledge, that has preoccupied thinkers for millennia.

These are not empirical but **conceptual** questions and because philosophy is centrally concerned with the critical analysis of concepts it is an indispensable discipline for psychiatry, alongside the brain sciences.

CAUSES, REASONS AND ACTIONS

In giving accounts of human behaviour, we use two kinds of explanation, one in terms of **causes** and the other in terms of **reasons**. For instance, we explain a knee jerk causally in terms of a reflex arc but we explain voting for a political party in terms of reasons for our choice. There may be complex chains of neural causation underlying the latter, but we do not consider them relevant. With actions of intermediate complexity, eg hysterical paralysis or the motor symptoms of schizophrenia, both kinds of explanation may be appropriate.

553

Psychiatry is concerned with **actions**, that is with behaviours imbued with meaning, motive and intended consequences, rather than mere movements. There is a tendency to revert to the language of causes when dealing with psychopathology, but from his own point of view, the sufferer from mental illness continues to act for reasons.

Psychoanalysis, with its concept of **unconscious reasons**, has extended the realm of reasons beyond that of ordinary common sense.

Furthermore, the criteria for mental disorder are drawn from the realm of reasons, eg the irrationality of delusions or the incongruity of abnormal mood states. These criteria are **normative**, ie they depend on following or transgressing rules.

The relationship of reasons and causes is controversial. Most contemporary theories of mind are materialist, at least in assuming that mental events depend closely on neural events. If beliefs and desires are physically encoded in the brain, this allows them a causal role in our behaviour (**intentional causation**). On the other hand, it has been argued by Donald Davidson (1917–2003) that there can never be lawful relationships between the chain of rational causes and that of physical causes.

Controversy persists as to whether mind language (reasons) can ever be reduced to brain language (causes) and whether the private experiences of consciousness can ever be understood in terms of physical events. If such **reductionism** is doomed to failure, we are left with some form of **property dualism**, ie the belief that while brain and mind are not different substances we will always experience them in different ways and need different languages to describe them. This is different from the **substance dualism** of Descartes (1596–1650) who maintained that mind and body were completely different entities (see below).

FACTS AND VALUES

Science is concerned with **facts**, while disciplines such as ethics and aesthetics are concerned with **values**. A strong case can be made that clinical practice is also unavoidably concerned with values (see below), but clarity of thinking is best served by keeping the realms of fact and value distinct.

Factual statements are marked by verbs such as '**is**', while value statements are marked by words such as '**ought**' and '**should**'. Factual adjectives are descriptive, while evaluative adjectives are typified by words such as 'good', 'bad', 'beautiful' or 'ugly' which do not describe features of people and things so much as express our reactions to them. If we believe that such reactions can be generalised into universal judgements, evaluative language also has the function of **commending** them to others.

A principle going back to David Hume (1711–1776) states that one cannot logically derive an 'is' from an 'ought'. Large red sweet apples may generally be accounted 'good' but their goodness does not follow logically from their descriptive properties: one may legitimately disagree without violating any of the laws of logic.

THE CONCEPTS OF ILLNESS AND DISEASE

In physical medicine, the concepts of illness and disease are often not distinguished and are generally thought to be unproblematic. Medicine is preoccupied with problems of specific diagnosis rather than with the idea of illness in general.

By contrast, in psychiatry, the notion of illness has been the subject of fierce controversy. This debate has tended to swing between two extreme positions which can for convenience be labelled **normativism** and **naturalism**.

Strong normativism is the idea that the attribution of mental illness amounts to nothing more than a value judgement based on the transgression of social rules. It is epitomised by the view of Thomas Szasz that so-called mental illness is a myth, because illness implies an abnormality of the body and no such abnormality is present in mental illnesses, which are characterised essentially by 'problems in living'.

Other writers concede that the attribution of disorder, including physical disorder, contains a necessary normative element, but for this to constitute illness or disease, factual criteria must also be satisfied. This might be described as **weak normativism**. Christopher Boorse has argued that **disease** is a matter of fact but **illness** is a matter of value: illnesses are those changes in the organism which we care about because they cause us problems. Thus, for Boorse, illness is a sub-set within the wider category of disease.

This relationship has been reversed by K. W. M. Fulford who argues that our logical starting point is essentially the diagnosis of illness which is value laden: we start by inferring that there is something wrong with the patient, which Fulford calls **action failure** and may or may not then discover organic causes which account for his condition, making it a disease.

Naturalism takes the view that one can define disease in an entirely factual way without using any terms implying judgements of value. R. E. Kendell argued that mental disorders, like physical illnesses, were essentially 'deviations from the biological norm which place the individual at a reproductive disadvantage'. The crucial point for psychiatry is that such deviations are essentially of **function** rather than **structure**. The issue is then whether function and **dysfunction** can be defined in a value-free way. The naturalist's tactic in general has been to argue that words which appear evaluative, such as good, bad, useful, dysfunctional etc, can all be understood in a Darwinian sense as favourable to survival or not and thus can be converted into purely factual terms. Their opponents maintain that even these concepts conceal covert value judgements.

Whatever the merits of these arguments about whether the diagnosis of illness or disease **logically entails** a negative value judgement, there is no doubt that attribution of mental disorder **conventionally implies** one. If the patient's mental state were just descriptively different, it would not constitute a disorder. We diagnose disorder when the patient's altered state is perceived as a problem, which involves an evaluation.

DEFINITION AND CLASSIFICATION

Just as the concept of mental illness in general has been subject to criticism, so has the definition of individual disease entities and their classification, including the two main systems, the fourth edition of the Diagnostic and Statistical Manual of Mental Disorders (DSM-IV) and the International Classification of Disease (ICD-10).

It is a scientific ideal that concepts and their definitions should correspond to entities in the real world, sometimes called **natural kinds**. Such definitions, which try to capture the essence of the thing described, have been called **essentialist**. There are however, difficulties with this idea, because our conception of a natural kind is liable to change with advances in knowledge and the notion of something persisting in the world independently of our shifting conceptions presents problems of how we could know about it. Does the 'real' essence of water, for instance, inhere in its wetness, transparency etc or in the fact that we now know it to be H_2O? If we are to define something **ostensively**, by pointing and naming as we teach words to children, what features are we to point to?

A solution is the principle of an **operational definition**, which is acknowledged to be provisional but heuristically useful, in other words it helps to advance our understanding until it is replaced by something more satisfactory. While our understanding of the fundamental causes of mental disorder remains rudimentary, we are obliged to use definitions of this sort. In so far as they are simply convenient labels or names, one can call this approach **nominalism**, in contrast to **essentialism**.

The aspiration of psychiatric classifiers in recent decades has been to classify by cause where causes are known, but otherwise to construct descriptive, value-free categories which do not assume underlying causes. It is assumed that a system based on such categories will aid the search for causal explanations and that it may need to be modified as such explanations emerge.

Problems arise from the dual character of the classificatory scheme (cause and description), from the fact that there are fundamental differences in the nature of underlying causes (physical, psychological and social) and that the aspiration to be value-free is unrealistic, particularly in view of the social dimension, which is both causal and constitutive of mental disorder (see above).

It is a common error to **reify** disease entities, ie to treat them as real things in the world rather than the provisional concepts outlined above.

PSYCHIATRY AND THE MEDICAL MODEL

Critics of psychiatry have often made the so-called **Medical Model** the target of their strictures. Though there is no universal definition of what constitutes the medical model, it seems to comprise the following elements:

- There is something wrong with the **individual's** mental state.
- The problem is properly construed as one of **illness** or **disease** (see above).
- The issue is primarily a matter of **fact**.

- Scientific medicine provides the best framework of understanding.
- The individual cannot help being the way they are.
- Doctors are best equipped to understand the phenomena.
- Doctors are best equipped to treat the problem.
- The authority of psychiatrists derives from this expertise.

The model thus comprises scientific, moral and social elements which are mutually supportive. These elements are **positivist**, ie based on the assumption that all true knowledge is based on the methods of the natural sciences. All have been called into question by alternative models of mental disorder.

- There has been increasing scepticism, despite the theoretical and practical triumphs of science, that one can delineate a single route to truth called the scientific method, even in the physical sciences.
- Despite the hopes of nineteenth-century positivists, it now seems doubtful that the **social sciences**, which are also fundamental to psychiatry, can ever be reduced to the same terms as the natural sciences. This is not just because of the complexity of the variables involved but is also because the entities studied by social scientists, eg money, marriage or crime, are themselves social constructions imbued with meaning; they are not independent features of the world.
- Social scientists are inclined to see the problems called mental disorders as features of social systems rather than individuals.
- Psychology contains two broad traditions, that of the **objective psychologies**, such as behaviourism and cognitive science, which aspire to the condition of the natural sciences and that of the **subjective psychologies**, such as psychoanalysis, which generally speaking do not, despite Freud's early hopes.
  - In so far as it is concerned with meanings rather than causes, **psychodynamics** has been described as **hermeneutic**, hermeneutics being the study of the interpretation of texts. This links with an increasing interest in **narrative** as a way of understanding the patient's predicament which gives weight to subjective meaning.
  - We all have a '**theory of mind**' and are experts in understanding each other's behaviour in terms of beliefs, desires, intentions and other mental states. Although derided by some as 'folk psychology', this serves us well in daily life and can be seen as the foundation of more sophisticated psychological theories.
- Scientific models of Man are **deterministic**. However, we experience ourselves as **agents**, ie as initiators of **actions** (see above) and attribute agency to others, whether or not we have freedom in any ultimate sense. This continues to be true for people who suffer from mental disorder. Humanistic and existential psychologies stress the importance of **agency** and it is central to any **moral** model of mental disorder. The perception of the afflicted person as **agent** shifts them out of the role of **patient** with its implied passivity. This in turn alters the traditional doctor–patient relationship towards something closer to a partnership of equals.
- Anti-psychiatrists reject the notion of mental illness as a contradiction in terms, eg Szasz (see above). Even more radical is the view that mental 'disorder' is not necessarily a problem at all, except in so far as it is rejected by society. It might even confer benefits such as the gift of special spiritual insight. It is now hard to defend

scientific psychiatry as having a unique, privileged status in the understanding of mental disorder. This is not to accept an uncritical relativism in which anything goes, nor to reject the relevance of physical and biological facts. The aim must be the best 'fit' between the perspectives of patient and professional, taking both facts and values into account.

Some alternative models of mental disorder are:

- psychodynamic
- cognitive
- behavioural
- family and systemic approaches
- humanist/existential
- moral
- sociological, eg deviance and labelling theory
- quasi-medical theories from non-Western healing traditions.

DELUSION, TRUTH AND RATIONALITY

Delusion is of central importance in psychiatry and poses the problem of finding reliable boundaries between rational and irrational thinking and of defining criteria for truth. Both have proved elusive.

For many years, the psychiatric concept of delusion was strongly influenced by the views of the psychiatrist/philosopher Karl Jaspers (1883–1969). He believed that true delusions, which he distinguished from delusion-like ideas, were derived in a radically different way from normal beliefs. According to Jaspers, ordinary beliefs, delusion-like ideas and over-valued ideas are all formed in a psychologically understandable way with which others can empathise. Delusions on the other hand arise **de novo** from a sudden perception of meaning which is unique to the patient and which is not understandable to others. Another way of putting this is to say that delusions imply a special **process** different in kind from normal psychological **developments**. Although the conventional definition of a delusion is a fixed false belief, for Jaspers the truth or falsehood of the idea takes second place to its mode of derivation. In short, delusion is characterised by its **form** rather than its **content**.

Problems arise because not all ideas derived from 'a sudden perception of meaning' are false: they may turn out to be true, as in the classic example of 'pathological' jealousy which turns out to be well founded.

It may be impossible to distinguish sudden creative insights or 'brainwaves' from delusions in Jaspers' sense, because they derive similarly from 'a sudden perception of meaning'. Conversely, there are many people who embrace beliefs, apparently derived in 'normal' ways, which seem to others just as fantastic or absurd as the delusions of psychotics.

Different cultures have radically different ideas of 'reality', eg belief in magic or witchcraft. Although non-veridical in Western terms, these can no longer be dismissed as the products of 'primitive' or 'irrational' thinking.

Within philosophy, there has been progressive disappointment in the hope of a 'sure-fire' epistemology (theory of knowledge) giving certain access to the truth, through reason, logic or experience. Psychology has failed to delineate any specific cognitive fault characteristic of deluded patients and, as we have just seen, there is no clear relationship between the truth or falsehood of beliefs and the way they are derived.

Such difficulties, together with the behaviour of deluded patients, whose actions are often inconsistent with their professed beliefs, have led to the suggestion that delusions are not primarily beliefs at all. Berrios has described them as 'empty speech acts'. What they share with normal beliefs is that they are **reasons for actions** and Fulford has suggested that their salient characteristic is that of being **inadequate reasons for action**. This entails a judgement of value because reasons, as opposed to causes, can be described as right or wrong. The evaluative aspect of delusions is evident in fixed **judgements of value** unacceptable to anyone else (like those in psychotic depression) which we still call delusions though they are not factual beliefs.

ETHICS AND PSYCHIATRY

The main strands of ethical theory are covered in Chapter 10.

Paternalism

The issue of paternalism towards alert, adult patients is peculiar to psychiatry. Up to a point it can be defended on the same grounds as we defend compulsion in the case of children or demented people, ie the absence of **capacity**. In such circumstances, common law sanctions the imposition of treatment on a non-consenting patient on the principle of serving their best interests. However, many patients detained under mental health legislation seem to have capacity, raising the question of whether the ethical basis for their detention is the same as for others. The issue turns on whether delusion and lack of insight are properly regarded as cognitive deficits or as being in a category of their own which entails a special kind of **value judgement**, based on the failure of **rational action** (see above).

Such considerations make psychiatric ethics more extensive than general medical ethics, where the issue of illness is normally considered a matter of fact and values only enter the picture when we are trying to decide what to do about it. An alternative view is that diagnosis always involves an element of value judgement, even in physical disease (see above). The difference is that the value judgements we make in physical medicine generally command wide consensus (eg that pain or death are bad), whereas there is more often room for dissent in psychiatry: what is normally called depression, for example, might be considered 'appropriate' in the context of grief. Judgements often have to be made as to whether emotional reactions are 'excessive', 'disproportionate' or 'inappropriate' to the social context, all of which involve values.

Psychiatric diagnosis

The ethical dimension of psychiatric **diagnosis** means that we have extended moral commitments (obligations) to patients. We need to take account of their framework of values and cultural beliefs, not just to establish that their experiences are descriptively abnormal for their peer group, but to understand how they evaluate them 'from the inside'. This obligation to respect the patient's view of the world takes its place alongside other professional duties such as those of competence, skill, care and confidentiality.

PHILOSOPHY OF SCIENCE

There is no doubting the cognitive and instrumental success of the natural sciences over the past three centuries. Science has made possible a cumulative and coherent body of knowledge which commands consensus and which has enabled powerful prediction and manipulation of the physical world, underpinned by theory.

It has traditionally been held that this success depends on the application of a special scientific method which demarcates science from non-science and which ensures progressive approximation to the truth. The delineation of such a method and its justification as a uniquely valid way of getting at truth (its **epistemology**) has become increasingly controversial. There are questions about the reality of postulated entities which can never be directly observed (eg electrons, quarks or the unconscious): these questions relate to the **ontology** of science, the problem of what is really there. They divide **realists** from **instrumentalists**, who conceive of theories as useful means of ordering and predicting observations rather than approaches to an unseen reality.

In the social sciences and psychology, doubt has been expressed that the methods of natural science can legitimately be applied in areas characterised by meaning, value and subjectivity. There is now a widespread perception that all knowledge is **perspectival**. An observer's position is defined by class, race, gender etc. It is doubtful whether one can realistically aspire to the objective 'view from nowhere' which is science's traditional vantage point.

Induction and deduction

Francis Bacon (1561–1626), the father of scientific method, described the process of **induction**, whereby knowledge is acquired through the collection of large bodies of facts, from which regularities, generalisations and laws are derived. Traditionally contrasted with **deduction**, which starts from general principles and derives conclusions by formal logic.

Induction is an empirical process. English empiricists, such as Locke and Hume, believe that all knowledge is derived from experience. Nevertheless, as Hume pointed out, induction cannot logically guarantee knowledge. The fact that the sun has risen every morning to date makes it highly likely that it will do so tomorrow but cannot make it certain.

Hypothetico-deductive method

Data are gathered in the light of theories and used to test hypotheses. The hypothetico-deductive method formalises this process. From a particular hypothesis deductions are drawn which form the basis for predictions. Experiment or observation then puts these predictions to the test so that they are confirmed or refuted.

Verificationism

Verificationism emphasises the importance of confirming hypotheses. The **logical positivists** held that the meaning of a proposition lay in its means of verification. The only meaningful statements were those provable by logic and mathematics or supported by empirical data from the natural sciences.

Falsificationism

This was introduced by Karl Popper (1902–1994), who pointed out that no amount of positive observations can conclusively confirm a hypothesis, whereas one negative observation can conclusively refute it. The first black swan to be observed overturned the generalisation 'all swans are white', which had apparently been confirmed by all observations up to that point. For Popper, a 'good' theory was one which was amenable to falsification and science proceeded by imaginative conjecture and experimental refutation. The truth can be approached by refining theories through processes of refutation and revision.

The application of such a method need not be confined to the natural sciences and Popper, himself, discussed how the principle of falsification might be applied to the social field. Its application to psychiatry was canvassed by Eliot Slater, among others, and it remains one of the best-known philosophical ideas among psychiatric researchers.

Critics of Popper point out that contrary observations do not, in fact, overturn a theory in the way that he claimed because all theories are underdetermined by data. In short, it is always possible to preserve a hypothesis by questioning other assumptions (eg the accuracy of instruments or the veracity of observers), even though this may lead to far-fetched conclusions. Theories are never tested in isolation but as part of a complex web of mutually supportive ideas.

Abduction

Abduction is a term coined by Charles Peirce (1839–1914), the originator of pragmatism. Abduction accepts a conclusion on the grounds that it best explains the available evidence. This has been called **inference to the best explanation**. The theory of evolution, for example, is not amenable to conclusive confirmation or refutation in our present state of knowledge but appears to fit the observed facts better than rival explanations.

Social constructionism

Knowledge cannot be divorced from social context and relationships, particularly power relationships which play as large a part in 'hard' science as in the social sciences and humanities. This perspectival view was shaped by Marxist theorists of the Frankfurt school and, later, by feminism. It is in opposition to any scientific method, which would claim a monopoly of the truth.

Thomas Kuhn (*The Structure of Scientific Revolutions*, 1963) had a profound effect on our perception of the scientific enterprise. A social historian, he in effect 'sociologised' the scientific method by focusing on how science is actually carried out, rather than its logical justification. Kuhn maintained that, in a given field of enquiry, research proceeds according to a guiding paradigm or accepted theoretical model. This is normal science. Most research results can be fitted into this paradigm, but with time anomalous results accumulate until they cannot be accommodated within it. At this point the paradigm breaks down with a consequent **paradigm shift**, eg the shift from Newtonian to Einsteinian physics or the arrival of plate tectonics in the earth sciences. The new paradigm then becomes dominant until it is overthrown in its turn. The choice of paradigm is not determined by logic or reason and paradigms are therefore incommensurable.

Scepticism about scientific method, expressed most thoroughly in Paul Feyerabend's *Against Method* (1975) is matched by widespread scepticism about the possibility of any absolute foundations for knowledge in general, which finds expression in **Post-modernism** and **Cognitive Relativism**. Anyone acquainted with the successes of science is likely to find such a view unreasonably nihilistic. Nevertheless, the delineation of just how science delivers its results and how they can be justified has proved remarkably elusive.

BRAIN AND MIND IN PSYCHIATRY: THE MAIN PHILOSOPHICAL POSITIONS

Historical theories

Substance dualism

Substance dualism is classically associated with Descartes ('Cartesian'). **Mind** and **Matter**, including body and brain, are conceived as radically different substances, matter being extended in space and multifarious, while mind occupies no space and is unified. Descartes believed that these entities interacted through the mediation of the pineal gland, the only unpaired cerebral structure. A sophisticated version of substance dualism can be found in *The Self and Its Brain* (Popper & Eccles, 1977) but it has few modern defenders.

Property dualism

Mind and **Matter** are not different substances but events referred to in mental or physical terms are so different, descriptively, that we cannot translate one into the other.

Psychophysical parallelism

Mental and physical events proceed exactly in parallel but without any causal interaction between them. This theory originated with Gottfried Leibnitz (1646–1716).

Epiphenomenalism

Mind is real, it arises in virtue of brain activity, but is of no causal relevance. Mind is a mere accessory, comparable to the noise emitted by a machine.

Idealism

All reality is fundamentally mental in nature. This is included, for completeness, as the polar opposite of materialism. It does not sit easily with the modern scientific world view.

Contemporary theories of mind

Materialistic monism

This is the basis of most contemporary theories; it holds that while there may be mental events, descriptively speaking, there is no such thing as a mental substance separable from the brain.

Logical behaviourism

Mental states are best conceived of as dispositions to behave. Thought, for example, is conceived of as inner speech. In *The Concept of Mind* (1949), Gilbert Ryle deployed this model to dispose of such hallowed concepts as the Cartesian ego ('The Ghost in the Machine').

Reductionism

Experiences we call mental are all capable of being expressed in physical terms, rather as the phenomena of heat can be expressed in terms of the kinetic energy of molecules or those of genetics in terms of DNA sequencing.

Eliminative materialism

A more radical position, asserting that mental language and concepts such as belief, desire and intention will eventually be bypassed altogether and consigned to history, together with such notions as phlogiston or the life force. A completed neuroscience will enable us to eliminate mind language altogether in favour of brain language, not merely to translate the former into the latter. Typically the proponents of this view (eg Paul and Patricia Churchland) refer to mental language as 'folk psychology'.

Identity or dual aspect theory

Brain and mind are literally identical, being different aspects of the same thing, perceived respectively from a third-person viewpoint or subjectively from within. Criticised on the grounds that the conscious events referred to in mental language (eg pains or desires) are totally different from the events described when looking at the brain (eg electric discharges or the release of neurotransmitters).

Anomalous monism

This was regarded by its originator, Donald Davidson, as a form of identity theory. Brain states and mind states may be identical but the causal laws which determine a succession of brain states are different from those which lead from one mental state to another. Hence there cannot be lawful relations between them, leading to the label 'anomalous'.

Functionalism

- This is currently the most widely accepted doctrine among cognitive scientists; it is strongly influenced by information technology and artificial intelligence.
- It stresses the programs involved in cognitive processes rather than the 'hardware' which instantiates them.
- In its strongest form it maintains that whether the 'hardware' consists of neurones or artificial components is irrelevant.
- Critics have pointed out that while functionalism can explain cognitive performance, it fails to account for the subjective phenomena of consciousness, sometimes known as **qualia**, eg my own particular experience of seeing a colour.
- John Searle has argued that while functionalism can explain grammar it cannot explain semantics, ie the brain's grasp of meaning.

Such categorical labels do not exhaust the possible positions that can be taken in the **Mind–Brain** debate, nor is it always possible to classify a given theory in such terms. The term 'Mind' has several overlapping implications including the capacity for thought, the fact that mental life is somehow 'about' the world (technically known as **intentionality**), consciousness, the capacity for self-awareness and the special qualities of subjective experience unique to the individual (qualia). A theory may explain some of these attributes but not others.

Some philosophers, eg Colin McGinn and Thomas Nagel, maintain that consciousness is irreducible and will remain mysterious. This position is rejected as defeatist by those such as Daniel Dennett who believe that consciousness can be explained in non-mysterious terms drawn from Darwinian biology and cognitive science.

A BRIEF HISTORY OF MODERN PSYCHIATRY: NAMES, DATES AND EVENTS

Modern psychiatry, its concepts, institutions and techniques, is largely a creation of the past two centuries. The word '**psychiatry**' dates from the 1840s and for several decades thereafter its practitioners were more commonly referred to as 'alienists', ie specialists in those alienated from their reason. Foucault (1926–1984) criticised psychiatry for precluding the possibility of a dialogue with 'unreason' in the wake of the Enlightenment, implying that our modern conception of mental illness is largely the creation of psychiatrists. However, madness has always been with us and a medical model has always had a place alongside moral, psychological and supernatural explanations.

Hippocrates believed that mental disorders had natural causes and advocated humane treatment including rest, exercise and dieting. He classified mental illness into categories that included mania, melancholia and phrenitis.

It is often assumed that during the **Middle Ages** the field was dominated by supernatural theories such as demonic possession. Even then, at least some of the insane were regarded as sick and, like other sick people, were looked after in institutions run by the Church, eg Bethlem Hospital in London (later Bedlam), founded in 1247, and the village of Gheel in Flanders.

Despite the witch craze, there were still physicians who defended naturalistic explanations of mental illness, eg the Swiss **Paracelsus**. At the end of the sixteenth century Johann Weyer argued that witches were actually mentally disturbed people in need of medical treatment.

For many centuries the theory of the four humours, formulated by **Galen**, held sway, giving place in the eighteenth century to the idea of nervous illness. At the beginning of the nineteenth century, the psychoses were generally attributed to psychological causes while the neuroses, as the word literally implies, were thought to be physical affections of the nerves. By 1900, under the influence of organic psychiatrists on the one hand and the early pioneers of dynamic psychiatry on the other, the implications of these categories were almost exactly reversed.

Unfortunately, even when the insane were regarded as sick, they were typically subjected to barbarous and degrading treatment, either in the guise of therapy or simply in attempts to subdue their frenzied and unmanageable behaviour. Modern psychiatry starts with attempts to manage the problem in less punitive and restrictive ways.

- **1789** Vincenzo Chiarugi (Florence): humane management and minimal restraint.
- **1793** Pinel orders the fetters to be struck off the lunatics in the Bicetre Hospital, Paris.
- **1796** The quaker, William Tuke founds the Retreat hospital in York.
- **1843** Dorothea Dix (USA) campaigns for a more humane approach to the mentally ill.
- **1843** Daniel McNaghten acquitted of the murder of Edward Drummond on the grounds of insanity. He is confined in Bethlem and later in Broadmoor.
- **1845** Lunacy Act ushers in the Asylum Era in Britain, replacing private mad-houses.

565

- **1852** Morel (France) makes the first reference to 'dementia praecox'. (Later (1857) he introduces the theory of degeneration, which has dire consequences.)
- **1856** John Connolly at Hanwell describes the abolition of all physical restraints and their replacement by 'moral' (ie psychological) treatment.
- **1863** Kahlbaum describes hebephrenia.
- **1867** Griesinger proclaims that mental illnesses are essentially brain diseases.
- **1869** Beard describes 'neurasthenia'.
- **1895** Freud and Breuer publish *Studies in Hysteria*.
- **1899** Emil Kraepelin's *Textbook* establishes the nosology which will dominate the next century.
- **1907** Alois Alzheimer describes the disease that bears his name.
- **1911** Eugen Bleuler's *Dementia Praecox or the Group of Schizophrenias*.
- **1913** Karl Jaspers' *General Psychopathology*.
    Noguchi and Moore demonstrate spirochaetes in the brains of general paretics.
- **1914–1918** World War One results in thousands of cases of 'shell shock', treated psychologically by W. H. R. Rivers and others.
- **1917** Wagner von Jauregg uses (malarial) fever treatment effectively in general paresis.
- **1919** J. B. Watson's *Psychology from the Standpoint of a Behaviourist*. He goes on to treat 'Little Albert', in whom he has induced an experimental neurosis.
- **1920** Tavistock Clinic opens in London for the treatment of neuroses.
- **1923** Maudsley Hospital is founded.
- **1926** Pavlov publishes *Lectures on Conditioned Reflexes*.
- **1930** Mental Treatment Act allows informal treatment, introduces outpatient services and re-names asylums 'mental hospitals'.
- **1933** Sakel introduces insulin coma for the treatment of schizophrenia.
- Hitler's rise to power uses the idea of degeneration to justify psychiatric euthanasia. The flight of psychoanalysts from Germany and Austria introduces a powerful analytic influence into American psychiatry, which lasts for three decades.
- **1934** Von Meduna uses camphor (later metrazol) to induce therapeutic convulsions.
- **1937** Cerletti and Bini use electroconvulsive therapy for the first time in Rome.
    Egas Moniz performs the first prefrontal leucotomy, leading later to its crude and undiscriminating use by Freeman and Watts in the USA.
- **1939** Joshua Bierer opens the first Day Hospital in London.
- **1939–1945** In World War Two psychiatric expertise is sought on military selection panels and in the treatment of nervous casualties.
    Northfield Experiment (British military hospital) introduces the principles of the Therapeutic Community.
- **1948** National Health Service: all British hospitals come under a single authority.
- **1949** Cade (Australia) discovers the anti-manic effects of lithium, later popularised by Baastrup and Schou in Denmark.
- **1950s** Open Door Policy spreads through British mental hospitals. Therapeutic Community approach is adopted at Dingleton, Fulbourn, Claybury etc.
- **1952** Chlorpromazine is used in France by Delay and Deniker after its discovery by Laborit.
    H. J. Eysenck publishes the first of several sceptical papers on the effects of psychoanalytic treatment.

- **1953** Imipramine is introduced (Kuhn).
- **1955** Mental hospital numbers peak in UK and US, before starting to decline.
- **1958** Joseph Wolpe publishes *Behaviour Therapy by Reciprocal Inhibition*.
- **1960** Thomas Szasz's *Myth of Mental Illness* and R. D. Laing's *The Divided Self* give theoretical impetus to the Anti-psychiatry movement.
- **1961** Tooth and Brooke predict a drastic decline in mental hospital populations; this influences Enoch Powell, who presses for their closure and the transfer of psychiatric beds to District General Hospitals. In the USA, the Report of the Joint Commission on Mental Illness and Health leads to the creation of Community Mental Health Centres (with little effect on major mental illness).
- **1963** Valium (diazepam) is launched.
- **1967** Report of an inquiry into maltreatment at Ely hospital, Cardiff; the first of several mental hospital scandals in Britain.
  Aaron Beck publishes on cognitive theory and therapy of depression.
- **1970** Wing and Brown's *Institutionalism and Schizophrenia* showed the influence of social stimulation on psychotic symptoms.
- **1975** Better Services for the Mentally Ill defines a future pattern of District General Hospital beds supported by community services provided by local authorities. The Butler Report points to inadequate facilities for mentally abnormal offenders and leads to the establishment of medium-secure units.
- **1976** Johnstone and Crowe demonstrate enlarged ventricles in schizophrenia.
- **1978** Influenced by Basaglia and others, Italy passes Law 180 closing its mental hospitals to new admissions, and sets up a new network of community services, with controversial results. Most developed countries pursue a policy of de-institutionalisation with varying degrees of success.
- **1980** DSM-III signals a shift from psychodynamic to descriptive and biological psychiatry.
- **1987** Prozac (fluoxetine) is launched.
- **1988** Kane's trial of Clozapine in treatment-resistant schizophrenia; other 'atypical' neuroleptics follow.
- **1989** Spokes Report into the case of Sharon Campbell (who killed her social worker) highlights the problems of community care and leads to the Care Programme Approach.

Chapter 28

Clinical Information Management

Sarah Price

CONTENTS

Clinical Information Management

CLINICAL GOVERNANCE

Patient care within the National Health Service (NHS) involves many different professionals. Effective clinical governance requires the following:

- adequate and secure record keeping
- information sharing and communication
- access to health records
- confidentiality.

To maintain best practice and clinical effectiveness, it is necessary to have up-to-date evidence-based research. Government NHS Executive initiatives express their aim to give all health professionals 'timely, accurate and appropriate access to the mental health information they need'. Further research and ongoing audit of current practice are also necessary.

HEALTH RECORDS

Anything written by a health-care professional about a person's physical or mental health constitutes a health record. Within mental health services this includes records made by doctors, nurses, psychologists, occupational therapists, art therapists, psychotherapists and physiotherapists.

Paper records

Entries in a patient's notes are the basis of communication between professionals about that patient's care. They may also be referred to by a court as the record of treatments and consultations that have occurred. Records should therefore be:

- clearly written
- dated
- signed (with printed name)
- concise and inclusive.

Note-keeping may vary between disciplines and may involving entries in different sections of a file, or the keeping of separate files. It is important to be familiar with the whereabouts of the various sources of information. Many Trusts now use one file in which consecutive entries are made by all disciplines involved. This gives ease of access to information and helps to minimise duplication.

Currently most hospital records are held on paper, giving rise to various potential problems:

- notes go missing
- duplication of records occurs
- incompleteness
- confidentiality: it is easy to borrow/photocopy notes but a computer system would require a user password
- bulk and storage increases with the increased population having chronic diseases.

Computer records

In contrast, many general practitioners' surgeries now operate a 'paperless' system, entering all records directly onto a computer system. It is an expressed aim of the Government to provide a paperless record-keeping system across the NHS.

Hospital computer systems use the local area network (LAN) to link computers within a department allowing sharing of information and standardisation of certain documents (eg discharge letters to general practitioners). The wide area network (WAN) links all the hospital's computers to a central computer which runs the patient administration system. The patient administration system contains administration software and stores basic details on all patients (name, date of birth, address, general practitioner, hospital number, etc). Other computers in the hospital can extract any of this information through the network.

Data security operates on two levels:

- Each user has an assigned password and access to different files can be restricted to certain users.
- Each workstation (computer terminal) within the network is linked to a file server. This is a centralised computer in which data from all the other computers are stored. The file server is attached to an uninterrupted power system which will keep it running in the event of a power failure. The information generated on all workstations is downloaded to, and stored on, the file server which can be isolated and kept in a secure environment.

Common uses for computer networks in hospitals are:

- managing appointment systems
- communicating pathology results
- providing monthly reports to the Department of Health on activity within the Trust.

Information is often communicated throughout a hospital trust computer network by means of an 'intranet', a system by which small networks can make use of web technology.

SHARING INFORMATION AND DATA SECURITY

Clinicians have a duty to share information with other professionals to provide optimal care and avoid errors. Information must be stored safely and only passed to those who are permitted access. Health-care professionals communicate about patient care by means of:

- entries in notes
- telephone calls
- written letters
- computer data, eg blood results
- fax, email
- information shared in multidisciplinary and Care Programme Approach (CPA) meetings.

Why share information?

Information is shared:

- to deliver optimal care and treatment
- to improve quality of care
- to monitor and protect patient health
- for risk assessment and management
- for teaching, training, research and audit
- at the request of the patient/another
- for disclosure, eg to police/court.

Maximising data security in daily practice

- Passwords and identification are required to gain access to the computer system.
- Identify the person requesting information.
- Attach confidentiality statements to emails, faxes and post.
- Document all information that has been shared and state with whom.
- Do not make computer screens visible to people passing by.
- Limit information written in view, eg whiteboards in Emergency Departments.
- Information is only shared on a 'need to know' basis, giving the minimum needed for the purpose, ie:
  - WHO wants the information?
  - WHY do they need it?
  - WHEN do they need it?
  - WHAT information do they need?
  - HOW should it be shared?

ACCESS TO HEALTH RECORDS

It is good practice to share written information with patients during the course of their treatment. In many cases, Trust policies state that patients should receive copies of all letters written by health-care professionals about their care.

Under the Access to Health Records Act 1990, it is possible for patients to have access to, read, obtain a copy of and be given an explanation of their medical notes. This applies to all records made since 1st November 1991 and any records prior to this that are needed for later records to be properly understood. Patients can apply to have entries in their records corrected should they consider the information to be inaccurate.

Seeking access

Access can be sought by:

- the patient
- an executor for a deceased person
- person(s) acting as parent(s) to a child
- anyone appointed by the court to manage a patient's affairs
- any person who has the patient's written consent.

Withholding information

Information can be withheld if:

- it was obtained from, or relates to a third party where specific consent from the third party for the patient to see that information has not been obtained
- it might lead to serious mental or physical harm occurring to the patient or another person
- it was recorded prior to 1991 (see above).

Caldicott Guardian

The responsibility for ensuring that correct access to health records is available is the Caldicott Guardian. Within each Trust this person is a senior health professional, eg the medical director. They oversee how staff use personal data and ensure that patients' rights to confidentiality are respected. The Caldicott Guardian may delegate responsibility for the management of access to health records to one of the hospital managers.

The process

- Written application for access goes to manager.
- Manager seeks written authorisation from lead clinician involved with that patient's care.

- Manager ensures that material for which access is denied is removed from notes.
- Patient has access to notes, usually in the presence of a health-care professional.

CONFIDENTIALITY

The Declaration of Geneva (1947) established a Common Law duty of confidence with regard to information recorded in patient health-care records. This duty applies even after the patient is dead:

It is generally recognised that, in caring for a patient's needs, information will be shared with other members of the immediate health-care team and that certain other people (eg secretaries typing letters and other administration staff) will also have access to that information. There may also be requests for information from 'staff of other agencies contributing to a patient's care' (Department of Health, 1996). An example would be a request from a housing association for information about a patient who was applying for housing.

It is good practice to inform patients on first meeting about the processes of sharing information, as there can be a tension between the need to share information to maintain quality of care and a patient's expectation that information pertaining to them will be kept confidential. The Common Law duty of confidentiality is based on legal precedent, requiring that 'unless there is a statutory/legal requirement or a sufficiently robust public interest, patient information should only be used for the purposes that the patient has been informed about and has consented to, either implicitly or explicitly.' It is also imperative that patients are made aware that, under certain circumstances, where other moral or legal obligations may become relevant, confidentiality cannot be absolute.

Disclosure to third parties/breach of confidentiality

Records can be disclosed:

- with the patient's consent, preferably in writing. A discussion about the reasons for disclosure is important, furnishing the patient with all the facts about how the information will be used and giving them an opportunity to object. Leaflets in waiting rooms and hospitals with information about situations in which information might be shared are good practice. The Data Protection Act (1998) refers to this as 'fair processing information'.
- where, for whatever reason, the patient is deemed incapable of consenting but sharing the information is deemed to be 'in the patient's best interests'.
- in the interest of others. The doctor has a duty to protect the public (see Table 28.1).

W. vs Egdell, 1990

'Rarely, disclosure may be justified on the grounds that it is in the public interest which, in certain circumstances such as, for example, investigation by the police of a grave or very serious crime, might override the doctor's duty to maintain his patient's confidence'. This case referred to a patient in a special hospital. Dr Egdell prepared a report for a Mental Health Review Tribunal on the instruction of the patient's solicitor and stated that the patient presented a high risk to the public. This opinion was not matched in a report by the patient's RMO. The patient's solicitor decided not to submit Dr Egdell's report to the Mental Health Tribunal but Dr Egdell was so concerned about the patient's risk to the public that he disclosed the report to the hospital authorities without the patient's consent. The judge ruled that in this case the public interest overrode the patient's right to confidentiality.

Tarassof vs Regents of the University of California

In this case, which involved a stalker, the judge ruled that 'If the counsellor knows or has reason to know of probable harm to another identifiable person or the property of another identifiable person, a warning must be issued if the client's behaviour cannot be controlled'.

Table 28.1 'In the interest of others'

Legislation covering disclosure

The following legislation covers disclosure:

- Notification of Births and Deaths NHS Act 1977
- Abortion Regulations 1991
- Notification of Communicable Diseases Public Health Act 1984
- Serious Accidents under the Health and Safety at Work etc Act 1974
- Mental Health Act 1983
- AIDS Control Act 1987
- Prevention of Terrorism Act 1989
- Road Traffic Act 1988
- Children's Act.

Disclosure ordered by the court

Disclosure can be ordered by the court for:

- report to the Judge or Chairman of the Court
- report to the Coroner
- release of information to the police at the order of a Circuit Judge.

Discretionary disclosure

Discretionary disclosure is used:

- when there is risk of serious harm to a third party
- when the patient is at risk of abuse and unable to give consent for disclosure
- when the information relates to a serious crime, eg murder
- when the patient is a health professional and a doctor has concerns over their fitness to practice, that they might pose a danger in relation to patient care
- when fitness to drive is a concern (see Chapter 10).

AUDIT

Audit serves to maintain and improve good practice in health care by comparing clinical care and service provision against standards drawn from evidence-based practice.

A good audit should be:

- short
- simple
- relevant.

Results should be:

- simple
- clear-cut
- practical with regard to implementing change.

Prior to execution an audit proposal should be submitted to the Trust Audit committee and possibly to an Ethics committee.

THE AUDIT CYCLE

It is important to complete the audit cycle which should be a continual process over time to monitor the effects of change.

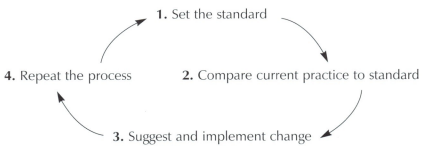

Figure 28.1 The audit cycle

ACCESS TO MEDICAL AND RESEARCH INFORMATION

Over recent years there has been a rapid growth in medical knowledge, particularly in research literature. No longer does medical-school learning form the knowledge-base needed for a lifetime of clinical practice. Textbooks are no longer sufficient. Information is widely available in the plethora of medical journals and, to both doctors and patients, on the world wide web. Today's clinicians are required to be lifelong learners.

Better availability of relevant clinical information serves to improve the treatment of patients and the efficiency of clinical practice. Research shows that requirements for information arise regularly when clinicians see patients. For every patient seen a clinician can generate at least one question:

- usually about treatment, with medication or otherwise
- often complex and multidimensional
- most questions go unanswered
- answers are sought from textbooks or colleagues but both can be inaccurate or outdated
- most questions can be answered from electronic sources.

Evidence-based practice

Hailed as 'bridging the gap between practice and research', evidence-based practice entails using the best evidence currently available when making decisions about the care of patients. Basic elements are as follows:

- define, precisely, a clinical question (eg Is drug X less likely than drug Y to produce extrapyramidal side effects (EPSEs) when used to treat psychosis?)
- structure the question, extracting keywords (X, Y, psychosis, EPSEs)
- search electronic databases (eg Medline, EMBASE, psychlit) using keywords as search terms
- obtain relevant journal articles
- appraise evidence critically (see Chapter 17)
- apply valid, relevant evidence to own clinical practice.

The Cochrane Collaboration

There is much evidence relating to all fields of medical practice, only a fraction of which can be found by an average searcher:

- not all research is published in English
- reviews that have not been prepared systematically may be unreliable
- some of the evidence is unpublished
- some evidence is less easily accessible
- finding and appraising all available evidence is a huge undertaking.

Founded in 1993, the Cochrane Collaboration is an independent, international organisation, giving up-to-date information on valid, reliable medical research.

The Cochrane Library is published quarterly and available on the internet (www.cochrane.org/reviews/clibintro.htm), and on CD-ROM, and is currently the best single source of reliable evidence about health care. It consists of regularly updated databases of evidence-based medicine, including the Cochrane database of systematic reviews. These review the effectiveness of treatments in given situations, allowing immediate access to best current evidence-based practice.

Other resources

Other sources of information are:

- specific journals (eg the *Journal of Evidence-based Mental Health*)
- bulletin boards on various websites. Some useful ones are:
  - www.cebm.net
  - www.bmjjournals.com
  - www.bmjpg.com
  - www.cochrane.org
  - www.nimh.nih.gov
  - www.nice.org.uk
- NICE (National Institute of Clinical Excellence) guidelines (www.nice.org.uk).

Chapter 29

Leading and Managing Service Development and Delivery

Steve Onyett

CONTENTS

Leading and Managing Service Development and Delivery

LEADERSHIP AND MANAGEMENT

Management, or **transactional leadership** (Bass, 1996) emphasises organising and planning the use of resources, dealing with problems as they emerge and monitoring the progress of activities directed at achieving predictable outcomes and specified objectives.

Transformational leadership (Bass, 1996) goes beyond management to encompass challenging the status quo to create new visions and scenarios, initiating new approaches and stimulating the creative and emotional drive in individuals to innovate and deliver excellence. Transformational leadership is associated with the commitment, effort, performance, innovation, harmony and job satisfaction of those being lead; the financial performance of the organisation; and performance in the public sector.

Both leadership for service development ('change that is an improvement') and the management of service delivery are essential.

Charismatic:	Providing highly esteemed **role models**, whom followers strive to emulate, who align others around a vision, common purpose and mission.
Inspirational:	Providing **meaning** and **optimism** about the mission and its attainability.
Intellectually stimulating:	Encourages followers to question basic assumptions, and to consider problems from new and unique perspectives.
Individually considerate:	Works with those being lead, diagnosing their needs; transcends their self-interests, enhances their expectations and **develops their potential**.

Table 29.1 Dimensions of transformation leadership (adapted from Bass *et al.*, 1996)

Many of the qualities highlighted above are also features of clinical practice valued by service users (see commentaries on the recovery approach; eg Stewart, E. & Kopache, R. (2002) *Use of the Ohio Consumer Outcomes Initiative to Facilitate Recovery: Empowerment and Symptom Distress*. http://www.mhrecovery.com/Boston%20Poster%20full%20version%20PDF.pdf).

It is also important to stress that the human qualities that are required for effective service improvement and day to day management overlap considerably: 'the real skill is in **being**

transactional (ie setting objectives, planning, providing feedback, etc) **in a transformational way**' (Alimo-Metcalfe and Alban-Metcalfe).

Studies of leadership qualities

The few studies on how leadership and management behaviours and attitudes translate into valued outcomes for users and carers has been dominated by US researchers, and is based almost exclusively on the study of white males.

In the UK, a factor analytical study of around 1100 National Health Service (NHS) managers and 1500 local government managers highlighted the qualities identified in Table 29.2. As the authors state: 'The emphasis in this model is not on heroism, but on serving and enabling others to lead themselves. It is not about being an extraordinary person, but rather a somewhat ordinary, humble, or at least open, accessible, and transparent individual who displays integrity and consistency' (Alimo-Metcalfe and Alban-Metcalfe).

Leading and developing others	
Genuine concern for others' wellbeing and development	Genuine interest in staff as individuals; values their contributions; coaches and mentors; develops their strengths
Empowers, delegates, develops potential	Trusts staff to take decisions/initiatives on important matters; delegates effectively; develops staff's potential
Accessible, approachable, in-touch	Approachable and not status-conscious; accessible and keeps in-touch
Encourages questioning, and critical and strategic thinking	Encourages questioning traditional approaches to the job; encourages new approaches/solutions to problems; encourages strategic thinking
Personal qualities	
Transparency, honesty, and consistency	Honest and consistent in behaviour; more concerned with the good of the organisation than personal ambition
Integrity and openness to ideas and advice	Open to criticism and disagreement; regards values as integral to the organisation
Decisive, risk-taking	Decisive when required; prepared to take difficult decisions, and risks when appropriate
Charismatic and in-touch	Inspirational; exceptional communicator; inspires others to join them
Analytical and creative thinker	Capacity to deal with a wide range of complex issues; creative in problem solving

Table 29.2 *continued opposite*

Leading the organisation

Inspirational communicator, networker and achiever	Inspiring communicator of the vision of the organisation/service to a wide network of internal and external stakeholders; gains the confidence and support of various groups through sensitivity to needs, and by achieving organisational goals
Clarifies individual and team direction, priorities, and purpose	Clarifies objectives and boundaries; team-orientated to problem solving and decision-making, and to identifying values
Unites through a joint vision	Has a clear vision, which various internal and external stakeholders are engaged in developing; draws others together in achieving the vision
Creates a supportive learning and self-development environment	Supportive when mistakes are made; encourages critical feedback of him/herself and the service provided
Manages change sensitively and skilfully	Sensitivity to the impact of change on different parts of the organisation; maintains a balance between change and stability

Table 29.2 The Alimo-Metcalfe leadership qualities

Leadership in the NHS

The *NHS Leadership Qualities Framework*, being promoted within the NHS, is similar although its evidence base is weaker (see www.NHSLeadershipQualities.nhs.uk).

Personal qualities

Self-belief	The inner confidence that you will succeed and can overcome obstacles to achieve the best outcomes for service improvement
Self-awareness	Knowing your own strengths and limitations and understanding your own emotions and the impact of your behaviour on others in diverse situations
Self-management	Being able to manage your own emotions and be resilient in a range of complex and demanding situations
Drive for improvement	A deep motivation to improve performance in the health service and thereby to make a real difference to others' health and quality of life

Table 29.3 *continued overleaf*

Personal integrity	A strongly held sense of commitment to openness, honesty, inclusiveness and high standards in undertaking the leadership role
Setting direction	
Seizing the future	Being prepared to take action now and implement a vision for the future development of services
Intellectual flexibility	The facility to embrace and cut through ambiguity and complexity and to be open to creativity in leading and developing services
Broad scanning	Taking the time to gather information from a wide range of sources
Political astuteness	Showing commitment and ability to understand diverse groups and power bases within organisations and the wider community, and the dynamic between them, so as to lead health services more effectively
Drive for results	A strong commitment to making service performance improvements and a determination to achieve positive service outcomes for users
Delivering the service	
Leading change through people	Communicating the vision and rationale for change and modernisation, and engaging and facilitating others to work collaboratively to achieve real change
Holding to account	The strength of resolve to hold others to account for agreed targets and to be held accountable for delivering a high level of service
Empowering others	Striving to facilitate others' contribution and to share leadership, nurturing capability and long-term development of others
Effective and strategic influencing	Being able and prepared to adopt a number of ways to gain support and influence diverse parties with the aim of securing health improvements
Collaborative working	Being committed to working and engaging constructively with internal and external stakeholders

Table 29.3 The NHS Leadership Qualities Framework

Effective leadership and management

These frameworks stress the importance of working through others, being able to see the world through their eyes and accept their concerns, agendas and perspectives, and of working with their ideas. Team-working and influencing feature strongly, requiring removal of barriers to communication and innovation, whether between individuals at different levels, different teams and departments, or outside stakeholders and partners. This emphasis on endless reciprocal relationships underpins a shift away from leadership and management being about the behaviours of particular individuals in senior positions, to the creation of organisational cultures in which everyone, including users and their supports, are supported in being as effective as they can be. Thus the explicit link made, for example, in the Leadership Centre's *Effective Teamworking and Leadership in Mental Health* programme, between leadership qualities and the predictors of effective team-working. This is even more important when recognising that the best leadership in organisations rarely resides at the top tier (see below).

Another theme is the encouragement of questioning, challenging of the status quo, and creating new 'mental models'. This requires an environment in which new ideas are truly valued, and the inevitable mistakes are exploited as learning opportunities.

What constitutes effective leadership and management is bound by context and the task at hand. Staff in public sector organisations experience Government's emphasis on a multitude of targets, and an overriding concern with minimising and managing the risks involved in working with complex systems and distressed individuals. At a local level this can make it more difficult to demonstrate the values espoused in the above frameworks, encouraging an archetypal managerial or transactional mode of behaviour. This may also disadvantage women, who are rated as significantly more transformational on most dimensions, regardless of the gender of the rater.

Other key facts about leadership:

- There is a strong association between the leadership style of top managers and the culture of the organisation. This is not always to the good. A review of leadership research in the USA found that regardless of site, 60–75% of employees reported that the worst or most stressful aspect of their job was their immediate line manager. These people will often have advanced on the basis of their competence in transactional rather than transformational leadership. The attitudes of top managers are the most formidable and ubiquitous barrier to successful leadership initiatives.
- Leadership behaviours impacting most strongly on factors that predict effectiveness (eg job satisfaction, motivation, reduced stress) are the areas where managers generally display the poorest performance (Alimo-Metcalfe *et al.*).
- In an analysis of the top three tiers of NHS management (chief executive and board-level managers; non-board-level directors and heads of service, and senior managers), the bottom tier was most transformational and the penultimate tier least transformational.

SERVICE DELIVERY THROUGH TEAMS

A team is: 'three or more people employed by an organisation who see themselves as a group, are seen by others in the organisation as a group and who depend on each other for resources ... to accomplish a task or set of tasks' (Shea & Guzzo).

Most service delivery in the NHS is achieved through some form of team-working. The maxim of form needing to follow function is particularly relevant to teams. A constant question to ask is: 'Is this the most effective way of generating actions that are based upon high-quality decision-making'. Teams should be used when team-working is required.

Effective community mental health teams enjoy (Borrill *et al.*, 2000– see Table 29.4):

- few part-time workers
- positive team climate (vision, high participation, an expectation of excellence and support for innovation)
- a single, clear leader
- relatively low stress levels.

The biggest contributor to poor functioning of teams is unclear team objectives, associated with absence of a clear team leader or co-ordinator or with conflict about leadership.

The left-hand column of Table 29.4 describes those factors that have been shown to be linked to ratings of team effectiveness in the NHS (Borrill *et al.*, 2000). The right-hand column underlines the linkage of these to leadership qualities described above.

Factors promoting effective team-working in the UK public sector	Effective leadership qualities in the UK public sector
Clear, shared objectives with feedback on performance	A clear vision, developed by engaging various internal and external stakeholders. Invests the time to gather information from a wide range of sources.
	Inspiring communicator of the vision of the organisation/service to a wide network of internal and external stakeholders; gains their confidence and support of various groups through political astuteness – being sensitive to their needs.
	Clarifies objectives and boundaries; team-orientated to problem solving and decision-making, and to identifying values.
	Ability to draw people together with a shared vision.
Participation: team member interaction, communication of information, influence over decision-making	Trusts staff to take decisions/initiatives on important matters; delegates effectively. Genuine concern for others' wellbeing, their development and their contribution.

Table 29.4 *continued opposite*

	Accessible, approachable and flexible. Charismatic in staying in close contact with others and encouraging their participation.
Focus on quality: critical evaluation of performance, constructive controversy, commitment to improving quality	Committed to making service performance improvements with a determination to achieve positive outcomes for users.
	Encourages challenges to the status quo. Supports a developmental culture – taking risks and modelling expression of dissatisfaction. Supportive when mistakes are made but holds people to account where required; encourages critical feedback of him/herself and the service provided.
	Analyses and thinks creatively with a wide range of complex issues.
Support for innovation: social support and practical support (time, resources, effort, co-operation)	Leads change through others – engages and facilitates others to work collaboratively to achieve real change.
	Being prepared to take action now.
	Being able and prepared to adopt a number of ways to gain support and influence diverse parties with the aim of securing health improvements.
	Committed to working and engaging constructively with internal and external stakeholders.
	Transparency. That aspect of integrity concerned with honesty and consistency. Placing the good of the organisation above personal gain.

Table 29.4 Factors promoting effective team-working in relationship to leadership qualities

Effective teams are also viable over the long-term. Staff in effective teams have better mental health than those working in looser groups or working individually (perhaps because of greater role clarity, better peer support, and the buffering effect of working in teams against a poor organisational climate or conflict).

The best mental health of team members is found in teams with:

- clarity of objectives
- good participation
- commitment to quality
- support for innovation.

WORKING WITH THE WIDER SYSTEM

Meaningful change needs (Plsek, 2002):

- **leadership**
- **improvement science**: the study and practice of enhancing the performance of processes and systems of work
- **care delivery systems**: the practical realities and future possibilities of how care is experienced by professionals, patients and the public.

Key qualities of a successful service improver (Plsek, 2002) are:

- sees whole systems and any counter-intuitive linkages within them
- brings in the experiences and voice of patients, clients, carers and staff
- seeks to translate evidence into practice
- exposes processes to mapping, analysis and redesign
- applies engineering concepts of flow, capacity, demand, and waste-reduction
- encourages flexible, innovative rethinking of processes and systems
- facilitates active local improvement, innovation and reflective practice
- sets up measurement to demonstrate impact and gain insight into variation
- works constructively with the human dimension of change
- sustains past improvement and drives for continuous improvement
- spreads improvement ideas and knowledge widely and urgently.

Key resources to explore

- **www.nimhe.org.uk** National Institute for Mental Health in England: archive of policies and frameworks, recent publications, downloads of Mental Health Policy Implementation Guide updates.
- **www.doh.gov.uk** Department of Health:
  - click on **Publications** for searches of circulars and press releases
  - **www.doh.gov.uk/mentalhealth/index.htm** for information specific to mental health.
- **www.scmh.org.uk** Sainsbury Centre for Mental Health
- **www.cgsupport.org** The Clinical Governance Support Team
- **www.modern.nhs.uk/improvementguides** The Modernisation Agency has a range of service improvement guides aimed at supporting local services in service improvement. Strategic Health Authorities (StHAs) and some primary-care trusts (PCTs) have Directors of Modernisation, with Service Improvement Managers offering expertise of service improvement techniques. Increasingly such roles are also being created at provider level.
- For more general background on the NHS see *The NHS Explained* on **www.nhs.uk/thenhsexplained/default.asp**

PCTs and commissioning

Commissioning is 'the assessment of health needs, the development of strategies to meet those needs, the purchasing of services for users and the monitoring of the quality of the services provided'.

Shifting the Balance of Power (Department of Health, 2001) continued the drive towards a primary care-led NHS where the resources for the bulk of health service commissioning lies with PCTs. The PCTs catchment population forms the basis around which partnership working, planning and co-ordinated service delivery takes place.

Key players in the PCT are:

- chief executive
- Chair of Professional Executive Committee (usually a general practitioner)
- (lay) Chair of the PCT Board.

The driving force of the PCT is the **Professional Executive Committee**, comprising local clinical staff (general practitioners, community nurses, allied health professionals, senior PCT managers), who are often receptive to other frontline staff and their ideas.

The Professional Executive Committee reports to the **PCT Board**. Without its support direct approaches to the PCT Board are likely to fail. Targeting this group is important in securing additional resources for mental health services.

Specialist commissioning is needed for local processes for bidding for capital developments and commissioning services that require highly specialist skills or serve small, widely dispersed populations with particular needs. This includes prison and secure services, eating disorder services, mother and baby provision, services for people with head injury, sensory impairment, etc. Procedures and protocols ensure that residents with specific needs are properly assessed, responded to, and reviewed (and that connections are maintained with their local supports where possible).

Performance management

The Department of Health is concerned with modernising the NHS and social care, as well as with improving public health. It develops policies, sets standards and monitors performance through inspection bodies such as the **Commission for Healthcare Audit and Inspection** (CHAI: incorporating CHI and some functions of the existing Audit Commission, and Mental Health Act Commission) and the **Commission for Social Care Inspection**, which replaces the Social Services Inspectorate.

The **star-rating system**, giving organisations between zero and three stars according to their performance against key government targets, is the key process for performance-managing PCTs, local authorities and health- and social-care providers. Projects that tie in with improving a star rating will have better prospects than those that do not. Local authorities are also required to conduct regular 'Best Value' reviews for particular care groups. These are intended to secure continuous improvement of the service taking account of efficiency, effectiveness and economy with the needs of service users as the driving force (see www.bvpi.gov.uk).

Another form of performance management specific to mental health is the **local imple-mentation planning** ('traffic lighting') process which has taken place annually since 1999 when the **National Service Framework for Mental Health** was published. Mental health services have their own annual process of **service mapping**, measuring activity across a range of service areas, and **finance mapping** which records the joint actual and intended spend. Service mapping information is available on the Durham University website (follow links from www.doh.gov.uk/servicemapping/) and the social-care benchmarking information is available through www.doh.gov.uk/paf.

Local implementation teams

Local implementation teams were established to drive the implementation of the National Service Framework, meeting the requirements of performance management alongside developing and improving services. They bring together the key players in effective commissioning: PCTs, local authorities, users and their supports, and providers in statu-tory/voluntary sectors.

Local implementation teams vary in their delegated authority to make decisions on behalf of the commissioning agencies (see Cameron, 2003).

Strategic health authorities

Health communities covered by local implementation teams produce **local delivery plans**, with 3-year funding allocations to be agreed by the StHA. The StHA combines the local delivery plans for each PCT to form the **annual delivery plan** for the whole StHA catchment. The StHA will include a manager with responsibility for mental health.

Social-care funding sources

Local authority resources for adult mental health services are:

- **Mental Health Grant** (100% targeted to meet National Service Framework priorities)
- **Mental-Illness-Specific Grant** (70% grant, requiring 30% matched funding from the local authority)
- **Carers' Grant** (aimed at stimulating diversity/flexibility of provision to provide carers' breaks.

Clinical governance

A framework through which NHS organisations are accountable for continually improving the quality of their services and safeguarding high standards of care by creating an envi-ronment in which excellence in clinical care will flourish.

Provides an opportunity for frontline staff to become involved in planning and developing services. For information on clinical governance and the **Clinical Governance Support Team**, go to www.modern.nhs.uk and click on 'clinical governance'.

Corporate governance

System by which an organisation is directed and controlled so as to achieve its objectives and meet standards of accountability and probity. This is achieved in the NHS through **controls assurance** which includes **corporate risk management** and **organisational control** with means to ensure effectiveness of the direction and control.

Other concepts

- **Organisational culture**. The way in which an organisation discharges its business, values staff and clients; the way people within the organisation think, feel and act. Difficult to change but central to effective working.
- **Organisational development**. See www.investorsinpeople.co.uk and www.doh.gov.uk/workdevcon/
- **Human resources management**. Management of workforce, includes:
  - ○ health and safety
  - ○ motivation morale and discipline
  - ○ recruitment
  - ○ working conditions (EEC Working Time Directive).
- **Finance management**. Resource planning, cost estimation, budgeting and control of finances.
- **Resource management**. Process of formal appraisals to identify productivity and areas for improvement.
- **Risk management**. Similar to clinical risk management but reviewing the risks (financial, legal, business etc) to the organisation.
- **Project management**. Process by which all solutions and services are delivered on time and specification.

Other agencies

It is important to investigate the following services in your local area so as to be able to discuss how they function:

- social services
- housing services
- leisure services
- user and carer organisations
- advocacy
- police and criminal justice systems (see Chapter 21).

CLINICIANS WITHIN MANAGED HEALTH-CARE SYSTEMS

Time

Time is the enemy of most clinicians given the requirements of service delivery, planning, CPD, study leave, meetings, college work and the myriad other activities. Inadequate time management can lead to burn-out. Recent initiatives around appraisal, job-planning and working time directives have begun to address some of these. There is an expectation that all new consultants will have access to a mentor who will help with time management among other issues.

Meetings management

Effective meetings have

- a clear purpose
- members who can contribute
- an agenda circulated in advance
- a descriptive, prioritised and timed agenda
- a minute-taker who is not the chair
- participants who respect each other and participate
- a clear chairman who facilitates discussion, sums up and generates actions
- brief minutes, highlighting actions and circulated promptly.

Problems can be:

- non-participation
- offering premature 'solutions'
- dominating personalities
- individuals with hidden agendas or 'hobby-horses'.

Styles of management can be:

- advisory
- bargaining
- collegiate
- commanding
- committee.

Personal responsibility and accountability

The responsibilities of doctors are covered by the General Medical Council (www.gmc-uk.org).

Training and RITA process

Details can be found in a PDF version of the Royal College of Psychiatrists' Trainees' Handbook, which can be downloaded from www.rcpsych.ac.uk.

Avoiding burn-out

Burn-out among senior psychiatrists is being recognised, belatedly, as a serious issue. Factors such as work stress, lack of facilities, emotional pressure, time pressure, threats of inquiries, loss of research time, lack of job satisfaction etc, contribute to a picture of stress symptoms, emotional difficulties, avoidance of the work situation and interpersonal difficulties, possibly leading to mental illness.

Strategies to avoid burn-out include job planning to ensure that the work is appropriate, moving jobs occasionally, ensuring study and research time is taken, sabbaticals, adequate staffing levels and non-punitive methods for dealing with adverse incidents.

Role of Royal College of Psychiatrists

The 'College' is the professional and educational body for psychiatrists in the UK and Republic of Ireland. Full details of its activities can be found on www.rcpsych.co.uk.

Its history is as follows:

- **1841**. Association of Medical Officers of Asylums and Hospitals for the Insane (became the Medico-Psychological Association) was formed.
- **1926**. This received the Royal Charter to become the Royal Medico-Psychological Association.
- **1971**. It received a supplemental Charter to become the Royal College of Psychiatrists.

It aims:

- to advance the science and practice of psychiatry and related subjects
- to further public education in psychiatry and related subjects
- to promote study and research work in psychiatry and all science, disciplines connected with the understanding and treatment of mental disorder in all its forms and aspects and related subjects and to publish the results of all such study and research.

(See www.rcpsych.ac.uk/college/about.htm)

FURTHER READING

This chapter has contained only a flavour of the many ideas and influences in NHS leadership management. In addition to the above websites, the following will help the reader to obtain a fuller understanding of these areas:

Alimo-Metcalfe, B. M. & Alban-Metcalfe, R. J. 2001. 'The development of a new transformational leadership questionnaire.' *Journal of Occupational and Organizational Psychology*, 74, 1–27.

Bass, B. M. 1997. *Transformational leadership*. Lawrence Erlbaum Associates.

Cameron, M. 2003. *Community renewal and mental health*. London: Kings Fund & NIMHE.

Department of Health. 2001. *Shifting the balance of power within the NHS*. London: Department of Health.

Lester, H. 2002. *The organisational development needs of PCTs in mental health commissioning and service provision*. Interdisciplinary Centre for Mental Health, University of Birmingham.

Onyett, S. R. 2003. *Teamworking in mental health*. (especially chapter 8) Basingstoke: Palgrave.

Plsek, P. 2002. *Framework for the Leading Modernisation Programme* (LMP). London: Modernisation Agency.

Scally, G. 1998. 'Clinical governance and the drive for quality improvement in the new NHS in England.' *British Medical Journal*, 317, 7150, 61–65.

Shea, G. P. 1987. 'Groups as human resources.' *Research in Personnel and Human Resources Management*, 5, 323–356.

Chapter 30

Cross-cultural Psychiatry

Sanju George

CONTENTS

Cross-cultural Psychiatry

CONCEPTUAL FRAMEWORK

Cross-cultural psychiatry can be defined as 'the study of the relationship between psychiatric disorders, psychological traits and characteristics of people, the cultures and societies they come from and the interaction between various factors arising from this'.

Cross-cultural studies, over the last few decades, have investigated:

- cultural variations in psychiatric disorders
- disorders unique to specific cultures (**culture-bound**)
- the cross-national validity of Western diagnostic categories
- designing culture-sensitive and valid assessment and diagnostic instruments.

Cultural factors are increasingly acknowledged to be important in the genesis of psychiatric symptoms, illness behaviour, symptom presentation, help-seeking behaviours, pathways to care and psychological and pharmacological treatments of mental illnesses. From a practical perspective, it is ever more important in today's multicultural society that mental-health professionals are in tune with the cultural beliefs and attitudes of patients and families.

Definitions of key concepts

- **Culture**: 'an organised group of ideas, habits and conditioned responses shared by members of a society'.
- **Race**: 'differences in the inherited (ie genetic) constitution of different groups within a species'.
- **Ethnicity**: 'the sense of belonging that binds certain individuals together' or 'a psychological sense of belonging, often cemented by similarities in physical appearance or social behaviour'.
- **Racism**: 'the belief that there is an inherent connection between perceived hereditary and cultural traits and that some groups are biologically superior to others'.
- **Prejudice**: 'the negative attitudinal and emotional set against an individual or group based on selected social or cultural characteristics'.
- **Culture shock**: 'occurs when the psychological cues that help an individual to function in society are withdrawn and replaced by new ones'. It is also defined as 'that terrible longing to be back home, to walk into that corner drugstore, to visit one's relatives and in general, to talk to people who really make sense' (Oberg, 1954).
- **Acculturation**: 'a cultural change, initiated by two or more cultural systems, whereby an individual selectively adopts cultural values from another culture (which tends to be dominant)'.

- **Racial discrimination**: 'attitudes and practices that are explicitly hostile to and denigratory towards people defined as belonging to another race'. Responses to discrimination include avoidance, aggression and acceptance.

Ethnic groups in the UK

Britain has a large and diverse ethnic population of around 5 million (8% of the British population). The approximate composition of the various ethnic groups is shown in Table 30.1.

White	92.1%
Indian	1.8%
Pakistani	1.3%
Bangladeshi	0.5%
Other Asian	0.4%
Black Caribbean	1.0%
Black African	0.8%
Black Other	0.2%
Chinese	0.4%
Other	0.4%
All minority ethnic groups	7.9% (4.6 million)
Total	100% (around 60 million)

Table 30.1 The approximate composition of the various ethnic groups according to the 2001 census

Geographical distribution

The geographical distribution within the UK of its ethnic population is:

- African and Caribbean predominantly in inner London
- Indian community in outer London (one-third), West Midlands and Leicestershire
- majority of Pakistanis in West Midlands and West Yorkshire.

MIGRATION, MIGRANTS AND REFUGEES

Migration is the process of social change whereby an individual moves from one cultural setting to another for the purposes of settling down either permanently or for a prolonged period.

Migrants migrate of their own choice and are more prepared, psychologically and practically, for the move.

Refugees are forced to flee to another country for their own safety and the whole process is usually unplanned and more difficult.

Motives for migration

People decide to migrate for a variety of reasons: social, political, economic, etc.

These motives for migration have been broadly grouped into 'push-factors' (the person is forced to leave one country as a result of social/economic/political problems) and 'pull-factors' (the person is attracted to move out of a country into another for positive reasons and/or aspirations).

Migration tends to be a stressful life event and can lead to a range of mental disorders.

Classification

Migrants have been classified into exiles, gastarbeiters and settlers.

- **Exiles** are those who flee their own country and seek refuge in a foreign country.
- *Gastarbeiters* are migrant workers who migrate from one place to another (usually rural to urban or underdeveloped to industrialised) in search of work.
- **Settlers** are different in that they move into a new country with the intention of settling there for good.

Despite such attempted distinctions, migrants do not always fit clearly into one category and may move from one to another.

Phases of migration

The process of migration can be conceptualised as occurring in three phases:

- **pre-migration**: the individual or family plans and prepares for the move
- **migration**
- **post-migration**: the individual attempts to integrate into the new country and is exposed to a range of positive and negative life experiences.

Mental health assessment of migrant and refugee patients

Points to explore when assessing the mental health of migrants and refugees include:

- reasons for migration
- pre-migration experiences
- reception by host society
- social support
- coping strategies
- employment/financial situation
- racial life events
- self-esteem
- cultural identity.

MENTAL ILLNESSES IN MIGRANT AND REFUGEE POPULATIONS: THE UK PERSPECTIVE

Some consistent findings have emerged in this area, a few of which are listed in the following sections.

Schizophrenia

The prevalence of schizophrenia in Britain's Afro-Caribbeans is 2–14 times that of Whites. Similar findings are seen in migrants from the Antilles to Holland, and in Norwegian migrants to the USA.

This migrant group also tends to have a relatively poorer outcome of schizophrenia, with more hospital re-admissions and more residual symptoms.

Though not unequivocal, it has been found that the rate of schizophrenia among Asians in Britain is the same as in Whites.

Various hypotheses have been put forward to explain the higher rates of schizophrenia among the British Afro-Caribbean population:

- racial discrimination
- misdiagnosis, methodological fallacies of these studies
- higher rates of social/economic deprivation
- higher rates of schizophrenia in the originating country
- those people with schizophrenic illness are predisposed to migrate.

None of the above explanations, on their own, satisfactorily explain this finding and research is ongoing.

Deliberate self-harm/suicide in Asians in the UK

Asian women have higher rates of attempted and completed suicide than Whites. The most often stated reason for the higher rates of deliberate self-harm and suicide in young Asian women is culture conflict.

Compared to the national average, Asian and Afro-Caribbean men have lower rates of suicide.

Higher suicide rates have also been found among the Irish in the UK.

Substance misuse

As in Whites, **cannabis** is the major illicit drug used by Afro-Caribbeans and young Asian men in Britain.

In the Somali community, **khat** use is particularly prevalent (khat is legal in Britain).

Akin to khat use by Somalis, Indians (especially older men), tend to chew **betel nuts/leaves** (not illegal in India or UK).

Alcohol consumption and alcohol-related problems are less among Afro-Caribbeans in the UK, compared to their White counterparts (similar findings are reported in men and women).

Sikh men were found to drink as much as, or more than, White men in the UK, and more than any other group. They tend to drink alone and are over-represented in alcohol-related hospital admissions as compared to White and Caribbean-born men.

The '**Pakistan holiday habit**' describes the fact that young men, while on holiday in Pakistan, pick up the habit of **heroin** use which, it is believed, later leads to heroin-dependence on their return to the UK.

Eating disorders

There are limited data available on the prevalence of eating disorders in migrant groups in the UK. Studies have found a higher prevalence of **bulimia nervosa** among second-generation Asian girls and a higher prevalence of **anorexia nervosa** among Egyptian girls in the UK.

Forensic psychiatry and ethnic minorities in the UK

An often quoted, and as yet incompletely understood finding is the over-representation of Afro-Caribbeans in the Criminal Justice System and Forensic psychiatry services in the UK. Possible explanations include:

- inherently increased crime rates in this group
- higher rates of socio-economic deprivation
- racial discrimination and stereotyping
- methodological artefacts.

UK research findings on this include the following:

- Among the prison population, Blacks were more likely to have psychotic disorders and less likely to have a diagnosis of personality disorder, neurosis and substance misuse (hard drugs) than Whites.
- There are more Afro-Caribbeans than Whites (with psychiatric disorders) presenting via the police, in secure psychiatric units and in prisons as mentally disordered offenders.
- Afro-Caribbeans tend to be diverted from custody less often and hence tend to be transferred to prison and inevitably then to hospital under part 3 of the Mental Health Act.
- Afro-Caribbean people are over-represented among psychiatric admissions with more being compulsorily detained under the Mental Health Act.
- Afro-Caribbean men were up to 25 times more likely (than Whites) to be detained under part 3 of the Mental Health Act.
- 20–30% of the population of regional and high security units are from ethnic minorities, most of them Afro-Caribbeans. Most Afro-Caribbean patients in Regional Secure Units and high-security units are detained with a diagnosis of schizophrenia. Fewer of them are given a diagnosis of psychopathic disorder as compared to Whites.

CULTURE AND SCHIZOPHRENIA

Schizophrenia and other psychiatric disorders exist all over the world, although its presentation could be modified by culturally determined factors. Since Kraeplin found cases similar to dementia praecox in Java at the beginning of the last century, cross-cultural research in schizophrenia has come a long way.

First, we will look at the two most important international studies on schizophrenia (World Health Organisation projects) and then focus on the cultural facets of epidemiology, phenomenology and outcome of schizophrenia and finally, look at some of the methodological limitations in such cross-cultural studies.

Cross-cultural studies in schizophrenia

The international pilot study of schizophrenia (IPSS, 1973).

The IPSS was an international, multi-centric epidemiological study of 1202 patients in nine countries (China, Columbia, Czechoslovakia, Denmark, India, Nigeria, former Soviet Union, UK and the USA). The main aims of the project were:

- to lay the foundations for future international epidemiological studies of schizophrenia
- to evaluate whether schizophrenia, as diagnosed by various psychiatrists across these cultures, would have similar signs and symptoms and, finally,
- to test the feasibility of such large-scale projects.

Its key findings were that:

- such a large-scale, multi-centric, international epidemiological study was feasible
- standardised instruments could be developed across all countries and investigators in these centres could be appropriately trained to make comparable assessments
- patients diagnosed with schizophrenia were similar across various centres (using a narrow definition of schizophrenia).

Follow-up of the original cohort demonstrated better overall outcome (clinical and social) for patients in developing countries compared to developed countries.

The study of determinants of outcome of severe mental disorders (DOSMeD)

This World Health Organisation co-ordinated international project was launched in 1978 to overcome some of the methodological limitations of the IPSS. It studied 1379 patients across 12 centres in 10 countries (six centres had participated in the IPSS study). Patients were recruited early in the onset of psychosis and half of the sample satisfied narrow diagnostic criteria for schizophrenia (CATEGO S+) and half met the broad definition of schizophrenia (CATEGO S, P, O).

The key findings were that:

- the incidence of narrowly defined cases of schizophrenia was similar across cultures and generally speaking these patients were very similar.

- patients from developing countries had better courses and outcomes of illness (on 2- and 5-year follow-up) than patients from developed countries.
- apart from the type of centre (developing vs developed), the only other significant determinant of outcome was the type of onset of psychosis (acute onset cases had better outcome than insidious onset cases).
- expressed emotion was shown to be a cross-culturally applicable concept and expressed emotion levels were lower in developing countries than developed ones.

Cross-cultural schizophrenia research: epidemiological findings

Studies have consistently found similar incidence and prevalence rates for schizophrenia across various parts of the world (range 1–2 per 1000 population).

No differences have been found in prevalence rates between developed and developing countries.

Cross-cultural schizophrenia research: phenomenological findings

- Schizophrenic symptoms and subtypes are broadly similar across cultures, but there are important differences as well.
- Delusions of the persecutory, grandiose and bizarre subtypes are more common among Asians and Africans.
- First-rank symptoms are reported to be less prevalent in non-Western societies.
- Paranoid schizophrenia was the commonest subtype in Western countries, whereas, catatonic and acute schizophrenic episodes were the commonest subtypes in developing countries.
- The positive–negative sub-syndromes of schizophrenia have been found in India, China and Nigeria, and are similar to those in the West.

Methodological limitations

Cross-cultural studies (especially the multi-centre, multi-national projects) are extremely difficult to conduct and are labour- and time-intensive. Despite deserving much credit, these projects have also been heavily criticised for methodological deficiencies, some of which include:

- a tendency to look for similarities rather than differences
- failure to incorporate potentially confounding cultural variables in the design of studies that evaluated the outcome of schizophrenia
- differing dropout rates across centres
- sample selection techniques, reliability of diagnosis
- cross-cultural validity of instruments (like the Present State Examination) and concepts (like expressed emotions) that originated in the West.

CULTURAL FACTORS IN PSYCHOPHARMACOLOGY

Cross-cultural psychopharmacology can be defined as 'the special area of pharmacology that deals with the variations in psychotropic drug responses in different populations and the contribution of pharmacological factors to such variations'.

Several interacting factors need to be considered in evaluating the role of culture in psychopharmacology.

Cultural influences

The range of culturally influenced social and environmental factors contributing to ethnic differences in response to drugs include:

- demographic factors: eg age, gender, race
- pharmacogenetic factors: eg enzymatic differences
- dietary factors/habits: eg diet, smoking, caffeine and alcohol intake, other drugs
- sociocultural factors: eg alternative treatment models, health and illness beliefs and explanatory models and expectations of treatment.

Pharmacogenetics: enzymatic differences

Cytochrome P450

The cytochrome P450 enzyme system, which has more than 20 isoenzymes, each coded for by a specific gene, plays a key role in the metabolism of various psychotropic medications.

- The proportion of **CYP 2Cmp** poor metabolisers in the population varies with ethnicity:
  - Whites, 3%
  - African-Americans, 18%
  - Asian and Japanese, 20%.
- **CYP 2D6** activity (involved in the oxidative metabolism of tricyclic antidepressants, selective serotonin reuptake inhibitors, typical antipsychotics, risperidone and clozapine) is lower in Asians compared to Whites.
- As compared to 3–5% Whites (poor metabolisers of **CYP2 C19**), 20% of East Asians are poor metabolisers.

Acetylation polymorphism

The rate of acetylation (rapid or slow) influences the metabolism of psychotropic medications and this varies considerably across ethnic groups:

The percentage of slow acetylators is:

- Asians, 5–20%
- African-Americans, 50%
- Whites, up to 65%.

ADH and ALDH polymorphism

Alcohol dehydrogenase (ADH) and aldehyde dehydrogenase (ALDH) enzyme activity varies across different cultures:

- 80–90% of Asians are extensive metabolisers with respect to a form of alcohol dehydrogenase (ADH2)
- 50% of Chinese and Japanese are deficient in ALDH (hence their low tolerance for alcohol); they have a high risk of rapid accumulation of acetaldehyde and a low risk of becoming dependent on alcohol.

Ethnic differences in therapeutic response and side-effects

Antipsychotics

- Asians were found to require lower doses of antipsychotics (in treatment of schizophrenia) and were more prone to extrapyramidal side-effects than Whites.
- Asian Americans have been shown to have higher blood levels of haloperidol and a larger prolactin response as compare to Whites.
- A shorter duration of peak plasma levels of haloperidol was demonstrated in Asians as against Whites.

Antidepressants

- Asians (compared to Whites) have higher plasma levels of tricyclic antidepressants, plasma peak levels are reached earlier (possibly because of slower hydroxylation) and clearance rates are slower.
- Asian, Chinese and African-American depressed patients were found to respond to lower doses of tricyclic antidepressants than Whites.
- African-Americans seem more prone to delirium (as a side-effect of tricyclic antidepressants) than other ethnic groups.
- African-American patients had 50% higher plasma nortryptilline levels than Whites.

Lithium

- African-Americans and Asians need lower doses of lithium than Whites (0.5–0.7 mEq/L vs 0.8–1.2 mEq/L).
- African-Americans as compared to Asians and Whites were noted to have a longer half-life of lithium and a higher red blood cell : plasma ratio (probably as a result of a deficiency in the Li–Na counter-transport protein).
- African-Americans are more prone to lithium-induced side-effects than Whites on similar doses.

Treatment compliance

Non-compliance to psychotropic medication is a major problem in psychiatric practice, with reported rates ranging from 20 to 80%.

A range of factors have been proposed to explain non-adherence to medication, among which the culturally relevant ones are:

- health beliefs of the patient
- clinician–patient relationship
- concurrent use of 'alternative medicine'
- diet
- placebo effect
- social support
- religious beliefs
- familial/societal attitudes.

A 2-year follow-up study of over 400 patients in South Africa showed varying rates of non-compliance for pharmacotherapies among different ethnic groups:

- Blacks, two-thirds
- Asian-Indian, one-half
- Whites, one-quarter.

Variations in placebo response to antidepressant treatment were demonstrated in a study in which Columbian patients responded better to placebo than did Whites and African-Americans.

With regards to compliance with psychotherapy, contrary to a commonly held notion, there is no specific evidence that 'ethnic-matching' of patient and therapist improves acceptance of therapy.

If patients fail to understand the rationale behind the specific model of psychotherapy, it can lead to non-acceptance of treatment.

Behavioural therapies have been noted to be more acceptable across cultures than psychoanalytical models of psychotherapy.

CULTURE-BOUND SYNDROMES

Long before the concept of culture-bound syndrome, as we understand it today crystallised, there were descriptions of these disorders. In 1770, Captain Cook described 'Amok'; 'Latah' was first noted by W. G. Ellis in a Singapore asylum in the late nineteenth century and Bonk, in 1895, described 'Koro' in Chinese living in Indonesia. The modern concept of culture-bound syndromes was first proposed by Yap in the 1950s.

The fourth edition of the Diagnostic and Statistical Manual for Mental Disorders (DSM-IV) defines culture-bound syndrome as 'recurrent, locality-specific patterns of aberrant behaviour and troubling experience that may or may not be linked to a particular DSM IV category'.

Anorexia nervosa, obesity and type A behaviour pattern have been proposed by some authors as Western culture-bound syndromes.

Exclusively 'Western' treatments (ie pharmacological interventions, psychotherapy etc) appear to have a limited role as compared to traditional folk-healing techniques. Results are better when these inputs are combined in a harmonious way to incorporate unique aspects of the patients' own culture and the families' and societies' culture-specific views of normality and illness.

Individual syndromes

- **Amok** is most commonly seen in young to middle-aged Malayo-Indonesian men. It is a dissociative episode, often preceded by a period of brooding or dysphoria and characterised by random, destructive, aggressive and even homicidal acts. This episode usually terminates in suicide or prolonged deep sleep. It has been found in association with acute and chronic psychosis and organic conditions like epilepsy, malaria and syphilis. Similar syndromes have been reported in Japan (**Imu**) and the USA (**Whitman syndrome**).

- **Koro**, or 'genital shrinking syndrome', is seen in South-East Asian men (rarely in females as a fear of retraction of nipples or labia). It is characterised by a sudden onset of intense anxiety and panic and a fear of retraction of penis into the abdomen and a fear of sterility and death. It is usually short-lasting and self-limiting and can, rarely, occur in epidemics. Patients (or they may get others to do it) may hold on to the penis and in some cases even apply clamps and strings to prevent retraction. In Chinese medicine, it is believed to be the result of a deficiency of 'Yang' and an excess of 'Yin', while psychoanalysts view this as Oedipal castration anxiety.

- **Latah** is a culture-bound syndrome of Malays and South-East Asians; it is more common in middle-aged females of lower socio-economic status. Its chief symptoms include an exaggerated startle response, echopraxia, echolalia, command obedience, coprolalia, hyper-suggestibility and trance-like behaviour. It is usually triggered by unexpected visual perceptions, touching, tickling etc. Synonyms for this syndrome include **Menkeiti** (Siberia), **Baah-ji** (Thailand) and **Silok** (Philippines).

- **Dhat** is mostly seen in young Indian men. Presenting symptoms are weakness, fatigue, poor concentration, vague somatic complaints, anxiety/dysphoria and guilt about masturbation. Patients attribute these symptoms to imagined loss of semen/sperm in urine. Dhat syndrome is also known as **Shen-K'uei** (China) and **Sukra prameha** (Srilanka).

- **Pibloktoq**, also known as 'Arctic Hysteria', is described in Arctic Eskimos (mostly in young women). It is characterised by a prodromal phase of brooding and confusion, followed by an episode of violent excitement (lasting about 30 minutes), with the patient tearing off clothing, rolling in snow, dangerous behaviour and coprophagia. The episode usually terminates in seizures and coma (lasting up to 12 hours). The aetiologies proposed are physical deprivation, psychological factors and hypervitaminosis A.

- **Brain fag** was first described by Prince in Nigerian students. It is more common in males and is now seen in West African students at home and abroad. Chief complaints include general bodily aches, difficulties in thinking, concentrating and remembering, fatigue, eye pain, excessive tearing and excessive sleepiness. It is believed to be the result of the stress of the Western educational style and overlaps considerably with anxiety and depressive syndromes.

- **Hwa-byong** is seen mainly in Korea and means 'illness of anger' (repressed). The major complaints include pressure in the chest, mass in the epigastrium, insomnia and fear of impending death.
- **Ataque de Nervious** is seen in Puerto Ricans and Latinos. It means 'attack of nerves' and is most common in women aged over 45. It is precipitated by grief and other acute stressful life events and is characterised by uncontrollable shouting, trembling, dizziness, bodily aches and a range of emotional symptoms.
- **Shenjing Shuairuo** is reported only in mainland China. In Chinese, Shenjing means 'nervous system' and Shuairuo means 'weakness'. It presents with symptoms akin to neurasthenia, such as tiredness, poor concentration, loss of sleep and appetite, headaches and irritability.
- Other culture-bound syndromes include: **Falling out**, **Windigo psychosis**, **Susto**, **Zar**, **Ghost sickness**, **Bilis**, **Colera**, **Spell**, **Rootwork**, **Locura** and **Mal de ojo**.

FURTHER READING

Bhugra, D. & Bhui, K. 2001. *Cross-cultural psychiatry: A practical guide*. London: Arnold.

Bhugra, D. & Cochrane, R. 2001. *Psychiatry in multicultural Britain*. London: Gaskell.

Fernando, S. 2002. *Mental health, race and culture*. New York: Palgrave.

Foster, G. M. 1973. *Traditional societies and technological change*. New York/London: Harper and Row.

Gaw, A. C. 2001. *Concise guide to cross-cultural psychiatry*. Washington, DC: American Psychiatric Publishing, Inc.

Leff, J. 1988. *Psychiatry around the globe*. London: Gaskell.

Rack, P. 1982. *Race, culture and mental disorder*. London and New York: Tavistock/Routledge.

Cross-cultural psychiatry papers in *Advances in Psychiatric Treatment* (1997–2003) *Cultural Psychiatry: International Perspectives*. (Sept 2001). The Psychiatric Clinics Of North America.

Selected Bibliography

Alimo-Metcalfe, B M. & and Alban-Metcalfe, R J. 2001. 'The development of a new transformational leadership questionnaire.' *Journal of Occupational and Organizational Psychology*, 74, pp 1–27.

Baddley, A D. & Hitch, G J. 1974. 'Working memory.' In G H Bower (ed). *The psychology of learning and motivation: Advances in research and theory*, Vol 8. New York: Academic press.

Bandura, A. 1963. 'Influence of models' reinforcement contingencies on the acquisition of imitative responses.' *Journal of Personality and Social Psychology*, 1, pp 859–595.

Bandura, A. 1977. *Social learning theory*. Prentice Hall. Upper Saddle River, New Jersey.

Bass, B M. 1997. *Transformational leadership*. Lawrence Erlbaum Associates. New Jersey.

Bowlby, J. 1952. *Attachment and loss*. Vol 1 *Attachment*. Hogarth Press, London.

The British Psychological Society. 1998. *Code of conduct, ethical principles & guidelines*. The BPS Society, Leicester.

Broadbent, D. 1958. *Perception and communication*. Pergamon.Oxford, England.

Brown, G W. & Harris, T O. 1978. 'Life-events and psychiatric disorders. 1.Some methodical issues.' *Psychological Medicine*, 3, pp. 74–87.

Bruner, J S. & Goodman, C D. 1967. 'Value and need as organising factors in perception.' *Journal of Abnormal and Social Psychology*, 42, pp. 33–44.

Cameron, M et al. 2003. *Community renewal and mental health: Strengthening the links*. King's Fund and NIMHE. London.

Cattell, R B. Eber, H W. & Tatsuoka, M M. 1970 *Handbook for the Sixteen Personality Factor Questionnaire*. Champaigne, IL: Institute for Personality and Ability Testing.

Cooper, P J., Murray, L., Wilson, A., & Romaniuk, H. 2003. 'Controlled trial of the short- and long- term effect of psychological treatment of post-partum depression. 1. Impact on maternal mood.' *British Journal of Psychiatry*, Vol 182, pp. 412–419.

Costa, P T & McCrae, R R. 1992. 'Four ways five factors are basic.' *Personality and Individual Differences*, 13(6), pp. 653–665.

Crick, F. & Mitchison, G. 1983. 'The function of dream sleep'. *Nature,* vol. 304. pp. 111–14.

Crowder, R G. 1976. *Principles of learning and memory*. Lawrence Erlbaum Assoc Inc., Hillsdale, NJ, USA.

Cameron, M. 2003. *Community renewal and mental health: Strengthening the links*. King's Fund & NIMHE, London.

Department of Health. 2001. *Shifting the balance of power within the NHS*. Department of Health, London.

Evans, J. Heron, J. Francomb, H. *et al*. 2001. 'Cohort study of depressed mood during pregnancy and after childbirth.' *British Medical Journal*, vol. 323, pp. 257–60.

Falloon, I. 1988. *Handbook of behavioural therapy (The caring professions*. Taylor & Francis Books Ltd., London.

Foucault, M. 1965. *Madness and civilisation*. New York: Random House, New York, NY, USA.

Foucault, M. 1976. *The Birth of the clinic*. Tavistock, London.

Foulkes, D. 1990. 'Dreaming and consciousness.' *European Journal of Cognitive Psychology*, vol. 2, pp. 39–55.

Friedman, T. & Gath, D. 1989. ' The psychiatric consequences of spontaneous abortion.' *British Journal of Psychiatry*, vol. 155, pp. 810–30.

Gibson, J J. 1966. *The senses considered as perceptual systems*. Houghton Mifflin, Boston, MA, USA.

Gregory, R L. 1970. *The intelligent eye*. McGrawHill, New York, NY, USA.

Hobson, J A. & McCarley, R W. 1977. 'The brain as a dream state generator: An activation synthesis hypothesis of the dream process.' *American Journal of Psychiatry*, vol. 134, pp. 1335–48.

Kanner. 1943. 'Autistic disturbances of affective contact.' *Nervous Child*, vol. 2, pp. 217–50.

Kinsey, A. Pomeroy, W. & Martin, C. 1948. *Sexual behaviour in the human male*. W B Saunders, Philadelphia, PA, USA.

Kleineman, A. 1988. *The illness narratives: Suffering, healing and the human condition*. Basic Books, New York, NY, USA

Kohler, W. 1925. *The mentality of apes*. Harcourt Brace World, New York, NY, USA.

Lewis, G. Hawton, K. & Jones, P.1997. 'Strategies for preventing suicide.' *British Journal of Psychiatry*, 171, 351–354.

Mann, S A. & Cree, W. 1976. 'New long stay psychiatric patients: A national sample survey of 15 mental hospitals in England and Wales 1972/3.' *Psychological Medicines*, 6, 603.

Mechanic, D. 1968. *Medical sociology*. 2nd ed. New York: Free Press

Neisser, U. 1976. *Cognition and reality*. W H Freeman. San Francisco.

Odegaard, O. 1932. 'Emigration and insanity.' *Acta Psychiatrica Scandanavica,* 53, 129–136.

Paykel, E S. et al. 1980. 'Life events and social support in puerperal depression.' *British Journal of Psychiatry.* Apr; 136: 339–46.

Plsek, 2002. Framework for the Leading Modernisation Programme (LMP). London: Modernisation Agency.

Richman, N. Stevenson, J. & Graham, P. 1982. *Preschool to school: a behavioural study.* Academic Press, London.

Rutter, M. Tizard, J. & Whitmore, K. 1970. *Education, health and behaviour.* Longman, London.

Rutter, M. Cox, A. Tupling, C. Berger M. & Yule, W. 1975. 'Attainment and adjustment in two geographical areas.' *British Journal of Psychiatry* 126: 493–509.

Shea, G P. 1987. Groups as human resources . *Research in Personnel and Human Resources Management,* 5, 323–56.

Tarrier, N. et al. 1988. 'The community management of schizophrenia: A controlled trial of a behavioural intervention with families to reduce relapse.' *British Journal of Psychiatry,* 153, 532–42.

Thompson, C. et al. 2000. 'Effects of a clinical-practice guideline and practice-based education on detection and outcome of depression in primary care: Hampshire Depression Project randomised controlled trial.' *Lancet,* 355, 185–91.

Thornicroft, G. & Tansella, M. 2000. *The Mental Health Matrix: A Manual to Improve Services.* Cambridge University Press, Cambridge.

Use of the Ohio Consumer Outcomes Initiative to Facilitate Recovery: Empowerment and Symptom Distress

Wilkinson, R G. 1996. *Unhealthy Societies: The Afflictions of Inequality.* Routledge. London.

Wing, J K. & Brown. 1976. *Institutionalism and schizophrenia.* Cambridge University Press.

Wing, J K. & Morris, B. 1981. *Handbook of psychiatric rehabilitation.* Oxford University Press.

Witkin, H A. 1967. 'A cognitive style approach to cross cultural research.' *International Journal of Psychology,* 2, 233–50.

Zola, K. 1973. 'Pathways to the doctor: from person to patient.' *Social Science and Medicine.* 7, 677- 89.

Index